Interventions f...
Amphetamine M...

Interventions for Amphetamine Misuse

Edited by

Richard Pates

BSc, D. Clin Psy
Department of Health Sciences,
University of Wales Institute, Cardiff, UK

and

Diane Riley

PhD
Toronto, Ontario, Canada

WILEY-BLACKWELL

A John Wiley & Sons, Ltd., Publication

Addiction **Press**

Library of Congress Cataloging-in-Publication Data

Interventions for amphetamine misuse / edited by Richard Pates and Diane Riley.
    p. ; cm.
  Includes bibliographical references and index.
   ISBN 978-1-4051-7558-6 (pbk. : alk. paper)   1. Amphetamine abuse.   I. Pates, Richard.
II. Riley, Diane M. (Diane Mary), 1953-
   [DNLM: 1. Amphetamine-Related Disorders–therapy.   2. Amphetamine-Related Disorders–complications.   3. Amphetamine-Related Disorders–epidemiology.   4. Amphetamines–therapeutic use.   5. Cross-Cultural Comparison. WM 275 I61 2010]
   RC568.A45I58 2010
   362.29'9–dc22

                                                                          2009007670

A catalogue record for this book is available from the British Library.

Set in 10/12.5 pt Sabon by Aptara® Inc., New Delhi, India
Printed and bound in Malaysia by KHL Printing Co Sdn Bhd

1   2010

CONTENTS

CONTRIBUTORS

Anjalee Cohen
PhD
Brain and Mind Research Institute, University of Sydney, Australia

Paul E. A. Glaser
MD, PhD
Department of Behavioral Science (College of Medicine), Department of Anatomy and Neurobiology (College of Medicine), Department of Pediatrics (College of Medicine), University of Kentucky, Lexington, Kentucky, USA

Jean-Paul Grund
PhD
CVO-Addiction Research Center, Utrecht, The Netherlands

Robert Heimer
PhD
Department of Epidemiology and Public Health, Yale University, New Haven, Connecticut, USA

Zoe Hildrey
BSc
Community Addiction Unit, Cardiff, UK

Kevin S. Irwin
MA, PhD
Community Health Program, Tufts University, Medford, Massachusetts, USA

Kerstin Käll
MD, PhD
Beroendekliniken, Universitetssjukhuset, Linköping, Sweden

Catherine McGregor
MPsych (Clin), PhD
Policy, Strategy and Information, Drug and Alcohol Office, Lawley, Western Australia

Jan K. Melichar
BSc, MB, BS, MRCPsych, MD
Bristol Specialist Drug Service, AWP NHS Trust, University of Bristol, Bristol, UK

David J. Nutt
DM, FRCP, FRCPsych, Fed Med Sci
Department of Community Based Medicine, University of Bristol, Bristol, UK

Richard Pates
BSc, D. Clin Psy
Department of Health Sciences, University of Wales Institute, Cardiff, UK

Richard A. Rawson
PhD
Integrated Substance Abuse Programs (ISAP), Semel Institute for Neuroscience and Human Behavior, David Geffen School of Medicine, UCLA, Los Angeles, California, USA

Diane Riley
PhD
Toronto, Ontario, Canada

Craig R. Rush
PhD
Department of Behavioral Science, Department of Psychiatry, and Department of Psychology, University of Kentucky, Lexington, Kentucky, USA

Akihiko Sato
BA, MA, PhD
Faculty of Letters and Graduate School of Social and Cultural Sciences, Kumamoto University, Kumamoto, Japan

James Shearer
BA, Grad Dip (Econ)
The Langton Centre, Sydney, Australia

Janie Sheridan
PhD, FRPharmS
School of Pharmacy, Faculty of Medicine and Health Science, The University of Auckland, Auckland, New Zealand

Alyson Smith
BSc, MA, PGCE, PhD, DClinPsych
School of Health Sciences, University of Wales Institute, Cardiff, UK

William W. Stoops
PhD
Department of Behavioral Science (College of Medicine), University of Kentucky, Lexington, Kentucky, USA

Sophie E. Thomas
BSc
Community Addictions Unit, Cardiff, UK

Andrea R. Vansickel
MA
Department of Behavioral Science (College of Medicine), Department of Psychology (College of Arts and Sciences), University of Kentucky, Lexington, Kentucky, USA

Chris Wilkins
PhD
Centre for Social and Health Outcomes, Research and Evaluation (SHORES), Massey University, Auckland, New Zealand

Tomas Zabransky
MD, PhD
First Medical Faculty, Psychiatric Clinic, Centre for Addictology, Charles University, Prague, Czech Republic

DEDICATION

This book is dedicated to my wife, Gemma, and my beautiful daughter, Cleo, for keeping me sane and alive during the past two years.

Richard Pates

ACKNOWLEDGEMENTS

We thank all the contributors who have given their time and extensive knowledge to help produce this book, to Gemma Wallace for her help in preparing the manuscript and to Katrina Hulme-Cross for her patience and wisdom in getting this book into production.

Chapter 1

INTRODUCTION

Richard Pates and Diane Riley

Amphetamine-type substances (ATS) are the second most commonly used drugs in the world (UNODC, 2007). Their use occurs across Europe, North America, Asia and Australasia, and in many places the use of these drugs can be problematic. The chapters in this book describe the nature of this drug, the effects of the drug and patterns of use in various parts of the world. Despite the widespread use of the drug and the problems that it may cause, there seems to be little consensus on effective treatment. One of the aims of this book is to review this international evidence and try to draw together examples of good practice. Opiates such as heroin and morphine are drugs which cause problems in many parts of the world, and there is now a widespread consensus on how effective treatment can be managed, usually by using substitute medication such as methadone. There is no similar pharmacological answer for the amphetamine group of drugs as yet, despite the magnitude of the problems they cause. Whether this is because there is no similar option for amphetamines compared to heroin or because the impetus to develop pharmacological treatments has not been seen to be of sufficient importance is open to debate.

The majority of amphetamine users are polydrug users. Benzodiazepines may be used to self-medicate amphetamine-related problems, and they are commonly used by amphetamine users (Darke et al., 1994). Heroin is also used by stimulant users to self-medicate (Hando et al., 1997), and there are reports of a significant association between daily alcohol intoxication and methamphetamine smoking (Furr et al., 2000). This means that polydrug use (and interactions with medications such as those for HIV) always needs to be considered as a possibility when considering interventions for amphetamine users (Baker et al., 2004).

Where and when did the problem arise?

As we will see in many of the chapters in this book, ATS have been regarded in different ways across the decades. They have been seen as drugs which are useful in times of war for keeping troops alert, as drugs used by both the Allies and Axis countries during the Second World War and still used today, as a useful tool for doctors, nurses, students, truck drivers and others to stay awake during long shifts, and as a partying drug for many young people to keep them awake during the long hours of pleasure.

Bett in 1946 suggested that there were at least 39 clinical uses for amphetamine, including treatment for epilepsy, schizophrenia, morphine and cocaine addiction, behavioural problems in children, and migraine. In America, at least, it had become widely accepted at that time by the medical profession as a useful drug. These days the clinical uses of ATS are very few, partly because of the lack of evidence of many of the conditions that were supposedly helped by the drug and also by the recognition of the drug's dependence potential and long-term psychological effects.

The Benzedrine inhaler was introduced in 1932 (Grinspoon and Hedblom, 1975) and this became a popular way of treating both the effects of asthma and even head colds, as one of the effects of amphetamine is to dilate the nasal and bronchial passages. The use of Benzedrine from these inhalers became an early form of the illicit use of amphetamine. In 1946, Harry 'The Hipster' Gibson recorded a song called 'Who Put the Benzedrine in Mrs Murphy's Ovaltine' (http://mog.com/dermahrk/blog_post/134472; accessed 16 August 2008), which was a humorous take on the effects of taking Benzedrine and the supposed benefits it gave the user. The song was banned from broadcasting in 1947 and Gibson was blacklisted by the music industry. This indicates the fact that the drug use was in the public consciousness in the middle of the twentieth century.

Jack Kerouac's novel *On the Road* written in 1951 and published in 1957 was a defining novel of the 'beat generation'. This remarkable book, written almost as a stream-of-consciousness novel about a journey across America, was written under the influence of Benzedrine, and the phrenetic tone of the novel gives the reader the impression of that speed culture.

In the 1990s the emergence of methamphetamine as a potent, smokeable form of the drug was seen as the latest 'scourge' blighting our society following the warnings that we had about the dangers of crack cocaine in the late 1980s. Methamphetamine has clearly become a drug of choice in some areas and has been associated with violent motorcycle gangs, both on the west coast of North America and in New Zealand, and concern has been registered about the dangerous amateur laboratories producing the drug. These laboratories are dangerous both because of the potential for violent explosions during the production of the drug and because of the toxic by-products of the drug.

What are the dangers?

Is amphetamine really a 'scourge' or is current concern about it just another moral panic? It is, after all, part of the same drug family that until the 1960s was widely prescribed as a tonic and a slimming aid by general practitioners in many countries including the UK and America. Many drugs have this Jekyll-and-Hyde history of being thought to be useful and benign in the early days but become diabolic in their reputation as time passes and the true or other effects of the drug are known. One difficulty in labelling a drug as 'dangerous' is that for many occasional users there have been no ill effects. A study by Pates and Mitchell (1996) surveying the use of the drug in South Wales in the UK found that some people used very small amounts, taken orally, on an occasional basis and experienced few problems with it. Other people surveyed were injecting up to 14 g/day and experiencing a host of psychological effects as a consequence.

What is clear is that these drugs, which have been used routinely by many people for purposes of alleviating fatigue in a work situation or for recreational purposes often without report of problems, are not benign. Chapter 2 of this book describes the physical effects and damage that may result from amphetamine use and Chapter 3 describes the psychological and psychiatric effects of the drug. One of the reasons that amphetamine use has not attracted as much publicity or been taken as seriously as other drugs such as heroin or cocaine (or even ecstasy) is that overdose from amphetamine use was rare (Pates, 1994), particularly in areas where the less potent amphetamine sulphate was in common use. With an increase in the use of methamphetamine, however, more concern has been expressed about the potential for fatalities from the use of this more potent form of amphetamine.

Kaye et al. (2008) reported on a survey of methamphetamine-related deaths in Australia. They comment that shift in the mid-1990s from the production and supply of amphetamine (sulphate) to that of the more potent methamphetamine has produced an increase in amphetamine-related problems. Examining the case notes of 371 individuals where coroners had decided that methamphetamine was a listed cause of death, they found that the great majority of deaths were accidental (only 14% being suicides). In the cases they reviewed, methamphetamine use or toxicity was identified as the direct cause of death, as an antecedent cause in 11% of the cases and as a significant contributory factor in 16% of cases. Cardiovascular problems were noted in more than half of the cases for which autopsy reports were available, the most common type of cardiac pathology being cardiac artery atherosclerosis. Cerebrovascular problems were found in 20% of the cases where autopsy findings were available, and non-traumatic cerebral haemorrhage was noted in half of these cases. Women were four times as likely as men to have had a cerebral haemorrhage. Kaye and colleagues comment that these deaths are not typically cases of death among young naive users. They also comment that there does not appear to be a clear dose–response relationship for methamphetamine toxicity.

In a study using electrocardiograms (ECG) obtained during screening in a previous trial, Haning and Goebert (2007) demonstrated that methamphetamine users showed abnormalities. They found that 36% of those studied had abnormal ECG results. The most frequent abnormality was a high frequency of prolonged QT intervals (the QT interval represents the interval of ventricular contraction or systole), 'which has implications for health of the myocardium, as the delay in the ventricular contractions may indicate cardiomyopathy or other cardio toxic injury' (p. 72). This is further evidence of the physical effects of methamphetamine.

Sexual risks of using amphetamine

The chapters in this book give descriptions of the problem of ATS use in various parts of the world. A number of papers have been published looking at its use among various groups. For example, in a study of methamphetamine use and HIV risk in South Africa, Simbayi et al. (2006) surveyed 441 men and 521 women about their sexual behaviour and drug use; 18% of men and 12% of women had used methamphetamine. Methamphetamine use was associated with being male, having multiple sexual partners and having unprotected sexual intercourse. Condoms were used in less than half of the incidents of sexual intercourse. The authors comment that the association between methamphetamine use and sexual risk practices could fuel the spread of HIV infection in a part of the world where infectivity is already high. They also comment that although methamphetamine users were more likely to use condoms than other drug users, they were also more likely to exchange sex for money or goods. In a national study of young Americans, Iritani et al. (2007) looked at, among other things, criminality and sexual risk associated with methamphetamine use. They found that the unadjusted odds ratio showed that methamphetamine use among men was associated significantly with having more than one sexual partner, inconsistent or no condom use and regretting a sexual situation. The odds ratios were higher for women than for men, and there was a strong relationship between methamphetamine use, sexual risk behaviour, inconsistent or no condom use and regretting a sexual situation. When these odds ratios were adjusted to include sociodemographic characteristics, other illegal drug use and novelty-seeking behaviour, the odds ratio was no longer significant. The sociodemographic variables showed that men were twice as likely as women to be drug users, and Hispanics and Afro-Americans were much less likely to use drugs than white people but Native Americans were 4.2 times as likely to use as white people. Methamphetamine users were more likely to smoke cigarettes and use marijuana, cocaine and/or intravenous drugs in the previous year. Novelty-seeking behaviour was measured by Cloninger's Tridimensional Personality Questionnaire.

Halkitis et al. (2007) sought to understand the popularity of methamphetamine in the gay male community in New York. Using a longitudinal study for over a year where 450 club drug-using gay and bisexual men were assessed by quantitative measure, they found that the use of methamphetamine in this group is a multifaceted behaviour. This behaviour was driven by a desire to heighten sensations, especially in relation to sexual experience, as well as to overcome painful emotions. Methamphetamine is perceived to have aphrodisiac by-qualities and is often used to enhance and prolong sexual activity. In another study, Bolding et al. (2006) examined the use of crystal methamphetamine and its association with high-risk sexual behaviour among gay men in London. They surveyed 388 HIV-positive gay men attending HIV clinics, 266 HIV-negative gay men attending clinics for HIV testing, and 1592 gay men using gyms. They found that the percentage of men who had used methamphetamine in the last 12 months varied by sample (HIV treatment 12.6%, HIV testing 8.3% and gyms 19.9%). The majority of the men used methamphetamine only once or twice a year, but most methamphetamine users had taken other recreational drugs, and the users of methamphetamine plus other drug were more likely to report high-risk sexual behaviour than either other drug users or non-drug users. It is interesting to note that methamphetamine appears to be popular amongst the gay male population especially in Britain.

Shoptaw and Reback (2007) reviewed the evidence regarding the prevalence of methamphetamine use amongst men who have sex with men and evaluated the factors that contribute to methamphetamine use and the potential for sexual transmission of HIV and other infectious diseases. They found that methamphetamine use is prevalent among men who have sex with men in the USA, Australia and in the UK and the use of methamphetamine may range from recreational through to chronic use and addiction. They found that the data indicated that the men who use this drug engage in concomitant HIV-related sexual behaviour. They also found that men who have sex with men using methamphetamine probably have higher rates of infection with HIV and syphilis than men who have sex with men who do not use the drug.

Will precursor regulation work?

Because most methamphetamine is made in 'kitchen' laboratories (i.e. non-pharmaceutical environments, often by amateurs) questions have been raised about whether controlling the precursors or substances required to make methamphetamine would reduce the supply of the drug. For example, in the USA, regulation of bulk ephedrine and pseudoephedrine was introduced in 1989, regulation of products containing ephedrine as the single active ingredient in 1995 and regulation of products containing pseudoephedrine in 1997. These were aimed at limiting access of these drugs to large-scale producers. Regulations aimed at small-scale producers were introduced on ephedrine products that included more than one medicinal ingredient in 1996 (Cunningham et al., 2008).

Cunningham et al. (2008) investigated whether the suppression of these substances affected the routes of administration of these drugs and thereby the relative potential risk of different routes. Using non-coerced admissions into treatment as a population sample, they found that admissions for snorting, smoking, swallowing and injecting initially rose sharply and then dropped when the 1995 regulations were introduced and snorting dropped after the 1997 regulations were introduced. Admissions for smoking showed a resurgence after the 1996 regulations and continued rising to higher levels than in 1995, and has continued to rise thereafter. This is interesting research because it used time series and a powerful quasi-experimental design to examine the effects of policy on drug use.

McKetin (2008) has suggested that as regulation of precursor chemicals in the developed world becomes more stringent the responsibility for controlling and policing chemical diversion may shift to the developing world which may have limited capacity to manage these problems. This could alter the relative availability of various drugs in different geographical areas of the world. As McKetin points out this may also increase levels of harm in these countries.

The chapters of this book closely examine the issues surrounding amphetamine use and the interventions provided to treat people with amphetamine-related problems. Inevitably, there will be omissions in terms of countries and some of the issues around the use of amphetamine. We have tried to be as comprehensive and inclusive as possible.

References

Baker, A., Gowing, L., Lee, N. K. and Proudfoot, H. (2004) Psychosocial interventions for psychostimulant users. In: Baker, A., Lee, N. K. and Jenner, L. (eds), *Models of Intervention and Care for Psychostimulant Users*, 2nd edn. National Drug Strategy Monograph Series No. 51. Australia: Commonwealth of Australia, pp. 63–84.

Bett, W. R. (1946) Benzedrine sulphate in clinical medicine: a survey of the literature. *Postgraduate Medicine Journal* 22: 205–218.

Bolding, G., Hart, G., Sherr, L. and Elford, J. (2006) Use of crystal methamphetamine among gay men in London. *Addiction* 101(11): 1622–1630.

Cunningham, J. K., Liu, L. M. and Muramoto, M. (2008) Methamphetamine suppression and route of administration: precursor regulation impacts on snorting, smoking, swallowing and injecting. *Addiction* 103(7): 1174–1186.

Darke, S., Ross, J. and Cohen, J. (1994) The use of benzodiazepines among regular amphetamine users. *Addiction* 89: 1683–1690.

Furr, C. D. M., Delva, J. and Anthony, J. C. (2000) The suspected association between methamphetamine 'ice' smoking and frequent episodes of alcohol intoxication: data from the 1993 National Household Survey on Drug Abuse. *Drug and Alcohol Dependence* 59: 89–93.

Grinspoon, L. and Hedblom, P. (1975) *The Speed Culture: Amphetamine Use and Abuse in America*. Cambridge, MA: Harvard University Press.

Halkitis, P. N., Mukherjee, P. P. and Palamar, J. J. (2007) Multi-level modelling to explain methamphetamine use among gay and bisexual men. *Addiction* 102(Suppl 1): 76–83.

Hando, J., O'Brien, S., Darke, S., Maher, L. and Hall, W. (1997) *The Illicit Drug Reporting System (IDRS) Trial: Final Report*. NDARC Monograph No. 31. Sydney: National Drug and Alcohol Research Centre.

Haning, W. and Goebert, D. (2007) Electrocardiographic abnormalities in methamphetamine users. *Addiction* 102(Suppl 1): 70–75.

Iritani, B. J., Hallfors, D. D. and Bauer, D. J. (2007) Crystal methamphetamine use among young adults in the USA. *Addiction* 102(7): 1102–1113.

Kaye, S., Darke, S., Duflou, J. and McKetin, R. (2008) Methamphetamine related fatalities in Australia: demographics, circumstances, toxicology and major organ pathology. *Addiction* 103(8): 1353–1360.

Kerouac, J. (1957) *On the Road*. New York: Viking Press.

McKetin, R. (2008) Methamphetamine precursor regulation: are we controlling or diverting the drug problem? *Addiction* 103(4): 521–523.

Pates, R. (1994) Speed on prescription. *Druglink* 9(3): 16–17.

Pates, R. M. and Mitchell, A. (1996) Amphetamine use in South Glamorgan. *Journal of Substance Misuse* 1(3): 165–173.

Shoptaw, S. and Reback, C. J. (2007) Methamphetamine use and infectious disease-related behaviours in men who have sex with men: implications for interventions. *Addiction* 102 (Suppl 1): 130–135.

Simbayi, L. C., Kalichman, S. C., Cain, D., Cherry, C., Henda, N. and Cloete, A. (2006) Methamphetamine use and sexual risks for HIV infection in Cape Town, South Africa. *Journal of Substance Use* 11(4): 291–300.

United Nations Office on Drugs and Crime (UNODC) (2007) *2007 World Drug Report.* Vienna: United Nations Office on Drugs and Crime.

Chapter 2

THE PHYSICAL EFFECTS OF AMPHETAMINE USE

Zoe Hildrey, Sophie E. Thomas and Alyson Smith

Introduction

Amphetamines are synthetic stimulants and are taken either legally for medicinal reasons or illegally for recreational use. Internationally, the Convention of Psychotropic Substances classifies amphetamines as Schedule II drugs or Schedule I drugs if prepared for injection. Amphetamines are prescribed to treat sleep disorders, such as narcolepsy (Szabadi, 2006), and attention deficit/hyperactivity disorder (ADHD) (Biederman et al., 2005), to aid in street amphetamine dependence (White, 2000) and as a diet suppressant (Colman, 2005). They can also be used to augment antidepressant therapy in treatment resistant (Carlson et al., 2004).

Amphetamines are available in crystalline form, tablet form or as a powder. They can be ingested in many ways: snorted, swallowed, smoked, injected or dissolved in a drink. In this chapter, the word amphetamines will be used to describe all types of amphetamines, methylamphetamines or methamphetamines, used medicinally, and all other types of illegal amphetamine, for example, speed.

The effect of using amphetamines will usually persist for up to 6 hours (Tyler, 1998). The main effects of the drug are increased heart rate and breathing rate, increased wakefulness, suppressed appetite and feelings of well-being, exhilaration, power and confidence (Tyler, 1998). Some users may also experience a dry mouth, hallucinations, sweating and increased urinary frequency. The user may have an increased sexual drive, making them more likely to participate in risky sexual behaviours (Semple et al., 2004).

As the effects of the drug wear off, fatigue often follows. It is thought that amphetamine withdrawal peaks within 24 hours of the last dose (McGregor et al., 2005). This is characterised by increased sleeping and eating. Dysphoria and depression-related symptoms such as inactivity can occur. Anxiety, tension, agitation, vivid dreams, craving, poor concentration, and irritability may also be experienced.

In this chapter, we focus on the many long-term consequences of amphetamine use. See Table 2.1 for an overview. Anorectic, neurotoxic and smoking effects are discussed as well as effects on sleep, heart, teeth and unborn babies. Links with human immunodeficiency virus (HIV), ADHD and Parkinson's disease are addressed.

Table 2.1 Physical effect of amphetamines.

Addiction	Amphetamine users are at risk of dependence, reflected by increased tolerance to the drug and both physical and psychiatric withdrawal symptoms. Injecting amphetamine or smoking crystal methamphetamine sharply increases the risk of dependence.
Effects on sleep	Short-term use induces wakefulness and reduces the need for sleep. Long-term use reduces total and REM sleep time. On withdrawal hypersomnia is likely, followed by poor sleep patterns.
Anorectic effects	Amphetamines are an appetite suppressant, producing marked decrease in food intake on the first day of administration. However, a dose-dependent tolerance develops.
Risks associated with route of administration	Injecting is associated with risks of blood-borne viruses (BBV) and vein damage. Smoking is associated with an earlier onset of psychotic symptoms. Smoking and snorting can lead to nasal damage, particularly sinusitis, and can exacerbate asthma.
Oral damage	Amphetamine use can severely damage the mouth, causing tooth surface loss, flattening of the teeth, gingivitis and angular cheilitis, caused by bruxism and xerostomia.
Cardiac effects and stroke	Amphetamine use is a risk factor for heart problems such as cardiomyopathy, arrhythmia and myocardial infarction. Documented cases of amphetamine-induced stroke, both ischaemic and haemorrhagic.
Link with BBV	There is an association between amphetamine use and increasing incidence of HIV and HCV. Factors that contribute to this are risky sexual behaviours and unsafe injecting practices.
Prenatal effects	Amphetamine use could cause an unborn baby to be small for their gestational age, underweight or be delivered preterm. However, there are complex confounding variables, which make it hard to draw to any conclusions.
Neurotoxic effects	Amphetamine acts on monoamine neurotransmitters in the central nervous system. It is an indirect dopamine and serotonin agonist and can lead to extensive long-term neural damage.
Parkinson's disease	There is evidence to suggest that chronic amphetamine use may be a risk factor for the development of Parkinson's disease in later life.

Sleep problems

Amphetamines induce alertness and wakefulness (Pagel and Parnes, 2001; Smith, 2006), and reduce the desire for sleep (Srisurapanont et al., 1999). Consequently, they are sometimes prescribed to help with the symptoms of sleep disorders such as the daytime sleepiness present in narcolepsy (Szabadi, 2006). Although amphetamines have this valuable use, it is important to note that they can severely disrupt night-time sleep and act as a major risk factor for insomnia (Dollander, 2002). In a laboratory-based study of the effects of amphetamines on sleep, Comer et al. (2001) found that participants reported being significantly less satisfied with sleep, took longer to fall asleep and woke more through the night.

This stimulant-induced wake may be modulated by dopamine (Jankovic, 2002). Dopamine plays an important role in modulating sleep, and taking amphetamine increases the extracellular levels of dopamine (Wisor et al., 2001). The increased wakefulness may be caused by the amphetamine blocking dopamine re-uptake or by stimulating dopamine, or by both processes (Boutrel and Koob, 2004; Ebert and Berger, 1998).

Amphetamines are also known to reduce the total time spent in sleeping, reduce the total time spent in rapid eye movement (REM) sleep by up to 50% (Baekeland, 1967), and increase the time spent getting to REM sleep (Schafer and Greulich, 2000; Smith, 2006).

On withdrawal from amphetamines, there is an REM rebound where the total sleep time increases and the time to REM decreases. REM sleep gradually returns to normal after this rebound upon discontinuation of use (Baekeland, 1967). In addition to an REM rebound following withdrawal from amphetamines, hypersomnia is likely to set in. McGregor et al. (2005) report an acute phase and a sub-acute phase. During the acute phase of abstinence (1 week), the user may 'crash' and is likely to sleep for up to a few days. In the sub-acute phase, sleep time returns to normal, but the user may take longer to fall asleep. Increased night waking and low clear-headedness on waking may also be experienced (Smith, 2006).

Prolonged amphetamine use, medicinal or not, could induce a stimulant-dependent sleep disorder. However, it is possible that an underlying sleep disorder precipitated the stimulant use. Therefore, stimulant-dependent sleep disorder could be a consequence of amphetamine use or an inadvertent consequence of self-medication (Smith, 2006).

Anorectic

Due to their appetite-suppressing properties, amphetamine-based substances can be used on a short-term basis to treat obesity (Colman, 2005). They were commercially sold as appetite suppressants until recreational use began to increase in the late 1950s. It is due to these anorectic effects that there is a significant association between abuse of illicit drugs and the risk for eating disorders (Piran and Gadalla,

2007). Matsumoto et al. (2002) noted that amphetamine was being abused by a higher proportion of young females with eating disorders compared to women without eating disorders.

Studies have shown a marked decrease in food consumption after repeated administration of amphetamines, with intake being reduced by 35% compared to the baseline consumption. However after the first day of use, daily food intake gradually returned to baseline levels (Foltin, 1990; Kuo, 2003). Not only food intake but also caloric intake decreases (Comer et al., 2001), and in the initial period after amphetamine administration a reduction in drinking behaviour has also been observed (Hsieh et al., 2005).

The gradual reversion to normal food intake despite continued amphetamine use shows that individuals develop a tolerance to the anorectic effects. Development of tolerance is dose dependent; intake of food is directly proportional to the dose of amphetamine ingested (Foltin, 1989; Wolgin, 2004). Return to normal levels of food intake occurs more rapidly at lower rather than higher doses, and it has been reported that when treated with doses greater than 5 mg/kg tolerance does not develop and the anorectic effect persists (Kuo, 2003).

These anorectic effects are linked to neural activity in the brain, specifically dopamine activity. The co-activation of both D1 and D2 receptors plays a role in amphetamine-induced anorexia (Kuo, 2003). Activity of the orexigenic neuropeptide Y helps regulate feeding behaviour, and levels are altered after administration of amphetamine; therefore, it may play an important role in the anorexia observed (Hsieh et al., 2005; Kuo and Cheng, 2002).

Health risks associated with injecting, smoking and snorting

Amphetamine can be administered in several ways: orally, intravenously, smoking or snorting. The dangers of injecting are quite well known, with the risk of blood-borne viruses (BBVs) from sharing injecting equipment. Repeated injecting can cause veins to collapse and bad injecting practices can lead to sores and infections (Zule and Desmond, 1999).

Smoking amphetamine is the process by which the vapourised fumes are inhaled. This results in a less intense experience than injecting (Matsumoto et al., 2002), but reduces the risk of contracting HIV or hepatitis. However, it is connected with its own detrimental effects. Regular smoking of amphetamine can exacerbate asthma, induce sore throat and lead to a bloody sputum. It is also reported that individuals who smoke amphetamine experience psychotic episodes sooner than injectors or poly-administration users (Matsumoto et al., 2002).

Snorting is the ingestion of amphetamine powder through the nasal passage, and this method along with inhalation can cause a runny nose, lead to nasal ulcers and damage the epithelium and nasal septum (McCann and Ricaurte, 2000). In more chronic cases, this can lead to septum perforation and sinusitis. Sinusitis occurs when the membrane of the sinus cavity and sinus openings become inflamed, usually due to blockage of the sinus passage, and this prevents them from draining properly. Taking amphetamine can leave individuals more susceptible to infections due to the moist environment created by sinusitis.

Oral damage

Regular use of amphetamine can cause damage to the mouth and teeth. 'Meth mouth' refers to the blackening and staining of teeth, loss of tooth surface and general tooth decay, thought to be caused by amphetamine's acidic nature (American Dental Association Division of Communication, 2005). In a comparison of 13 amphetamine users with matched control subjects, it was found that amphetamine users had a greater severity of wear of their lower first molars and upper first molars than controls (Nixon et al., 2002). The lack of a significant difference in wear of anterior (front) teeth suggests that amphetamine users tend to clench or grind mainly on their posterior (back) teeth. In more severe cases, fine cracks were identified in posterior teeth, indicating that heavy and prolonged use could lead to erosion of these teeth (Nixon et al., 2002). It is thought that erosion of teeth in this manner is because use of amphetamine can cause bruxism and xerostomia.

Bruxism is a para-functional activity including clenching, bracing and grinding of the teeth (See and Tan, 2003). Bruxism is experienced by most individuals, to some degree, usually at night and is not detrimental; however, use of amphetamine causes bruxism for extended periods of time, and it has been observed for up to 48 hours after administration of amphetamine. Bruxism can cause chips in the teeth and flattening of the biting surface.

Xerostomia refers to the dryness of the mouth experienced by amphetamine users and is sometimes referred to as 'pasties'. Xerostomia reduces the amount of protective saliva from around the teeth and can lead to an increased number of cavities, decay around the gum line and possibly gingivitis (inflammation of the gums). Xerostomia can also lead to angular cheilitis (inflammation and cracking of the corners of the mouth) and has been shown to exacerbate candidasis (oral thrush), increasing the percentage area of lesions (Freire-Garabal et al., 1999).

Another cause of these symptoms is the duration of the effects of amphetamine (approximately 6 hours), which may lead to more extended periods of time where individuals do not brush their teeth, or possibly brush their teeth more vigorously, causing gum damage (American Dental Association Division of Communication, 2005).

Cardiac effects

Cardiomyopathy and myocardial infarction are recognised side effects of amphetamine use, although occurrence of these side effects is rare (Costa et al., 2001). An even less common outcome is death although there are some documented cases (Jacobs, 2006). Cardiomyopathy refers to a condition where the heart wall muscle is unusually enlarged or stiffened. It impairs the heart's ability to pump blood, which can result in congestive heart failure, an acute pulmonary oedema (rapid build up of fluid in the lungs) and arrhythmia.

Arrhythmia is when the muscle contraction of the heart is irregular; the resting heart rate is either too high (tachycardia) or too low (bradycardia). Tachycardia typically means a heart rate of above 100 beats per minute, indicating that the body needs more oxygen and nutrients. Bradycardia is when the resting heart rate is below 60 beats per minute, although individuals do not tend to become symptomatic until rate is below 50 beats per minute. Bradycardia can add to or lead to fatigue and can lead to hypotension (abnormally low blood pressure), and can progress to cardiogenic shock.

In a review of methamphetamine use and cardiovascular pathology, Kaye et al. (2007) concluded that users were at elevated risk of cardiac pathology. This risk was highest for chronic users and not restricted to the duration of drug use. Kaye et al. also found that methamphetamine use was 'likely to exacerbate the risk of cardiac pathology from other causes, and may therefore lead to premature mortality' (p. 102).

Drug abuse is recognised as a risk factor for stroke. In the USA, amphetamine use has been identified as the second most common cause of drug-induced stroke after cocaine (Centers for Disease Control and Prevention, 1995). A stroke is when the blood supply to part of the brain is cut off, causing brain cells to die. This can be caused by a blood clot that blocks the artery that carries blood to the brain (ischaemic stroke) or when there is a bleed in the brain (haemorrhagic stroke).

Amphetamine causes strokes through its effects on cerebral circulation, including vasculitis or vascular malformations. Administration of amphetamine causes blood vessels to narrow (vasoconstriction). Vasoconstriction is an important cause of both forms of stroke, as it causes a prolonged decrease in blood flow (Horita et al., 1953). This can lead to the blood supply being cut off, causing an ischaemic stroke, or the blood vessel becoming weakened leading to bulges that may burst, causing a haemorrhagic stroke.

Studies have found that elevation in blood pressure (hypertension), another effect of amphetamine, increases the risk of stroke (Perez et al., 1999; Westover et al., 2007). Hypertension is also significantly associated with death, in patients with haemorrhagic stroke. Myocardial infarction is significantly associated with death in ischaemic stroke patients (Westover et al., 2007). Intravenous methamphetamine use is the most common preparation of amphetamine that leads to stroke, but there are some documented cases of stroke after oral and intranasal amphetamine use (Perez et al., 1999; Ragland et al., 1993).

Amphetamine-induced stroke tend to occur within a few minutes or hours of administration (Kaku and Lowenstein, 1990; Kase, 1986). Westover et al.'s (2007) longitudinal study of all hospital admissions in Texas found the incidence of stroke amongst amphetamine users increased between 2000 and 2003 as did the rate of abuse of amphetamine. This study revealed a significant association between amphetamine use and haemorrhagic stroke, but not between amphetamine use and ischaemic stroke. Some cases of ischaemic stroke after amphetamine use have been recorded, but haemorrhagic stroke is more common (Perez et al., 1999).

The link with BBVs

Hepatitis C virus (HCV) is the most common chronic blood-borne infection and can lead to chronic liver disease, resulting in 8000 to 10 000 deaths a year in the USA (Williams, 1999). There is an association between amphetamine use and the increasing incidence of HIV and HCV infection. It is estimated that 55% of HIV patients have used amphetamines prior to diagnosis (Robinson and Rempel, 2006). This association may be due to the risky sexual behaviours and injecting practices that are linked with amphetamine use.

The primary route of transmission of HCV infection is injecting drug use. Gonzales et al. (2006) found that 15% of amphetamine users and 44% of injecting users were infected with HCV. Injecting increases the likelihood of contracting both HIV and HCV, as it allows for possible sharing of drug paraphernalia and other unsafe injecting practices (e.g. using an unsterilised needle). One report found that 52% of amphetamine injecting drug users had shared needles with one or two people and 11% with more than two people. It was also reported that 48% of the users never or only occasionally disinfected the needles that they used (Zule and Desmond, 1999). This indicates that over half of injecting amphetamine users are engaging in injecting practices that place them at risk of contracting HIV and HCV.

BBVs such as HCV can be sexually transmitted (Halfon et al., 2001). An amphetamine user who does not inject or who practices safer injecting is still four to six times more likely to engage in sexual activity with another injecting drug user (Krawczyk et al., 2006; Molitor et al., 1998), thus increasing the risk of contracting BBVs.

Evidence shows that amphetamine increases an individual's desire for sexual activity, with 65% of users reporting increased interest in sex (Semple et al., 2004). Individuals also report using amphetamine in order to enhance their sexual pleasure (Robinson and Rempel, 2006).

This increased desire for sexual activity may lead to amphetamine users engaging in more risky sexual activity such as not using a condom. Molitor et al. (1998) reported that amphetamine users were twice as likely as non-amphetamine users to have had sex with a prostitute or had sex in exchange for drugs.

Amphetamine users had a significantly higher number of casual or anonymous female sexual partners compared to non-amphetamine users (64.8%, 44.4%) (Krawczyk et al., 2006; Sattah et al., 2002). Semple et al. (2004) noted that male and female amphetamine users have three times as much vaginal sexual intercourse per month compared to national average. It was also recorded that they had lower rates of condom use, more anal and vaginal sex and higher rates of sexually transmitted infection (Baskin-Sommers and Sommers, 2006; Molitor et al., 1998) than their non-using counterparts, all of which are behaviours that increase the risk of contracting BBVs.

Despite the reported higher incidence of sexually transmitted infections amongst this population, recent amphetamine users were no more likely to have been checked for HIV or *Chlamydia* (Krawczyk et al., 2006) despite their increased risk of contracting these viruses; the reasons for this are unclear.

The evidence shows that amphetamine users are at a significantly increased risk of contracting BBVs, either through unsafe injecting practices or through engaging in risky sexual behaviour.

Prenatal effects

A number of physiological changes occur during pregnancy that can affect drug pharmacokinetics. These include increased cardiac output and renal function, increased body weight, high hormone levels and fluid retention, increased plasma volume and a decrease in plasma albumin and intestinal motility (Dean and McGuire, 2004). There are less than 25 proven teratogens amongst marketed drugs; this includes two psychostimulants: dexamphetamine and methylphenidate. Psychostimulants are thought to affect the fetus by blocking the neuronal re-uptake of catecholamines in the mother, resulting in cardiac stimulation and vasoconstriction. This leads to decreased uterine blood flow and a decrease in the transfer of oxygen and other nutrients to the fetus. In addition, psychostimulants act on serotonergic or noradrenergic transporters expressed in placental cells and may increase levels of monoamines and restricted blood flow to the placenta. Elevation of serotonin and noradrenalin levels can alter uterine contractility (Dean and McGuire, 2004).

A growing number of women of childbearing age are using amphetamines. Amphetamine use has an estimated prevalence of 7% in pregnant women in the UK (McElhatton, 2005; Sanaullah et al., 2006). In the National Household Survey on Drug Abuse conducted in the USA, 2.8% of pregnant women reported that they used illicit drugs, and one-tenth of these were using cocaine (Ebrahim and Gfroerer, 2003). In an Australian study describing characteristics of 96 infants born within a chemical dependence unit, 6% of mothers were using amphetamines alone and 66% were using injection drugs (Kelly et al., 2000). There are no Canadian data on stimulant use in pregnancy, with surveys either focusing on alcohol and tobacco use or combining street drugs as one category.

Prenatal exposure to amphetamines may affect children in two ways: directly from the drug or from its effects on the fetal environment. Furara et al. (1999) found that 25% of amphetamine users have underweight babies and 28.6% of babies delivered were preterm. However, the mother's nutritional status, social status and smoking habits were not taken into account. Amphetamine use has been associated with babies being small for their gestational age (Smith et al., 2003, 2006). White et al. (2006) report a rate of fetal loss in amphetamine users of 14.9% in comparison to 5% in the general population. Some other effects noted are clefting, cardiac anomalies and fetal growth retardation (Plessinger, 1998). The later adjustment of a child may also be affected by prenatal amphetamine exposure (Billing et al., 1988).

Discontinuing amphetamine use whilst pregnant may improve the health of the baby. Smith et al. (2003) found a lower birth weight and head circumference in women who took methamphetamine in all three trimesters compared to those who took amphetamines in the first two.

These studies highlight the worrying effects that prenatal amphetamine exposure can have on a child. However, most of the studies rely on self-reported drug use, have a lack of appropriate control groups and are confounded by environmental factors (Wouldes et al., 2004). Poly-drug use is common and many of these results may be attributable to the effects of other drugs such as nicotine.

Smoking is damaging to an unborn baby. After controlling for amphetamines, smoking was highly predictive of the baby having a lower birth weight, being smaller for its gestational age and having a smaller head circumference (Smith et al., 2003, 2006; White et al., 2006). Smoking has been shown to cause fetal growth restriction, and is associated with stillbirth, preterm birth and placental abruption (Cnattingius, 2004).

The Ovine Model suggests that these effects occur as both amphetamines and nicotine act as vasoconstrictors, decreasing the diameter of the blood vessels causing an increase in blood pressure (Stek et al., 1995). In combination with amphetamines, nicotine may have an additive effect. When more than one drug is used, it is difficult to establish which drug, or both in combination, was responsible for the observed effects. More research is required to improve our understanding of the effect poly-drug use has on the unborn child.

Mothers who use amphetamines are likely to have other problems as well, which will also affect an unborn child. These women may be young and come from a disadvantaged background (White et al., 2006). For example, they may be more likely to be single, have a lower socio-economic status, have a lower household income, be younger, seek less prenatal care and have fewer midwife visits (Smith et al., 2006). Mothers may have psychological problems, fewer years of education, a history of criminal activity and a history of physical and sexual abuse (Wouldes et al., 2004). These factors may predispose the developing fetus to the damaging effects of amphetamines (Plessinger, 1998). These complex confounding variables make it hard to isolate amphetamines as the cause of damage to an unborn baby. Therefore, no conclusions can be made with any confidence.

Amphetamines are excreted into breast milk, and depending on the dose, measurable amounts can be detected in the urine of the infant. In one study of 103 nursing infants whose mothers were taking amphetamines, no neonatal insomnia or stimulation was observed over a 24-hour period (Ayd, 1973). The decision to engage in or avoid breastfeeding should be influenced by an individual's pattern of drug use. It is best to avoid breastfeeding during periods of heavy psycho-stimulant use.

Attention deficit/hyperactivity disorder

Attention deficit/hyperactivity disorder (ADHD) and attention deficit disorder (ADD) are the most commonly diagnosed neurobehavioural disorders in children (Richters et al., 1995). One of the medicinal treatments for ADHD and ADD are amphetamines such as Adderall, Adderall XR, methamphetamine and mixed amphetamine salts extended release. Stimulants have a paradoxical calming effect, focus attention and improve executive function in patients with ADHD or ADD (Arnsten, 2006). These treatments have been found to be well tolerated and result in significant behavioural improvements (Ahman et al., 2001; Biederman et al., 2005).

The main side effects associated with amphetamine treatment are anorexia, insomnia and headaches (Efron et al., 1997; McGough et al., 2005). Brown et al. (2005) also report other mild side effects that are of short duration: motor tics, abdominal pain, irritability, nausea and fatigue. However, Ahman et al. (2001) report that some of the pre-existing symptoms of ADHD or ADD can be mistaken for side effects of the treatment. It is possible that people who abuse street amphetamine may be self-medicating to manage underlying symptoms of ADHD or ADD, which may have gone undiagnosed. The relationship between amphetamines and ADHD is addressed in more detail in Chapter 5.

Neurotoxic

Amphetamine acts on monoamine neurotransmitters in the central nervous system, by bringing about the rapid release of dopamine, serotonin and norepinephrine. The release of these neurotransmitters is caused by the redistribution of catecholamines from synaptic vesicles to cytosol (Wagner et al., 1980). After administration of amphetamine, there is an increase in the concentration of monoamines. After cessation of use, during the early withdrawal period, there is then a decrease in monoamines and in neurotransmitter release. These neurochemical changes are associated with the onset of depressive-like symptoms and decrease in individual's motivation (Barr et al., 2002).

Evidence shows that repeated administration of high doses of amphetamine results in extensive long-term neural damage, which can last up to 6 months after cessation of use (Barr et al., 2006; Dunn and Kilcross, 2006; Ernst et al., 2000; Wagner et al., 1980).

Amphetamine is an indirect dopamine agonist. It works by blocking dopamine transporters, which in turn inhibits dopamine re-uptake, resulting in an increase in extracellular dopamine levels (Kuo, 2003, 2005). Kuczenski et al. (1995) found that this was a dose-dependent relationship, with the duration of increase of dopamine being proportional to the dose of amphetamine administered. It has been found that repeated administration of D-amphetamine leads to a 30–60% decrease in dopamine terminal markers (Belcher et al., 2005) and a 55% decrease in density of dopamine uptake sites (Wagner et al., 1980). Decrease in dopamine has been observed in the nucleus accumbens, olfactory tubercle (Brunswick et al., 1992), striatum (Wagner et al., 1980) and the caudate (Brunswick et al., 1992; Kuczenski et al., 1995).

Amphetamine has a similar effect on the serotonergic system, causing long-term reduction in serotonin terminal markers and changes in levels of serotonin and serotonin transporter (Brunswick et al., 1992; Hanson et al., 2004; Robinson and Becker, 1986). Damage to the serotonergic system has been shown to be more diffuse than to the dopaminergic system, with hippocampal areas, parietal cortex and basolateral amygdaloid nucleus (Belcher et al., 2005; Brunswick et al., 1992).

Less is known about the effect of amphetamine-like substances on norepinephrine pathways. Some researchers have found a decrease in levels of norepinephrine transporter binding sites in the amygdaloid nucleus and dorsomedial hypothalamic nucleus (Brunswick et al., 1992). Conversely, Wagner et al. (1980) found no significant differences in norepinephrine in any of the brain regions studied including the caudate, midbrain and hypothalamus. A review of the literature indicated that the effect of amphetamine on norepinephrine may be dose dependent, with chronic administration of high doses of amphetamine leading to depletion of norepinephrine, but lower- and shorter-term use not affecting norepinephrine levels (Robinson and Becker, 1986).

Parkinson's disease

Parkinson's disease is a neurodegenerative disease where there is an inability to execute smooth bodily movements. This is caused by the degeneration of dopaminergic neurons, which leads to an insufficiency of dopamine (Wolters et al., 1995).

Long-term amphetamine use has also been found to be neurotoxic towards the brain's dopamine neurons (McCann and Ricaurte, 2004; Riddle et al., 2006) by destroying dopamine nerve fibres which leads to long-term dopamine depletion (Ricaurte et al., 1984). This irreversible loss of dopamine function may leave amphetamine users at risk of developing Parkinson's disease in later life (McCann et al., 1998). Garwood et al. (2006) found that 11% of patients with Parkinson's disease had a prolonged exposure to prescribed or street amphetamines prior to diagnosis. This suggests that amphetamine use could be a risk factor for the development of Parkinson's disease.

Evidence of neurotoxicity from amphetamines also comes from a main dopamine pathway, the nigrostriatal pathway (Hanson et al., 2004). The nigrostriatal pathway is a neural pathway connecting the substantia nigra with the striatum. It is part of a system called the basal ganglia motor loop, where a loss of dopaminergic neuronal markers has been found in chronic amphetamine users (Guilarte, 2001). The loss of dopaminergic neuronal markers is a main pathological feature of Parkinson's disease. This raises the possibility that amphetamine users may be at risk for the development of parkinsonism or neuropsychiatric conditions in which brain dopamine neurons have been implicated (McCann et al., 1998).

It has also been suggested that amphetamine use could produce structural changes beyond the dopamine system. A study by Iacovelli et al. (2006) shows that a novel change is made by amphetamine to a multi-enzymatic complex known as the ubiquitin–proteasome system, which is in the central nervous system. A dysfunction of the ubiquitin–proteasome system due to inherited mutations produces degenerative Parkinson's disease. This suggests that damage from amphetamine use is similar to processes that occur in degenerative diseases.

It is unclear as to whether chronic amphetamine use may cause a later onset of Parkinson's disease or just similar symptoms as a result of the dopamine loss. For example, Guilarte (2001) found that the neuronal marker VMAT-2 was changed in patients with Parkinson's disease but not in patients with chronic amphetamine use. This neuronal marker highlights terminal degeneration but is not affected by drugs prescribed to control Parkinson's disease symptoms, suggesting that damage by amphetamine use may only share similar pathways with Parkinson's disease.

There is evidence to suggest that chronic amphetamine use may be a risk factor for the development of Parkinson's disease in later life. Longitudinal studies are needed to determine the extent of this (McCann et al., 1998). Further evidence is needed in regard to whether biological changes and symptoms present in amphetamine users who have long-term dopamine depletion are identical to those in people with Parkinson's disease.

Conclusion

Amphetamine use results in many short-term physical effects. These are dose dependent and likely to discontinue after cessation of use. Upon administration, the need for sleep reduces and appetite is suppressed. An increasing dose is needed to maintain these effects. Otherwise, appetite and sleep patterns will return to normal. Smoking or snorting amphetamines could exacerbate asthma or oral thrush. It could also cause permanent damage to teeth.

Use can also lead to long-term diseases. Smoking amphetamine can lead to an earlier onset of psychotic symptoms. Injecting amphetamines increases the risk of contracting BBVs via unsafe injecting practices. The risk is further amplified by the effect of amphetamines, increased sexual drive, which could lead to risky sexual behaviours. There is evidence to suggest that chronic use may be a risk factor for the development of Parkinson's disease in later life due to dopamine depletion. The risk of stroke and heart problems such as cardiomyopathy, arrhythmia and myocardial infarction are significantly increased with amphetamine use.

There is some evidence suggesting that amphetamine use has a neurotoxic effect on an unborn baby. However, there are complex confounding variables that make it difficult to draw any conclusions. The main side effects associated with amphetamine treatment in people with ADHD are anorexia, insomnia and headaches.

References

Ahman, P. A., Theye, F. W., Berg, R., Linquist, A. J., Van Erem, A. J. and Campbell, L. R. (2001) Placebo-controlled evaluation of amphetamine mixture – dextroamphetamine salts and amphetamine salts (Adderall): efficacy rate and side effects. *Pediatrics* 107(1): E10.

American Dental Association Division of Communication (2005) Methamphetamine use and oral health. *Journal of American Dental Association* 136: 1491.

Arnsten, A. F. T. (2006) Stimulant: therapeutic actions in ADHD. *Neuropsychopharmacology* 31: 2376–2383.

Ayd, D. (1973) in Dean, A. and McGuire, T. *Psychostimulant Use in Pregnancy and Lactation in Models of Intervention and Care for Psychostimulant Users*, 2nd edn Baker, A., Lee, N. and Jenner, L. (eds), Monograph Series No. 51, Commonwealth of Australia 2004, pp. 35–50.

Baekeland, F. (1967) Pentobarbital and dextroamphetamine sulfate: effects on the sleep cycle in man. *Psychopharmacologia* 11: 388–396.

Barr, A., Paneka, W., MacEwan, G. W., Thornton, A., Lang, D. J., Honer, W. G. and Lecomte, T. (2006) The need for speed: an update on methamphetamine addiction. *Journal of Psychiatry and Neuroscience* 31(5): 301–313.

Barr, A. M, Zis, A. P. and Phillips, A. G. (2002) Repeated electroconvulsive shock attenuates the depressive-like effects of D-amphetamine withdrawal on brain reward function in rats. *Psychopharmacology (Berlin)* 159: 196–202.

Baskin-Sommers, A. and Sommers, I. (2006) The co-occurrence of substance use and high-risk behaviours. *Journal of Adolescent Health* 38: 609–611.

Belcher, A. M., O'Dell, S. J. and Marshall, J. F. (2005) Impaired object recognition memory following methamphetamine but not *p*-chloroamphetamine or D-amphetamine-induced neurotoxicity. *Neuropsychopharmacology* 30(11): 2026–2034.

Biederman, J., Spencer, T. J., Wilens, T. E., Weisler, R. H., Read, S. C. and Tulloch, S. J. (2005) Long-term safety and effectiveness of mixed amphetamine salts extended release in adults with ADHD. *CNS Spectrums* 12(20): 16–25.

Billing, L., Eriksson, M., Steneroth, G. and Rolf, Z. (1988) Predictive indicators for adjustment in 4-year-old children whose mothers used amphetamine during pregnancy. *Child Abuse and Neglect* 12: 503–507.

Boutrel, B. and Koob, G. F. (2004) What keeps us awake: the neuropharmacology of stimulants and wakefulness-promoting medications. *Sleep* 27(6): 1181–1194.

Brown, R. T., Amler, R. W., Freeman, W. S., Perrin, J. M., Stein, M. T., Feldman, H. M., Pierce, K. and Wolraich, M. L. (2005) Treatment of attention-deficit/hyperactivity disorder: overview of evidence. *Pediatrics* 155(6): 749–757.

Brunswick, D. J., Benmansour, S., Tejani-Butt, S. M. and Hauptmann, M. (1992) Effects of high-dose methamphetamine on monoamine uptake sited in rat brain measures by quantitative autoradiography. *Synapse* 11(4): 287–293.

Carlson, P. J., Merlock, M. C. and Suppes, T. (2004) Adjunctive stimulant use in patients with bipolar disorder: treatment of residual depression and sedation. *Bipolar Disorders* 6(5): 416.

Centers for Disease Control and Prevention (1995) Increasing morbidity and mortality associated with abuse of methamphetamine – United States, 1991–1994. *Morbidity and Mortality Weekly Review* 44: 882–886.

Cnattingius, S. (2004) The epidemiology of smoking during pregnancy: smoking prevalence, maternal characteristics and pregnancy outcomes. *Nicotine & Tobacco Research* 6(2): S125–S140.

Colman, E. (2005) Anorectics on trial: a half-century of federal regulation of prescription appetite suppressants. *Annals of Internal Medicine*, 143(5): 380–385.

Comer, S. D., Hart, C. L., Ward, A. S., Haney, M., Foltin, R. W. and Fischman, M. W. (2001) Effects of repeated oral methamphetamine administration in humans. *Psychopharmacology* 155(4): 397–404.

Costa, G. M., Pizzi, C., Bresciani, B., Tumscitz, C., Gentile, M. and Bugiardini, R. (2001) Acute myocardial infarction caused by amphetamines: a case report and review of the literature. *Italian Heart Journal* 2(6): 478–480.

Dean, A. and McGuire, T. (2004) Psychostimulant use in pregnancy and lactation. In: Baker, A., Lee, N. and Jenner, L. (eds), *Models of Intervention and Care for Psychostimulant Users*, 2nd edn. Monograph Series No. 51. Australia: Commonwealth of Australia, pp. 35–50.

Dollander, M. (2002) Etiology of adult insomnia. *Encephale* 28(6 Pt 1): 493–502.

Dunn, M. J. and Kilcross, S. (2006) Differential attenuation of D-amphetamine-induced disruption of conditional discrimination performance by dopamine and serotonin antagonists. *Psychopharamcology* 188: 183–192.

Ebert, D. and Berger, M. (1998) Neurobiological similarities in antidepressant sleep deprivation and psychostimulant use: a psychostimulant theory of antidepressant sleep deprivation. *Psychopharmacology* 140: 1–10.

Ebrahim, S. H. and Gfroerer, J. (2003) Pregnancy-related substance use in the United States during 1996–1998. *Obstetrics & Gynaecology* 101(2): 374–379.

Efron, D., Jarman, F. and Barker, M. (1997) Side effects of methylphenidate and dexamphetamine in children with attention deficit hyperactivity disorder: a double-blind, crossover trial. *Pediatrics* 100(4): 662–666.

Ernst, T., Chang, L., Leonido-Yee, M. and Speck, O. (2000) Evidence for long-term neurotoxicity associated with methamphetamine abuse: A 1H MRS study. *Neurology* 28(6): 1344–1349.

Foltin, R. W. (1989) Effects of anorectic drugs on topography of feeding behaviour in baboons. *Journal of Pharmacology and Experimental Therapeutics* 249(1): 101–109.

Foltin, R. W. (1990) Differential development of tolerance to the effects of D-amphetamine and flenfluramine on food intake. *Journal of Pharmacology and Experimental Therapeutics* 252(3): 960–969.

Freire-Garabal, M., Nunez, M. J., Balboa, J., Rodriguez-Cobo, A., Lopez-Paz, J. M., Rey-Medez, M., Suarez-Quintanilla, J. A., Millan, J. C. and Mayan, J. M. (1999) Effects of amphetamine on development of oral candidiasis in rats. *Clinical and Diagnostic Laboratory Immunology* 6(4): 530–533.

Furara, S. A., Carrick, P., Armstrong, D., Pairaudeau, P., Pullan, A. M. and Lindow, S. W. (1999) The outcome of pregnancy associated with amphetamine use. *Journal of Obstetrics and Gynaecology* 19(4): 377–380.

Garwood, E. R., Bekele, W., McCulloch, C. E. and Christine, C. W. (2006) Amphetamine exposure is elevated in Parkinson's disease. *Neurotoxicology* 27(6): 1003–1006.

Gonzales, R., Marinelli-Casey, P., Shoptaw, S., Ang, A. and Rawson, R. A. (2006) Hepatitis C virus infection among methamphetamine-dependent individuals in outpatient treatment. *Journal of Substance Abuse Treatment* 31: 195–202.

Guilarte, T. R. (2001) Is methamphetamine abuse a risk factor in Parkinsonism? *Neurotoxicology* 22: 725–731.

Halfon, P., Riflet, H., Renou, C., Quentin, Y. and Cacoub, C. (2001) Molecular evidence of male-to-female sexual transmission of hepatitis C virus after vaginal and anal intercourse. *Journal of Clinical Microbiology* 39(3): 1204–1206.

Hanson, G. R., Rau, K. S. and Fleckenstein, A. E. (2004) The methamphetamine experience: a NIDA partnership. *Neuropharmacology* 47(Suppl 1): 92–100.

Horita, A., West, T. C. and Dille, J. M. (1953) Cardiovascular responses during amphetamine tachyphylaxis. *Journal of Pharmacology and Experimental Therapeutics* 108(2): 224–232.

Hsieh, Y.-S., Yang, S.-F. and Kuo, D.-Y. (2005) Amphetamine, an appetite suppressant, decreases neuropeptide Y immunoreactivity in rat hypothalamic paraventriculum. *Regulatory Peptides* 127: 169–176.

Iacovelli, L., Fulceri, F., De Blasi, A., Nicoletti, F., Ruggieri, S. and Fornai, F. (2006) The neurotoxicity of amphetamines: bridging drugs of abuse and neurodegenerative disorders. *Experimental Neurology* 201: 24–31.

Jacobs, W. (2006) Fatal amphetamine-associated cardiotoxicity and its medicolegal implications. *The American Journal of Forensic Medicine and Pathology* 27(2): 156–160.

Jankovic, J. (2002) Emerging views of dopamine in modulating sleep / wake state from an unlikely source: PD. *Neurology* 58(3): 341–346.

Kaku, D. A. and Lowenstein, D. H. (1990) Emergence of recreational drug abuse as a major risk factor for stroke in young adults. *Annals of Internal Medicine* 113(11): Abstract.

Kase, C. S. (1986) Intracerebral haemorrhage: non-hypertensive causes. *Stroke* 17: 590–595.

Kaye, S., McKetin, R., Duflou, J. and Darke, S. (2007) Methamphetamine and cardiovascular pathology: a review of the evidence. *Addiction* 102: 1204–1211.

Kelly, J. J., Davis, P. G. and Henschke, P. N. (2000) The drug epidemic: effects on newborn infants and health resource consumption at a tertiary perinatal centre. *Journal of Paediatrics and Child Health* 36(3): 262–264.

Krawczyk, C. S., Molitor, F., Ruiz, J., Facer, M., Allen, B., Green-Ajufo, B., Lynch, M., Klausner, J. D., McFarland, W., Bell-Sandford, G., Ferrero, D. V., Morrow, S., Page-Shafer, K. and Lemp, G. (2006) Methamphetamine use and HIV risk behaviours among heterosexual men – preliminary results from five northern California countries, December 2001–November 2003. *Morbidity and Mortality Weekly Report* 55(10): 273–288.

Kuczenski, R., Segal, D. S., Cho, A. K. and Melega, W. (1995) Hippocampus norepinephrine, caudate dopamine and serotonin and behavioural responses to the stereoisomers of amphetamine and methamphetamine. *The Journal of Neuroscience* 15(2): 1308–1317.

Kuo, D.-Y. (2003) Further evidence for the mediation of both subtypes of dopamine D1/D2 receptors and cerebral neuropeptide Y (NPY) in amphetamine-induced appetite suppression. *Behavioural Brain Research* 147: 149–155.

Kuo, D.-Y. (2005) Involvement of hypothamlamic neuropeptide Y in regulating the amphetamine-induced appetite suppression in streptozotocin diabetic rats. *Regulatory Peptides* 127: 19–26.

Kuo, D.-Y. and Cheng, J.-T. (2002) Role of cerebral dopamine but not plasma insulin, leptin and glucocorticoid in the development of tolerance to the anorectic effect of amphetamine. *Neuroscience Research* 44: 63–69.

Matsumoto, T., Kamijo, A., Miyakawa, T., Endo, K., Yabana, T., Kishimoto, H., Okudaira, K., Iseki, E., Sakai, T. and Kosaka, K. (2002) Methamphetamine in Japan: the consequences of methamphetamine abuse as a function of route of administration. *Addiction* 97(7): 809–817.

McCann, U. D. and Ricaurte, G. A. (2000) Drug abuse and dependence: hazards and consequences of heroin, cocaine and amphetamines. *Current Opinion in Psychiatry* 13(3): 321–325.

McCann, U. D. and Ricaurte, G. A. (2004) Amphetamine neurotoxicity: accomplishments and remaining challenges. *Neuroscience and Biobehavioural Reviews* 27(8): 821–826.

McCann, U. D., Wong, D. F., Yokoi, F., Villemagne, V., Dannals, R. F. and Ricaurte, G. A. (1998) Reduced striatal dopamine transporter density in abstinent methamphetamine and methcathinone users: evidence from positron emission tomography studies with [11C]WIN-35,428. *The Journal of Neuroscience* 18(20): 8417–8422.

McElhatton, P. R. (2005) Drug abuse and pregnancy. *Clinical Toxicology* 43(5): 391.

McGough, J. J., Biederman, J., Wigal, S. B., Lopez, F. A., McCracken, J. T., Spencer, T., Zhang, Y. and Tulloch, S. J. (2005) Long-term tolerability and effectiveness of once-daily mixed amphetamine salts (Adderall XR) in children with ADHD. *Journal of American Academic of Child and Adolescent Psychiatry* 44(6): 530–538.

McGregor, C., Srisurapanont, M., Jittiwutikarn, J., Laobhripatr, S., Wongtan, T. and White, J. (2005) The nature, time course and severity of methamphetamine withdrawal. *Addiction* 100(9): 1320–1329.

Molitor, F., Truax, S. R., Ruiz, J. D. and Sun, A. K. (1998) Association of methamphetamine use during sex with risky behaviours and HIV infection among non-injecting drug users. *The Western Journal of Medicine* 168(2): 93–97.

Nixon, P. J., Youngson, C. C. and Beese, A. (2002) Tooth surface loss: does recreational drug use contribute? *Clinical Oral Investigations* 6: 128–130.

Pagel, J. F. and Parnes, B. L. (2001) Medications for the treatment of sleep disorders: an overview. *Primary Care Companion Journal of Clinical Psychiatry* 3(3): 118–125.

Perez, J. A., Asura, E. L. and Stategos, S. (1999) Methamphetamine-related stroke: four cases. *The Journal of Emergency Medicine* 17(3): 469–471.

Piran, N. and Gadalla, T. (2007) Eating disorders and substance abuse in Canadian women: a National Study. *Addiction* 102(1): 105–113.

Plessinger, M. A. (1998) Prenatal exposure to amphetamines. Risks and adverse outcomes in pregnancy. *Obstetrics and Gynaecology Clinics of North America* 25(1): 119–38.

Ragland, A. S., Ismali, Y. and Lasura, E. L. (1993) Myocardial infarction after amphetamine use. *American Heart Journal* 125(1): 247–249.

Ricaurte, G. A., Seiden, L. S. and Schuster, C. R. (1984) Further evidence that amphetamines produce long-lasting dopamine neurochemical deficits by destroying dopamine nerve fibers. *Brain Research* 303: 359–364.

Richters, J., Arnold, L., Jensen, P., Abikoff, H., Conners, C. K., Greenhill, L. L., Hechtman, L., Hinshaw, S. P., Pelham, W. E. and Swanson, J. M. (1995) NIMH Collaborative Multisite Multimodal Treatment Study of Children With ADHD, I: background and rationale. *Journal of American Academic of Child and Adolescent Psychiatry* 34: 987–1000.

Riddle, E. L., Fleckenstein, A. E. and Hanson, G. R. (2006) Mechanisms of methamphetamine-induced dopaminergic neurotoxicity. *The AAPS Journal* 8(2): E413–E418.

Robinson, L. and Rempel, H. (2006) Methamphetamine use and HIV symptom self-management. *Journal of the Association of Nurses in AIDS Care* 17(5): 7–14.

Robinson, T. E. and Becker, J. B. (1986) Enduring changes in brain and behaviour produced by chronic amphetamine administration: a review and evaluation of animal models of amphetamine psychosis. *Brain Research* 396(2): 157–198.

Sanaullah, F., Gillian, M. and Lavin, T. (2006) Screening of substance misuse during early pregnancy in Blyth: an anonymous unlinked study. *Journal of Obstetrics and Gynaecology* 26(3): 187–190.

Sattah, M. V., Supawitkul, S., Dondero, T. J., Kilmarx, P. H., Young, N. L., Mastro, T. D., Chaikummao, S., Manopaiboon, C. and van Grienscen, F. (2002) Prevalence of and risk factors of methamphetamine use in northern Thai youths: results of an audio-computer-assisted self-interviewing survey with urine testing. *Addiction* 97: 801–808.

Schafer, D. and Greulich, W. (2000) Effects of Parkinsonian medication on sleep. *Journal of Neurology* 247(4): IV24–IV27.

See, S.-J. and Tan, E.-K. (2003) Severe amphetamine-induced bruxism: treatment with botulinum toxin. *Acta Neurologica Scandanavia* 107: 161–163.

Semple, S., Patterson, T. L. and Grant, I. (2004) Determinants of condom use stage of change among heterosexually-identified methamphetamine users. *AIDS and Behaviour* 8(4): 391–400.

Smith, H. R. (2006) Stimulant-dependent sleep disorder. *Medlink Neurology*. Avialable at www.medlink.com.

Smith, L., Yonekura, M. L., Wallace, T., Berman, N., Kuo, J. and Berkowitz, C. (2003) Effects of prenatal methamphetamine exposure on fetal growth and drug withdrawal symptoms in infants born at term. *Developmental and Behavioural Paediatrics* 24(1): 17–23.

Smith, L. M., LaGasse, L. L., Derauf, C., Grant, P., Shah, R., Arria, M., Haning, W., Strauss, A., Grotta, S. D., Liu, J. and Lester, B. M. (2006) The infant development, environment and lifestyle study: effects of prenatal methamphetamine exposure, polydrug exposure and poverty on intrauterine growth. *Paediatrics* 118: 1149–1156.

Srisurapanont, M., Jarusuraisin, N. and Jittiwutikarn, J. (1999) Amphetamine withdrawal: II. A placebo-controlled, randomised, double-blind study of amineptine treatment. *Australian and New Zealand Journal of Psychiatry* 33: 94–98.

Stek, A. M., Baker, R. S., Fisher, B. K., Lang, U. and Clark, K. E. (1995) Fetal responses to maternal and fetal methamphetamine administration in sheep. *American Journal of Obstetrics and Gynaecology* 173: 1592–1598.

Szabadi, E. (2006) Drugs for sleep disorders: mechanisms and therapeutic prospects. *British Journal of Pharmacology* 61(6): 761–766.

Tyler, A. (1998) *Street Drugs*. London: Hodder and Stoughton.

Wagner, G. C., Ricaurte, G. A., Johnson, C. E., Schuster, C. R. and Seiden, L. S. (1980) Amphetamine induces depletion of dopamine and loss of dopamine uptake sites in caudate. *Neurology* 30: 547–550.

Westover, A. N., McBride, S. and Hayley, R. W. (2007) Stroke in young adults who abuse amphetamines and cocaine: a population based study of hospitalized patients. *Archives of General Psychiatry* 64: 495–501.

White, R. (2000) Dexamphetamine substitution in the treatment of amphetamine abuse: an initial investigation. *Addiction* 95(2): 229.

White, R., Thompson, M., Windsor, D., Walsh, M., Cox, D. and Charnaud, B. (2006) Dexamphetamine substitute-prescribing in pregnancy: a 10 year retrospective audit. *Journal of Substance Use* 11(3): 205–216.

Williams, I. (1999) Epidemiology of hepatitis C in the United States. *American Journal of Medicine* 107(6B): 2S–9S.

Wisor, J. P., Nishino, S., Sora, I., Uhl, G. H., Mignot, E. and Edgar, D. M. (2001) Dopaminergic role in stimulant-induced wakefulness. *The Journal of Neuroscience* 21(5): 1787–1794.

Wolgin, D. L. (2004) Tolerance to amphetamine hypophagia: a real time depiction of learning to suppress stereotypes. *Behavioural Neuroscience* 118(3): 470–478.

Wolters, E. C., Tissingh, G., Bergmans, P. L. and Kuiper, M. A. (1995) Dopamine agonists in Parkinson's disease. *Neurology* 45(3): S28–S34.

Wouldes, T., LaGasse, L., Sheridan, J. and Lester, B. (2004) Maternal methamphetamine use during pregnancy and child outcome: what do we know? *Journal of the New Zealand Medical Association* 117(1206): U1180.

Zule, W. A. and Desmond, D. P. (1999) An ethnographic comparison of HIV risk behaviours among heroin and methamphetamine injectors. *American Journal of Drug and Alcohol Abuse* 25(1): 1–12.

Chapter 3

THE PSYCHOLOGICAL AND PSYCHIATRIC EFFECTS OF AMPHETAMINES

Richard Pates and Diane Riley

Introduction

Amphetamines produce euphoria, mood elevation and a sense of well-being (Becker, 1999; de Wit et al., 2002). This is combined with an increase in energy and wakefulness, a reduction in fatigue and increased concentration and alertness (Chapotot et al., 2003). An increase in motor and speech activities can increase talkativeness (Higgins and Stitzer, 1989). Amphetamines can improve physical performance (Chandler and Blair, 1980), and performance of some mental tasks may also improve; higher doses or chronic use are associated with deficits in cognitive and motor performance (Ornstein et al., 2000; Rogers et al., 1999; Simon et al., 2000; Soetens et al., 1995; Wiegmann et al., 1996). At higher doses, euphoria becomes more intense, but adverse effects also increase. These include restlessness, tremor, changes in libido, anxiety, dizziness, tension, irritability, insomnia, confusion and aggression (Degenhardt and Topp, 2003). Teeth grinding may occur and may produce wearing of teeth (one reason some users wear baby suckers around their necks at raves) (McVinney, 2005; Richards and Brofeldt, 2000). Psychosis, delirium, auditory, visual and tactile illusions, paranoid hallucinations, panic stages and loss of behavioural control may occur (Angrist et al., 1974; Iwanami et al., 1994; Janowsky and Risch, 1979; Miczek and Tidey, 1989). Delusions of being monitored with hidden electrical devices are common. There can be a sense of 'bugs' that are felt and seen on the skin, leading to picking and scratching. Restless, jerky and tic-like movements are often present; experienced amphetamine users may describe the combination of paranoia and compulsive movements as 'tweaking' (Forster et al., 1999). Alterations in consciousness may occur (Nakatani and Hara, 1998).

Psychostimulants are associated with a range of mental health problems. Mental health effects appear to be more often documented for amphetamine users than cocaine and ecstasy users. After a binge, the 'crash' is characterised by depression, fatigue and sleeping difficulties. Depression and suicidal behaviour have been identified as significant risks during the crash period (Kamieniecki et al., 1998). In a review of adverse effects of psychostimulants, Kamieniecki and colleagues noted a particularly high prevalence of mental health symptoms among amphetamine users. Between 50 and 90% reported symptoms of depression, between 60 and 80% reported anxiety symptoms and between 30 and 80% had experienced symptoms of psychosis (Kamieniecki et al., 1998). There are several case studies of self-mutilation after amphetamine use; in each case this was attributed to psychosis (Israel and Lee, 2001). Self-mutilation behaviours have also been seen in animal studies (Kratofil et al., 1996). Kratofil and colleagues noted that the behaviour often involved religious, sexual and 'neurotic' themes, such as self-punishment and control. Self-mutilation included amputation of limbs or enucleation of eyes, genital mutilation, stabbing and cutting injuries. The behaviours appear to be relatively rare among women who use psychostimulants, but may be under-reported (Israel and Lee, 2001). Other psychological symptoms that have been noted as a result of psychostimulant use include agitation and anxiety, paranoia, hostility and aggression, confusion, delirium and hallucinations (especially auditory and tactile) (Baker and Dawe, 2005; Baker and Lee, 2003; Lee, 2004a).

Darke et al. (2008) reviewed the literature on both physical and psychological harm associated with methamphetamine use and concluded that rates of both depression and suicide among methamphetamine users are substantially higher than in the general population; both are associated with longer-use careers, more frequent use, dependence and injecting. They also found that the same was true of anxiety, with the same risk associations as depression and anxiety. Darke et al. found that violent behaviours appeared common in methamphetamine users, that psychosis may be accompanied by violent behaviours and that experimental work had shown that chronic use can increase aggressive behaviours and acute intoxication may enhance or augment aggressive responses when threatened or provoked.

Risks associated with high-dose use

Reports of violence and aggressive behaviour associated with amphetamine use have been increasing with increasing use of amphetamines and the availability of the more potent forms of methamphetamine (Lee, 2004a). The relationship between amphetamine use and violence is complex and in need of further research. Amphetamine-related violence is the result of the interaction between the drug, the individual concerned and context of use. Those thought to be more likely to become violent under the influence of amphetamines are people who have previously been violent, those who belong to an aggressive subcultural group, and those in a highly stimulating environment. Aggressive and violent behaviour is more likely to be seen in heavy users of amphetamines, those who inject and those experiencing paranoia or psychosis (Lee, 2004a).

When intensive use of psychostimulants stops, users experience what is known as a 'crash', which is a period of recovery that can last for a few days associated with dysphoria, hunger and fatigue. As use continues, the intensity of the crash increases, and users can experience sleep disturbances and depression, which is sometimes of a suicidal intensity. Deaths attributable to psychostimulant overdose are rare. Where people have died following use of psychostimulants, they have usually taken other drugs as well, most often opioids. In sufficiently high doses, methamphetamine can be lethal due to hyperthermia, convulsions, heart attack or stroke (Wray, 2000).

Risks associated with long-term use

Psychosocial

A clear dependence syndrome has been described, and dependence can be seen in heavy drug users who use drugs several times a week on a regular basis, especially if the usual form of use is injecting. Users who are dependent are likely to experience declining social functioning (Lee, 2004b).

Mental health problems

Intensive and long-term psychostimulant use can result in mental health problems such as psychosis and mood and anxiety disorders, which usually resolve when use stops (Lee, 2004b). Some people experiencing these mental health problems following psychostimulant use have symptoms prior to use. Psychostimulant use can act as a stressor or trigger for an underlying psychotic disorder that does not resolve after stopping use. The severity of mental health problems arising from psychostimulant use is related to the severity of dependence, frequency of use, and injecting as the usual route of administration; the transition to injecting is correlated with serious psychiatric symptoms (Lee, 2004b).

Intensive or prolonged psychostimulant use can produce a psychosis similar to that which occurs in non-drug-induced psychosis. The psychosis usually appears as a result of chronic high-dose use and usually disappears after drug use stops (Lee, 2004b). Symptoms may include hallucinations, paranoid delusions and un-controlled violent behaviour. Psychostimulant-induced psychosis is more common following amphetamine use than cocaine use, and this has especially been the case since the more potent forms of methamphetamine (ice and base) have become more available (Lee, 2004b). Risk of drug-induced psychosis increases as drug-use risk increases (high doses, chronic use and injecting) and as vulnerability to psychosis increases. Psychosis vulnerability increases if the user has had drug-related psychotic symptoms in the past, schizophrenia, paranoid disorder, brief reactive psychosis, mood disorder with psychotic features, or family history of serious mental illness. High rates of psychological problems, especially depression and anxiety, are seen with psychostimulant use. Other symptoms include panic, mania, hallucinations and paranoia and are more common following amphetamine use rather than cocaine use. This may be due to the longer half-life of methamphetamine or may reflect higher levels of pre-existing disorders in different groups of users (Lee, 2004b).

Chronic use of amphetamines can be associated with cognitive impairments. Block et al. (2002) compared the cognitive performance of adult drug users and non-using control subjects while controlling for subjects' intellectual abilities before the onset of drug use. In tests 2–3 weeks after the subject's last use of drugs, drug users scored lower than non-users on each of four achievement tests, as well as on tests of memory and abstraction ability. Stimulant users performed worse than polydrug users on three tests and worse than alcohol users on one test. Stimulant users whose major problem was with amphetamines did not differ in cognitive performance from problem cocaine users. When drug users who remained abstinent were compared with drug users who had not remained abstinent and to control subjects in performance during later retesting, tests showed relative improvements in abstinent drug users. Improvements with abstinence did not vary among stimulant, alcohol and polydrug users. Ernst et al. (2000) reported damage to the brains of methamphetamine users to be similar to that caused by stroke or Alzheimer's disease. Those who had used the most methamphetamine had the strongest indications of cell damage. It is not clear whether this damage reverses with abstinence and treatment.

Neurotoxicity

Neurotoxic risks associated with psychostimulant use may include short- and long-term disruption to brain neurotransmitters that can lead to hyperactivity, mental confusion, agitation, fever, tachycardia and tremor (known as the 'serotonin syndrome'), the effects of which can be fatal. Monoamine depletion can also lead to depressed mood, anhedonia and lethargy post-use ('come down'). Neurotoxic effects appear to persist for extended periods post-administration in animals (Parrott, 2002). To avoid neurotoxicity, users should limit their intake and be aware of possible signs of neurotoxic effects.

Early experience of amphetamine psychosis

The relationship between amphetamine use and psychosis has been known for years; for example see Sato, Chapter 11 in this book, with descriptions of amphetamine psychosis in post-war Japan, and Connell's classic monograph on amphetamine psychosis published in 1958 (Connell, 1958). In fact the earliest report of the potential for amphetamine-type substances (ATS) to produce psychosis was by Young and Scoville (1938), who reported that 2 out of 3 patients being treated for narcolepsy with Benzedrine developed a paranoid psychosis. They suggested that a latent paranoid tendency had produced the psychosis. The authors concluded that it might be better for such patients to endure narcolepsy rather than be treated with a drug which makes manifest their latent paranoia.

Grinspoon and Hedblom (1975) quote a number of early reports of ATS psychosis. Schneck (1948) described a case of psychosis in a prison inmate misusing Benzedrine inhalers. Monroe and Drell (1947), also studying penal inmates, found that of a population of 1200, 25% were misusing Benzedrine inhalers and 4 of these were paranoid and had hallucinations. Norman and Shea (1945) reported on a case of a 49-year-old man who was prescribed amphetamine sulphate by his doctor, and had escalated his dose and became severely paranoid with auditory and visual hallucinations.

Early searches for causation of amphetamine psychosis suggested that psychosis occurred in individuals who had 'susceptible personalities'. For example, Shorvon

(1945) described a fireman who went through the London Blitz and from 1940 until his hospitalisation took 125–150 mg of Benzedrine per day to help him through the extremely stressful work in which he was involved. He developed bad dreams, felt people were talking about him and became agitated and confused. Shorvon suggests that his pre-morbid personality was that of a psychopath.

Carr (1946) reported on a case of amphetamine psychosis attributed to the inhalation of methamphetamine. The patient was admitted to hospital following the use of five Methedrine inhalers to relieve nasal congestion; he was hallucinating and very anxious. After 7 days in hospital the symptoms remitted, but following a further dose of methamphetamine administered intravenously he again experienced hallucinations for several days. After discharge from hospital he once again used inhalers and again experienced a psychotic episode. Carr's view was that the pre-morbid personality of the patient predisposed him to a psychotic breakdown.

In 1954 Chapman contributed to the debate writing as follows:

> It is often difficult to say whether the misuse of amphetamine is symptomatic of an incipient psychosis or precipitated the psychosis in an emotionally unstable person.
> It has been suggested that amphetamine compounds, by inducing a state of distractible alertness, facilitate feelings of personal reference from the environment, and thus precipitate paranoid episodes in emotionally predisposed persons; whether the episode is transitory or becomes chronic would depend on the severity of the pre psychotic tendency toward paranoid, projective processes. (Chapman, 1954 quoted in Grinspoon and Hedblom, 1975, p. 116.)

The largest series of cases of psychosis due to amphetamine published up to 1954 (Herman and Nagler, 1954) observed seven instances of amphetamine psychosis and concluded the typical picture was a paranoid psychotic reaction with a minimal disturbance in the intellectual and cognitive functions. Many of the patients showed a number of abnormalities usually associated with psychopathology (quoted in Grinspoon and Hedblom, 1975, p. 116.)

Thus most of the references in the 1940s and 1950's suggest that amphetamine psychosis was an interaction between amphetamine and a pre-morbid personality. Exceptionally, Freyhan (1949) described a case of a man who, following the ingestion of three inhalers in 3 days developed feelings of persecution and a fear that he was about to be killed. Freyhan wrote that the patient was not pre-morbidly paranoid and that the fear and persecutory delusions might be the effect of the drug alone.

Current views

Symptoms of amphetamine psychosis closely mimic the symptoms of paranoid schizophrenia. Chen et al. (2003) reported on a sample of methamphetamine users who had developed psychosis. They found that 84.5% experienced auditory hallucinations, 71% experienced persecutory delusions, 62.8% experienced delusions of reference, 46.5% experienced visual hallucinations and 40.5% experienced delusions of influence. These are classed as positive symptoms; negative symptoms such as poverty of speech and flat affect were only experienced by 21.4% of psychotic amphetamine users in a study by Srisurapanont et al. (2003).

In individuals who have been diagnosed with schizophrenia the use of amphetamine can trigger psychotic episodes and intensify psychotic symptoms (Curran et al., 2004). Chen et al. (2005) found that relatives of methamphetamine users with a lifetime diagnosis of amphetamine-induced psychosis have a significantly increased risk of developing schizophrenia.

Does this mean that certain individuals are more likely to be predisposed to amphetamine induced psychosis? It is now well established that amphetamines may cause psychosis, and this is accepted by both the users and mental health professionals. Psychosis is usually preceded by paranoia that has been described (Anon., personal communication, 2003) by an experienced user as initially not being unpleasant: 'It gives an exciting edge to life'. Z. Hildrey, A. Smith, and R. Pates, unpublished data) quoted one amphetamine user as saying that 'I know people who can work off psychosis, they are not normal unless they are psychotic'. However, as the psychosis progresses the user loses touch with reality and starts to believe that what he or she is experiencing is real. Anon (personal communication, 2000), a chronic amphetamine user, described how he believed that his neighbours had bugged his house, implanting microphones in the wall. He brought into clinic the plaster he had removed from the walls in an attempt to find these bugging devices, which he was still convinced were present in the plaster debris. Following cessation of amphetamine use he acknowledged that this was a psychotic reaction.

It is also interesting to note from clinical experience that psychosis is not inevitable from heavy amphetamine use. Some users will have a psychotic episode after a small amount and others may use heavily for years and never have a psychotic episode; it does not appear to be dose related or temporally related to length of use. However, it is clear that amphetamine use dramatically increases the likelihood of experiencing psychotic symptoms. McKetin et al. (2006) reported that over one fifth of methamphetamine users had experienced clinically significant symptoms of psychosis in the past year. The also reported that dependent methamphetamine users were three times as likely to experience psychotic symptoms than their non-dependent counterparts and eleven times more likely as the general population. The authors commented 'that the prevalence of psychotic symptoms among methamphetamine users was alarmingly high in comparison with the general population even among methamphetamine users with no known history of schizophrenia or other psychotic disorders'.

Matsumoto et al. (2002) suggested that individuals who smoke amphetamine experienced their first psychotic episode significantly sooner than those who inject and that injecting amphetamine users experience significantly more auditory hallucinations than individuals who smoke amphetamine. Whether these differences are due to route of administration or individual susceptibility is not clear.

A systematic review of studies that investigated stimulant use and psychosis was conducted by Curran et al. (2004). They did this by a comprehensive review of the literature reviewing 54 papers. One of the theories that they were interested in was whether repeated low doses of stimulant lead to a sensitisation. Ellingwood and Kibley (1980) proposed that repeated low doses of a stimulant lead to changes in the central nervous system producing 'kindling' effect, a psychotic illness similar to schizophrenia. Curran and colleagues suggested that occurrence of this sensitisation has implications for treatment. They thought that early treatment and retention of stimulant users in mental health services would improve the mental health of these users. The aim of their study was to examine the evidence for sensitisation, and they hypothesised that stimulant psychoses could be divided into a response that was a toxic reaction to stimulant use and a chronic persisting response caused by long-term stimulant use. This was important an important distinction for it might help explain why some people react quickly to small doses and others only after long-term use.

Curran and colleagues concluded that although the papers they reviewed provided good evidence about the effect on pre-existing psychotic illnesses of stimulant use, the evidence for sensitisation was less convincing. They also found the evidence for the effect of antipsychotic medication in blocking the action of stimulants and preventing deterioration in psychotic illnesses was not borne out. They found that the presence of positive symptoms of schizophrenia gave an individual an increased likelihood of deterioration in their illness following a single dose of a stimulant drug.

The evidence reviewed by Curran and colleagues also showed that irrespective of their mental state a large enough dose of a stimulant can produce a brief psychotic reaction, probably lasting only a few hours, and in the majority of individuals this is self-limiting. Evidence of sensitisation was found only in two studies: one by Strakowski et al. (1997) who found that when two doses of a stimulant were given to volunteers free from psychosis, the second dose produced a greater psychotic response, which they suggest is a 'sensitised' response. The study sought to find a response to a repeated dose of stimulants. In the control group there was a greater response to the second dose of dexamphetamine than the first but participants with a pre-existing psychosis did not show a greater response to the second dose. In a study by Brady et al. (1991) stimulant users reported psychotic symptoms appearing with lower doses over a period of time.

Dalmau et al. (1999) conducted a study of psychosis rates among inpatients who used drugs and noted that psychosis rates were higher among patients who used cannabis or stimulants than those who used opiates. It was though that sensitisation may have been a contributory factor but not the only one It was suggested that one reason might be that opiate-dependent patients were admitted more frequently to the inpatient unit whereas stimulant users were more likely to be treated on an outpatient basis. The results hardly seem surprising given that both stimulants and cannabis (but not opiates) have been associated with the development of psychosis.

Evidence quoted by Curran and colleagues against the sensitisation hypothesis included Seibyl et al. (1993) who noted that in their study the onset of psychotic symptoms preceded stimulant use. Is this debate important? Curran and colleagues believe it is because of the relevance to clinical situations: clinicians need to plan treatment in the absence of an evidence base with a difficult client group. They conclude that in the absence of good evidence treatment should proceed on the basis of symptomatic treatment with antipsychotic drugs and the encouragement of abstinence from stimulants.

Psychostimulant withdrawal and detoxification

While the existence of a psychostimulant withdrawal syndrome is now well recognised, the literature pertaining to psychostimulant withdrawal is inconsistent and of mixed quality. In their review, Jenner and Saunders found that there are no studies that describe the natural history of methamphetamine withdrawal among dependent individuals and that the process is still poorly understood (Jenner and Saunders, 2004). There is some agreement that the psychostimulant withdrawal syndrome is unlike the withdrawal syndromes that occur in people who are dependent on CNS depressant drugs such as opioids or alcohol, the features of which are the opposite to those of the acute pharmacological effects of these drugs. In contrast, several features of the psychostimulant withdrawal syndrome actually mimic those of intoxication, particularly agitation and hyper-arousal.

Many users of psychostimulants will experience what is commonly called a 'crash' or brief period of recovery that may last for a few days following binge use. Jenner and Saunders point out that this recovery period does not in itself constitute a clinically significant withdrawal syndrome, but is a process of recovery from a period of CNS over-stimulation and is usually characterised by excessive sleeping and eating and irritability of mood. Such a recovery period may be compared to the experience of a 'hangover' from alcohol characterised by irritability, tiredness, headache and nausea, which is widely recognised as time-limited and not a withdrawal syndrome in itself. A withdrawal syndrome is a cluster of symptoms, lasting for a meaningful duration, which impairs functioning to a clinically significant degree. The presence of a withdrawal syndrome is not necessary for a person to meet criteria for dependence (which includes psychological factors). The roles that tolerance (neuroadaptation) and acute toxicity play in long-term withdrawal are also unclear.

The incidence, severity, course and subjective experience of the withdrawal syndrome depend on the following:

- the severity of dependence
- duration of use
- frequency of psychostimulant use
- potency of psychostimulant used
- duration of action of psychostimulant
- the presence of other physical or psychiatric disorders and
- psychosocial factors

According to Jenner and Saunders, during psychostimulant withdrawal, dominant signs of CNS hypoactivity such as lethargy, slowed movements and poor concentration are interspersed with agitation and insomnia; dysphoria and depression are also common. This is the result of depletion of monoamine neurotransmitter stores and alteration in brain structure identified by brain imaging studies of current and past methamphetamine users, the effect of which is slowed motor function and impaired memory (Jenner and Saunders, 2004; Cho and Melega, 2002).

Studies examining the natural history of amphetamine withdrawal are significantly fewer than those of cocaine withdrawal. Clinicians report that following cessation of daily use of amphetamine, users report fatigue and inertia, an initial period of hypersomnia followed by protracted insomnia and an onset of agitation, usually within 36 hours of cessation, that exists for between 3 and 5 days. The degree of mood disturbance ranges from dysphoria to severe clinical depression (Jenner and Saunders, 2004).

Conclusions

The evidence quoted above shows clearly that there is a relationship between amphetamine use and mental health problems, particularly psychosis. Amphetamine (and other stimulant related) psychoses typically remit after treatment with antipsychotic drugs and abstinence from the drug. The evidence seems clear that psychosis is experienced not just by those who are susceptible through pre-existing mental health conditions but also by those previously thought to have good mental health. Research is still needed on dose relationships between use and psychotic episodes and the characteristics of those who do become psychotic.

References

Angrist, B., Sathananthan, G., Wilk, S. and Gershon, S. (1974) Amphetamine psychosis: behavioral and biochemical aspects. *Journal of Psychiatric Research* 11, 13–23.

Baker, A. M. and Dawe, S. (2005) Amphetamine use and co-occuring psychological problems: review of the literature and implications for treatment. *Australian Psychologist* 40(2): 87–94.

Baker, A. and Lee, N. K. (2003) A review of psychosocial interventions for amphetamine use. *Drug and Alcohol Review* 22: 323–335.

Becker, J. B. (1999) Gender differences in dopaminergic function in striatum and nucleus accumbens. *Pharmacology Biochemistry and Behavior* 64(4): 803–812.

Block, R. I., Ermin, W. J. and Ghoneim, M. M. (2002) Chronic drug use and cognitive impairment. *Pharmacological Biochemistry and Behavior Journal* 73: 491–504.

Brady, K. T., Lydiard, R. B., Malcolm, R. and Ballenger J. C. (1991) Cocaine induced psychosis. *The Journal of Clinical Psychiatry* 52(12): 509–512. Quoted in Curran, C., Byrappa, N. and McBride, A. (2004) Stimulant psychosis: systematic review. *British Journal of Psychiatry* 185: 196–204.

Carr, R. B. (1946) Acute psychotic reaction after inhaling methylamphetamine. *British Medical Journal* 1: 1476.

Chandler, J. V. and Blair, S. N. (1980) The effect of amphetamines on selected physiological components related to athletic success. *Medicine and Science in Sports and Exercise* 12(1): 65–69.

Chapman, A. H. (1954) Paranoid psychosis associated with amphetamine usage: a clinical note. *The American Journal of Psychiatry* 111: 43. Quoted in Grinspoon, L. and Hedblom, P. (1975) *The Speed Culture: Amphetamine Use and Abuse in America*. Cambridge, MA: Harvard University Press.

Chapotot, F., Pigeau, R., Canini, F., Bourdon, L. and Buguet, A. (2003) Distinctive effects of waking EEG. *Psychopharmacology* 166(2): 127–138.

Chen, C., Lin, S., Sham, P., Ball, D., Loh, E. and Hsiao, C. (2003) Pre-morbid characteristics and co-morbidity of methamphetamine users with and without psychosis. *Psychological Medicine* 3(8): 1407–1414.

Chen, C., Lin, S., Sham, P., Ball, D., Loh, E. and Murray, R. (2005) Morbid risk for psychiatric disorder among the relatives of methamphetamine users with and without psychosis. *American Journal of Medical Genetics. Part B: Neuropsychiatric Genetics* 136B: 87–91.

Cho, A. K. and Melega, W. P. (2002) Patterns of methamphetamine abuse and their consequences. *Journal of Addictive Diseases* 21(1): 21–34.

Connell, P. H. (1958) *Amphetamine Psychosis*. Oxford: Oxford University Press.

Curran, C., Byrappa, N. and McBride, A. (2004) Stimulant psychosis: systematic review. *British Journal of Psychiatry* 185: 196–204.

Dalmau, A., Bergman, B. and Brismar, B. (1999) Psychotic disorders among in-patients with abuse of cannabis, amphetamine and opiates. Do dopaminergic stimulants facilitate psychiatric illness? *European Psychiatry* 14: 366–371. Quoted in Curran, C., Byrappa, N. and McBride, A. (2004) Stimulant psychosis: systematic review. *British Journal of Psychiatry* 185: 196–204.

Darke, S., Kaye, S., McKetin, R. and Duflou, J. (2008) Major physical and psychological harms of methamphetamine use. *Drug and Alcohol Review* 27(3): 253–262.

Degenhardt, L. and Topp, L. (2003) 'Crystal meth' use among polydrug users in Sydney's dance party subculture: characteristics, use patterns and associated harms. *International Journal of Drug Policy* 14(1): 17–24.

de Wit, H., Enggasser, J. L. and Richards, J. B. (2002) Acute administration of D-amphetamine decreases impulsively in healthy volunteers. *Neuropsychopharmacology* 27(5): 813–825.

Ellingwood, E. H. and Kibley, M. M. (1980) Fundamental mechanisms underlying altered behavior following chronic administration of psycho stimulants. *Biological Psychiatry* 15: 749–757.

Ernst, T., Chang, L., Leonido-Yee, M. and Speck, O. (2000) Evidence for long-term neurotoxicity associated with methamphetamine abuse: a 1H MRS study. *Neurology* 54: 1344–1349.

Forster, O. L., Buckley, R. and Phelps, M. A. (1999) Phenomenology and treatment of psychotic disorders in the psychiatric emergency service. *Psychiatric Clinics of North America* 22(4): 735–754.

Freyhan, F. A. (1949) Craving for Benzedrine. *Delaware State Medical Journal* 21: 151–156. Quoted in Grinspoon, L. and Hedblom, P. (1975) *The Speed Culture: Amphetamine Use and Abuse in America*. Cambridge, MA: Harvard University Press.

Grinspoon, L. and Hedblom, P. (1975) *The Speed Culture: Amphetamine Use and Abuse in America*. Cambridge, MA: Harvard University Press.

Herman, M. and Nagler, S. H. (1954) Psychoses due to amphetamine. *Journal of Nervous and Mental Disease* 120: 268–272. Quoted in Grinspoon, L. and Hedblom, P. (1975) *The Speed Culture: Amphetamine Use and Abuse in America*. Cambridge, MA: Harvard University Press.

Higgins, S. T. and Stitzer, M. L. (1989) Monologue speech: effects of D-amphetamine, secobarbital and diazepam. *Pharmacology Biochemistry and Behaviour* 34(3): 609–618.

Israel, J. A. and Lee, K. (2001) Amphetamine usage and genital self-mutilation. *Addiction* 97: 1215–1218.

Iwanami, A., Sugiyama, A., Kuroki, N., Toda, S., Kato, N., Nakatani, Y., Horita, N. and Kaneko, T. (1994) Patients with methamphetamine psychosis admitted to a psychiatric hospital in Japan. A preliminary report. *Acta Psychiatrica Scandinavica* 89(6): 428–432.

Janowsky, D. S. and Risch, C. (1979) Amphetamine psychosis and psychotic symptoms. *Psychopharmacology* 65(1): 73–77.

Jenner, L. and Saunders, J. (2004) Psychostimulant withdrawal and detoxification. In: Baker, A., Lee, N. K. and Jenner, L. (eds), *Models of Intervention and Care for Psychostimulant Users*. Monograph Series No. 52, Australia: Commonwealth of Australia, pp. 35–50.

Kamieniecki, G., Vincent, N., Allsop, S. and Lintzeris, N. (1998) *Models of Intervention and Care for Psychostimulant Users*. Monograph Series No. 32. Canberra: National Centre for Education and Training on Addiction.

Kratofil, P. H., Baberg, H. T. and Dimsdale, J. E. (1996) Self-mutilation and severe self-injurious behaviour associated with amphetamine psychosis. *General Hospital Psychiatry* 18(2): 117–120.

Lee, N. (2004a) Risks associated with psychostimulant use. In: Baker, A., Lee, N. K. and Jenner, L. (eds), *Models of Intervention and Care for Psychostimulant Users*. Monograph Series No 51, pp 35–50. Australia: Commonwealth of Australia.

Lee, N. K. (2004b) *Psychostimulants Information for Health Care Workers*. Melbourne: Turning Point Alcohol and Drug Centre.

Matsumoto, T., Kamijo, A., Miyaka, T., Endo, K., Yabana, T. and Kishimoto, H. (2002) Methamphetamine in Japan: the consequences of methamphetamine abuse as a function of route of administration. *Addiction* 97(7): 809–817.

McKetin, R., McLaren, J., Lubman, D. and Hides, L. (2006) The prevalence of psychotic symptoms among methamphetamine users. *Addiction* 101(10): 1473–1478.

McVinney, D. (2005) The pharmacology of crystal methamphetamine. *Presented at* Science and Response Conference. Salt Lake City, Utah.

Miczek, K. A. and Tidey, J. W. (1989) Amphetamines: aggressive and social behavior. In: Ashghar, K. and De Souza, E. (eds), *Pharmacology and Toxicology of Amphetamine and Related Designer Drugs*. NIDA Research Monograph No. 94. Rockville, MD: US Department of Health and Human Services, pp. 68–100.

Monroe, R. R. and Drell, H. J. (1947) Oral use of stimulants obtained from inhalers. *The Journal of the American Medical Association* 135: 909–914. Quoted in Grinspoon, L. and Hedblom, P. (1975) *The Speed Culture: Amphetamine Use and Abuse in America*. Cambridge, MA: Harvard University Press.

Nakatani, Y. and Hara, T. (1998) Disturbance of consciousness due to methamphetamine abuse. A study of 2 patients. *Psychopathology* 31(3): 131–137.

Norman, J. and Shea, J. T. (1945) Acute hallucinosis as a complication of addiction to amphetamine sulphate. *New England Journal of Medicine* 233: 270–271. Quoted in Grinspoon, L. and Hedblom, P. (1975) *The Speed Culture: Amphetamine Use and Abuse in America*. Cambridge, MA: Harvard University Press.

Ornstein, T. J., Iddon, J. L., Baldacchino, A. M., Sahakian, B. J., London, M., Everitt, B. J. and Robbins, T. W. (2000) Profiles of cognitive dysfunction in chronic amphetamine and heroin abusers. *Neuropsychopharmacology* 23(2): 113–126.

Parrott, A. C. (2002) Recreational ecstasy/MDMA, the sertonin syndrome, and serotonergic neurotoxicity. *Pharmacology, Biochemistry and Behavior* 71(4): 837–844.

Richards, J. R. and Brofeldt, B. T. (2000). Patterns of tooth wear associated with methamphetamine use. *Journal of Periodontology* 71(8): 1371–1374.

Rogers, R. D., Everitt, B. J., Baldacchino, A., Blackshaw, A. J., Swainson, R., Wynne, K., Baker, N. B., Hunter, J., Carthy, T., Booker, E., London, M., Deakin, J. F., Sahakian, B. J. and Robbins, T. W. (1999) Dissociable deficits in the decision-making cognition of chronic amphetamine abusers, opiate abusers, patients with focal damage to prefrontal cortex, and tryptophan-depleted normal volunteers: evidence for monoaminergic mechanisms. *Neuropsychopharmacology* 20(4): 322–339.

Schneck, J. M. (1948) Benzedrine psychosis: report of a case. *Military Surgeon* 102: 60–61. Quoted in Grinspoon, L. and Hedblom, P. (1975) *The Speed Culture: Amphetamine Use and Abuse in America*. Cambridge, MA: Harvard University Press.

Seibyl, J. P., Satel, S. L., Anthony, D., Southwick, S. M., Krystal, J. H. and Chaney, D. S. (1993) Effects of cocaine on hospital course in schizophrenia. *Journal of Nervous and Mental Diseases* 181: 31–37. Quoted in Curran, C., Byrappa, N. and McBride A. (2004) Stimulant psychosis: systematic review. *British Journal of Psychiatry* 185: 196–204.

Shorvon, H. J. (1945) Use of Benzedrine sulphate by psychopaths: the problems of addiction. *British Medical Journal* 2: 285–286.

Simon, S. L., Domier, C., Canell, J., Brethen, P., Rawson, R. and Ling, W. (2000) Cognitive impairment in individuals currently using methamphetamine. *American Journal on Addictions* 9(3): 222–231.

Soetens, E., Casaer, S., D'Hooge, R. and Hueting, J. E. (1995) Effect of amphetamine on long-term retention of verbal material. *Psychopharmacology* 119(2): 155–162.

Srisurapanont, M., Ali, R., Marsden, J., Sunga, A., Wada, K. and Monterio, M. (2003) Psychotic symptoms in methamphetamine psychotic in-patients. *International Journal of Neuropsychopharmacology* 6(4): 347–352.

Strakowski, S. M., Sax, K. W., Setters, M. J., Stanton, S. P. and Keck, P. E. (1997) Lack of enhanced response to repeated D-amphetamine challenge in first episode psychosis: implications for a sensitisation model for psychosis in humans. *Biological Psychiatry* 42: 749–755. Quoted in Curran, C., Byrappa, N. and McBride, A. (2004) Stimulant psychosis: systematic review. *British Journal of Psychiatry* 185: 196–204.

Wiegmann, D. A., Stanny, R. R., McKay, D. L., Neri, D. F. and McCardie, A. H. (1996) Methamphetamine effects on cognitive processing during extended wakefulness. *International Journal of Aviation Psychology* 64(4): 379–397.

Wray, J. (2000) Psychophysiological aspects of methamphetamine abuse. *Journal of Addictions Nursing* 12(3–4): 143–147.

Young, D. and Scoville, WB. (1938) Paranoid psychosis in narcolepsy and the possible danger of Benzedrine treatment. *Medical Clinics of North America* 22: 637–646.

Chapter 4

THE MECHANISMS OF AMPHETAMINE IN THE BRAIN

Jan K. Melichar and David J. Nutt

Introduction

Amphetamines are chemicals that act both centrally on the brain and peripherally on the heart, lungs and other parts of the body. This chapter outlines what is known about the mechanisms of action of these drugs in the brain, specifically concentrating on the actions that are thought to be important when amphetamines are misused.

The pharmacology of amphetamines

An understanding of the pharmacology of amphetamines gives insight as to the reasons they have become abused substances. Addictiveness depends on the actions and effects of a drug, the dose received and the rapidity of onset of effects.

Amphetamines are man-made chemicals, similar in structure to two of the brain's own chemical messengers, dopamine and norepinephrine. Dopamine is involved in the reward pathway, in memory and in a person's drive. Norepinephrine is involved in the brain in attention and mood modification. The actions and effects of amphetamines are discussed in more depth in section on 'Amphetamines – the cycle of use and the systems involved'; however, also important is the way in which amphetamines reach the brain (part of the pharmacokinetics, i.e. how the drug gets to and from its site of action).

The higher the dose of a drug, the more rapidly it reaches the brain, and the faster the onset of its effects, the more addictive it is likely to be. A substance user might experience this as a 'rush'. The route of administration of a psychoactive drug determines how quickly it reaches the brain. For example, intravenous injection or inhalation of a drug may achieve high concentrations in the brain quickly, and so drugs taken in these ways are more addictive than those taken by oral or intramuscular routes.

The other frequently abused stimulant, cocaine, can be used to illustrate these principles. Cocaine is least addictive when taken as coca leaves (taken orally and in small concentrations) compared to preparations with a faster onset of effects. In order of speed of onset of effects, these would be coca paste (taken orally but at higher concentrations), purified cocaine (although snorted, absorption is mostly oral, but with a far higher concentration of cocaine delivered) and lastly crack (this may be smoked or injected, and a large quantity of cocaine arrives rapidly in the brain).

In the case of amphetamine, tablets taken orally are less addictive than when they are crushed and snorted, smoked (methylamphetamine) or injected intravenously. Indeed, methamphetamine is a drug which causes concern in large part because, unlike amphetamine, it can be smoked (having a much lower melting point). There is thus a dramatic increase in the 'rush' and consequently the dependency that results (Schifano et al., 2007)

Reward pathways in the brain and the pharmacology of addiction

To understand how amphetamines act in the brain, it is necessary to understand how the brain system signalling reward works and the way in which addictive substances interact with it. This is extensively reviewed elsewhere (Kalivas and Volkow, 2005; Lingford-Hughes and Nutt, 2003), so only a brief summary is given here. The past decade has seen a great deal of research in this field. It is now clear that drug addiction has a biological basis: drugs such as amphetamine have biological effects on the brain, and once a person is addicted, this may drive much of their behaviour.

Indeed, although initial drug use is a voluntary behaviour, prolonged use changes the brain in fundamental and long-lasting ways. The changes usurp the normal brain circuitry related to motivation and free will. This occurs in stages and across many parts of the brain. The addicted person moves into a state of compulsive behaviour, which is resistant to change without treatment.

Previously, it was thought that the chief result of drug use was the release of the brain chemical dopamine, in a single region of the brain involved in reward and pleasure. Current research points to a more complicated picture. Dopamine is now known to also play a role in systems involved in memory and drive – the systems that let us develop memories that can alter behaviour – as well as movements and emotion.

Despite these other functions of dopamine, the principal pathway in addiction is the meso-cortico-limbic dopaminergic 'reward' pathway. This pathway is common to many addictive drugs including the amphetamines and is illustrated in Figure 4.1. The pathway arises in the brain stem (which controls the basic functions critical to life) in an area rich in dopamine-producing cell bodies, the ventral tegmental area (VTA). From the VTA, dopamine-rich neurones send projections upwards to reach the limbic system, a poorly defined area with much connectivity. Amongst other things, the limbic system is involved in reward and the perception of emotion. The primary component of the limbic system related to reward and goal-directed behaviour is the nucleus accumbens, where many of the VTA's projections release dopamine. From the nucleus accumbens (and directly from the VTA), there are further projections upwards to the higher centres of the brain, especially the

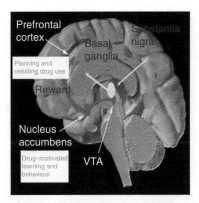

Figure 4.1 Diagrammatic representation of the dopaminergic reward pathway.

cerebral cortex. In particular, there are projections to the pre-frontal cortex, which is critical in planning and decision-making.

There have been numerous studies showing that this pathway is critical for the development of dependency. For example, if a rat has electrodes implanted to stimulate various parts of its brain, it will repeatedly press the lever stimulating the projections from the VTA. This has in turn been shown to be directly linked to increased levels of dopamine in the nucleus accumbens (Crow, 1972; Fiorino et al., 1993). Additional research has shown that in addition to these cells being more active and firing more frequently following reward, there is decreased firing when an animal is stressed or in withdrawal (Zacharko et al., 1987).

The site of amphetamine action

Many addictive drugs interact directly or indirectly with the dopaminergic reward pathway to cause an increase in the amount of dopamine released in the nucleus accumbens, as noted above. This increase can be anywhere between two and five times the amount that is released due to natural rewards such as eating and sex (Wise, 2002). Drugs of addiction achieve this in a variety of ways, whether by causing a direct release of dopamine or by preventing its normal recycling.

In the case of the amphetamines, it has been shown that there is a direct action on the dopamine neurones that arise from the VTA. In the absence of amphetamines, extracellular dopamine is taken up by a transporter in the neurone's cell membrane, which then carries the dopamine back into the cell, recycling it. Until recently, it was widely thought that the key action, in terms of dependency, was for amphetamines to simply block this re-uptake transporter site (Figure 4.2)

Recent work (Kahlig et al., 2005) has further refined this, by recording directly from these transporter sites in cell membranes in vitro. Their results seem to indicate that not only do amphetamines act by preventing the re-uptake of dopamine, but they also cause dopamine to be released by reversing the transporter system. In

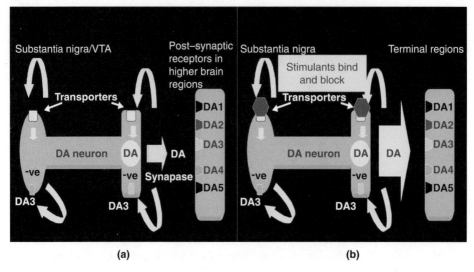

(a)   (b)

Figure 4.2 (a) Dopamine systems; (b) amphetamines blocking dopamine reuptake.

addition to this reversal, the transporter acts as a much faster channel and there is a more rapid efflux of dopamine. The experience is of increased pleasure and the effect is addiction.

Amphetamines – the cycle of use and the systems involved

Given that amphetamines cause a rapid rise in the amount of dopamine released in the nucleus accumbens, what are the consequences? Chronic excess stimulation of the dopamine reward pathway affects the functioning of the brain and causes a 'cycle of use' of amphetamines (Figure 4.3). Early on, when amphetamine is taken, vastly increased amounts of dopamine are quickly released. This mimics the events that occur in the nucleus accumbens following a behaviourally salient stimulus, that is something that is judged to be important, such as food or sex (Grace et al., 2007), when there is a large release of dopamine over a short period. Because amphetamines signal 'importance' and tap into learning and memory systems, there is then a great deal of reinforcement of the drug-using behaviour (Everitt and Wolf, 2002).

There is now a large body of evidence showing that the resultant repeated amphetamine use, and the accompanying repeated large releases of dopamine in the nucleus accumbens, can cause changes in the dopamine pathway (Hyman et al., 2006).

One of the critical consequences of this excessive dopamine release is that the balancing (homeostatic) mechanisms come into play. The brain adjusts to the overwhelming amount of dopamine being released in two principal ways: it reduces the amount of dopamine produced and/or reduces the number of receptors that

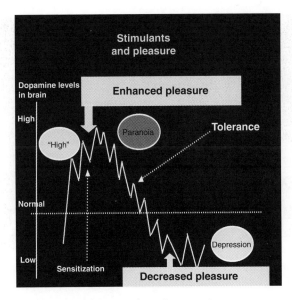

Figure 4.3 Stimulants enhance pleasure, then decrease it.

will respond to dopamine. Thus the amphetamine addict, having stimulated their brains so that the salience and importance of everything and anything to do with taking amphetamines is increased, finds that they get less and less pleasure from using amphetamines. Indeed, as Figure 4.3 shows, the drug users not only experience less pleasure (which they can temporarily compensate for by increasing dose), they eventually have so little rewarding effect from dopamine release that they feel depressed and flat. At this stage, the amphetamine is taken simply in order to feel normal. The paranoia often felt is not completely understood, although the same dopamine system has been implicated in the paranoid symptoms of schizophrenia (Featherstone et al., 2007).

Imaging studies using amphetamines

The neurobiology of amphetamines has in the main, been dissected out in preclinical and in vitro studies, due to the difficulty in studying the changes in the brain in man in vivo. However, some studies have used functional and pharmacological neuroimaging to extend our knowledge of these processes in humans. These help bridge the gap between the findings from the animal literature and the reality of clinical addiction.

Positron emission tomography is an important neuroimaging tool. It allows the measurement of neurochemical and metabolic processes in the living human and primate brain. There are several radioactively labelled molecules (ligands) that have been used to examine dopaminergic systems, looking at, for example, neuroreceptor numbers and dopamine levels.

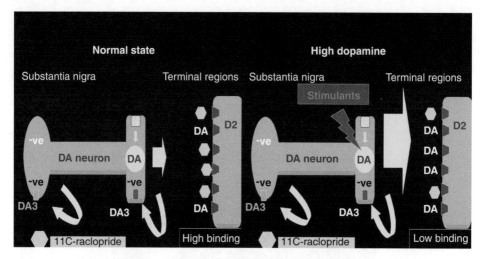

Figure 4.4 Measuring dopamine levels using [¹¹C]-raclopride positron emission tomography (PET).: (a) normal state and (b) high dopamine levels.

One of the first groups to use this technique extensively in man was Nora Volkow's group at the Brookhaven National Laboratory in New York. They used both amphetamines and cocaine in a variety of studies to look at both shorter- and longer-term consequences of drug use. Cocaine, although not an amphetamine, is a stimulant which activates similar dopaminergic pathways to amphetamine. Changes found following cocaine abuse are likely to be mirrored in the amphetamine-abusing population.

Volkow's group (Volkow et al., 1999a) administered increasing amounts of intravenous methylphenidate (which is structurally similar to amphetamine and acts in a similar way) to healthy, drug-naive volunteers to mimic the rapid onset effects of amphetamine (amphetamine itself was not given for ethical reasons). They scanned the subjects using a ligand/marker ([¹¹C]-raclopride) of dopamine D2 receptors: any increases or decreases of dopamine would be shown by a consequent change in the signal seen (Figure 4.4). As shown in Figure 4.5a, they found that increasing doses caused a reduced signal: the methylphenidate caused a dose-dependent change and hence an increase in the amount of dopamine. Furthermore, this increase directly correlated with the perceived reward or 'high' and 'rush' from the drug. A parallel study (Volkow et al., 1999b) also showed that the original baseline levels of dopamine D2 receptors predicted how pleasant (and reinforcing) the dose of methylphenidate would be (Figure 4.5b).

Work paralleling this in the primate has been done by Michael Nader's group (Morgan et al., 2002; Nader et al., 2006). Critically, they found that initial levels of D2 receptors predict the reinforcing nature of cocaine – the larger the receptor number, the lesser the reinforcement. Interestingly, this initial level of D2 receptors was directly correlated to the social status of the monkeys – those with a higher social status had more receptors and were less likely to self-administer cocaine

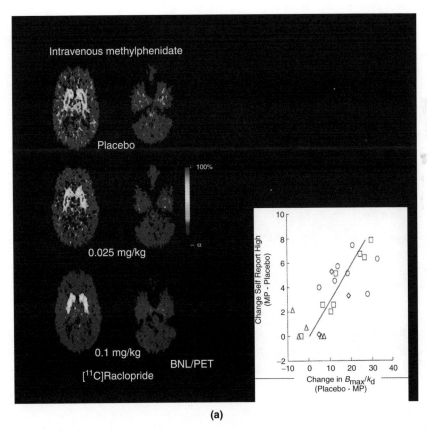

(a)

Figure 4.5 (a) Rewarding effects of psychostimulants correlate with increases in dopamine (taken from Volkow et al., 1999a); (b) perceived reinforcing benefits of psychostimulants predicted by baseline dopamine D2 receptor levels (taken from Volkow et al., 1999b). MP, methylphenidate; BNL, Brookhaven National Laboratory. B_{max}/K_d is a measure of D_2-receptor concentration used in PET neuroimaging. Circle, Square, Diamond, Triangle represent concentrations of methylphenidate given in mg/kg. Circle, 0.5 mg/kg; square, 0.25; diamond, 0.1; triangle, 0.025.

(they were able to 'just say no'). Lower social status monkeys were more likely to self-administer. In the follow-up study, monkeys were again allowed to self-administer cocaine – over the course of a year of self-administration, the amount they took inversely correlated, again, to initial D2 receptor levels. Over the course of the year, D2 receptor levels reduced by approximately 20% (perhaps reflecting, as shown earlier in Figure 4.3, the reduction in general pleasure seen in humans). When followed up for a further year of enforced abstinence, it is worth noting that in 60% of the monkeys, the D2 receptor levels returned to normal; 40% did not return to a 'normal' functioning dopaminergic system.

This and other works (see reviews by Dom et al., 2005; Volkow et al., 2004) have led to the understanding that stimulant drugs such as amphetamine elicit the biological sequelae of dependency through repeated excessive short-term bursts

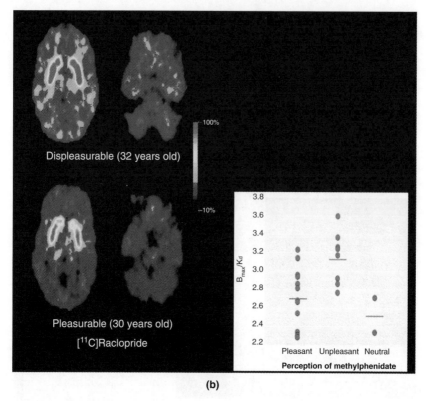

Displeasurable (32 years old)

Pleasurable (30 years old)

[^{11}C]Raclopride

(b)

Figure 4.5 (*Continued*)

of dopamine which alter the sensitivity of the brain to a variety of stimuli. The end result is that drug-specific stimuli have high importance and non-drug-related stimuli have less importance. Furthermore, there is evidence from the literature that, in part, there is a reduction in activity/blood flow of the orbitofrontal cortex, a key area thought to be involved in decision-making and inhibitory control. So, the drugs not only increase salience to drug-specific stimuli, but also reduce and disrupt the frontal inhibition which would reduce the desire to take drugs.

Model of addiction in terms of brain circuitry

We know that the action of amphetamines is to release excessive dopamine and that this drives a variety of changes in the brain, subverting the normal processes that are involved in reward, reward-related learning, memory and drive. This knowledge and information from neuroimaging studies have led to one model of addiction that summarizes the diverse evidence and knowledge (Volkow et al., 2003) and is shown in Figure 4.6.

These circuits work together and change with experience. Each is linked to an important concept: saliency (reward), internal state (motivation/drive), learned

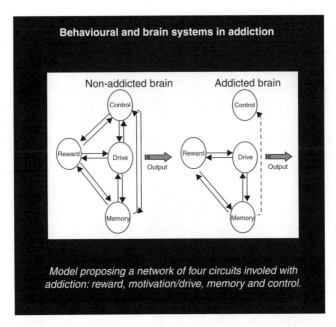

Figure 4.6 Model proposing a network of four circuits involved with addiction: reward, motivation/drive, memory and control.

associations (memory), and conflict resolution (control). During addiction, the enhanced value of the drug in the reward, motivation, and memory circuits overcomes the inhibitory control exerted by the prefrontal cortex, thereby favouring a positive-feedback loop initiated by the consumption of the drug and perpetuated by the enhanced activation of the motivation/drive and memory circuits.

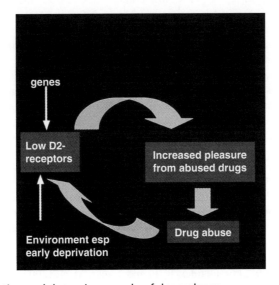

Figure 4.7 Addiction and dopamine: a cycle of dependence.

Summary

Amphetamines act by causing rapid supra-physiological increases in the levels of dopamine in pathways in the brain that are activated in reward and attention. Repeated activation of these pathways results in chronic changes to both this system and higher cortical systems to do with control/inhibition, especially in individuals who already have a low-functioning dopaminergic system (which may be a result of biological and/or environmental causes). Thus, in dependency, the underlying biological circuitry is primed to focus on drug-related stimuli with little active inhibition to prevent a drug-taking response (Figure 4.7). Some of the data do support the notion that even following a period of abstinence, individuals who will still find it difficult to resist will remain though the majority can, potentially, recover.

References

Crow, T. J. (1972) A map of the rat mesencephalon for electrical self-stimulation. *Brain Research* 36(2): 265–273.

Dom, G., Sabbe, B., Hulstijn, W. and van den Brink, W. (2005) Substance use disorders and the orbitofrontal cortex: systematic review of behavioural decision-making and neuroimaging studies. *British Journal of Psychiatry* 187: 209–220.

Featherstone, R. E., Kapur, S. and Fletcher, P. J. (2007) The amphetamine-induced sensitized state as a model of schizophrenia. *Progress in Neuropsychopharmacology Biological Psychiatry* 31(8): 1556–1571.

Everitt, B. J. and Wolf, M. E. (2002) Psychomotor stimulant addiction: a neural systems perspective. *Journal of Neuroscience* 22: 3312–3320.

Fiorino, D. F, Coury, A., Fibiger, H. C. and Phillips, A. G. (1993) Electrical stimulation of reward sites in the ventral tegmental area increases dopamine transmission in the nucleus accumbens of the rat. *Behavioural Brain Research* 55(2): 131–141.

Hyman, S.E., Malunka, R.C. and Nestler, E. J. (2006) Neural mechanisms of addiction: the role of reward-related learning and memory. *Annual Review of Neuroscience* 29: 565–598.

Grace, A. A., Floresco, S. B., Goto, Y. and Lodge, D. J. (2007) Regulation of firing of dopaminergic neurons and control of goal-directed behaviors. *Trends in Neuroscience* 30(5): 220–227.

Kahlig, K. M., Binda, F., Khoshbouei, H., Blakely, R. D., McMahon, D. G., Javitch, J. A. and Galli, A. (2005) Amphetamine induces dopamine efflux through a dopamine transporter channel. *Proceedings of the National Academy of Science of the United States of America* 102(9): 3495–3500.

Kalivas, P. W. and Volkow, N. D. (2005) The neural basis of addiction: a pathology of motivation and choice. *American Journal of Psychiatry* 162(8): 1403–1413.

Lingford-Hughes A. and Nutt, D. (2003) Neurobiology of addiction and implications for treatment. *British Journal of Psychiatry* 182: 97–100.

Morgan, D., Grant, K. A., Gage, H. D., Mach, R. H., Kaplan, J. R., Prioleau, O., Nader, S. H., Buchheimer, N., Ehrenkaufer, R. L. and Nader, M. A. (2002) Social dominance in monkeys: dopamine D2 receptors and cocaine self-administration. *Nature Neuroscience* 5(2): 169–174.

Nader, M. A., Morgan, D., Gage, H. D., Nader, S. H., Calhoun, T. L., Buchheimer, N., Ehrenkaufer, R. and Mach, R. H. (2006) PET imaging of dopamine D2 receptors during chronic cocaine self-administration in monkeys. *Nature Neuroscience* 9(8): 1050–1056.

Schifano, F., Corkery, J. M. and Cuffolo, G. (2007) Smokable ('ice', 'crystal meth') and nonsmokable amphetamine-type stimulants: clinical pharmacological and epidemiological issues, with special reference to the UK. *Annali Dell Istituto Superiore Di Sanita* 43(1): 110–115.

Volkow, N. D., Wang, G. J., Fowler, J. S., Logan, J., Gatley, S. J., Wong, C., Hitzemann, R. and Pappas, N. R. (1999a) Reinforcing effects of psychostimulants in humans are associated with increases in brain dopamine and occupancy of D(2) receptors. *Journal of Pharmacology and Experimental Therapeutics* 291(1): 409–415.

Volkow, N. D., Wang, G. J., Fowler, J. S., Logan, J., Gatley, S. J., Gifford, A., Hitzemann, R., Ding, Y. S. and Pappas, N. (1999b) Prediction of reinforcing responses to psychostimulants in humans by brain dopamine D2 receptor levels. *American Journal of Psychiatry* 156(9): 1440–1443.

Volkow, N. D., Fowler, J. S. and Wang, G. J. (2003) The addicted human brain: insights from imaging studies. *Journal of Clinical Investigation* 111(10): 1444–1451.

Volkow, N. D., Fowler, J. S., Wang, G. J. and Swanson, J. M. (2004) Dopamine in drug abuse and addiction: results from imaging studies and treatment implications. *Molecular Psychiatry* 9: 557–569.

Wise, R. A. (2002) Brain reward circuitry: insights from unsensed incentives. *Neuron* 36(2): 229–240.

Zacharko, R. M., Lalonde, G. T., Kasian, M. and Anisman, H. (1987) Strain-specific effects of inescapable shock on intracranial self-stimulation from the nucleus accumbens. *Brain Research* 426(1): 164–168.

Chapter 5

METHYLPHENIDATE FOR THE TREATMENT OF ADHD: CLINICAL EFFICACY, ABUSE POTENTIAL AND CONSEQUENCES OF USE

Craig R. Rush, Andrea R. Vansickel, William W. Stoops and Paul E. A. Glaser

Methylphenidate (Ritalin) is one of the most commonly prescribed psychoactive drugs in the USA and prescriptions for methylphenidate have increased in recent years (Robison et al., 1999). Methylphenidate is used primarily for the management of behavioural problems associated with attention-deficit/hyperactivity disorder (ADHD). ADHD is a psychiatric disorder that originates in childhood and often continues into adulthood. It has been estimated that between 3 and 10% of all children are affected by ADHD and that 33–66% of these children have ADHD symptoms into adulthood (Wender et al., 2001). The purpose of this chapter is to provide an overview of the clinical efficacy, abuse potential and consequences of use of methylphenidate.

Clinical efficacy of methylphenidate for treating ADHD

The efficacy of methylphenidate in the treatment of ADHD has been demonstrated for a range of behaviours across a variety of settings in a number of clinical trials (reviewed in Brown et al., 2005; Dodson, 2005; Faraone et al., 2006). Improvement of ADHD symptoms in children has been widely demonstrated on a number of outcome variables including the Conners' Rating Scales (clinician, parent and teacher rated versions), Child Behavior Checklist (CBCL) and behavioural observations (Brown et al., 2005). In an early placebo-controlled crossover trial, 12 boys demonstrated significant improvement on the Conners' Rating Scale, the Children's Checking Scale and sustained attention tasks during maintenance on methylphenidate relative to placebo (Anderson et al., 1981). These findings have been supported in placebo-controlled, parallel-group trials as well (Horn et al., 1991; Klein and Abikoff, 1997; Pliszka et al., 2000). In one trial, 58 children were maintained on placebo, methylphenidate or mixed amphetamine salts (Pliszka et al., 2000). Maintenance on the active drugs resulted in significant improvement in problem classroom behaviour and Clinical Global Impression (CGI) scores. Recently, the efficacy of methylphenidate in all types of ADHD (primarily inattentive, primarily hyperactive/impulsive and combined type) was examined (Barbaresi et al.,

2006). Overall, methylphenidate was effective regardless of the type of childhood ADHD.

As in children with ADHD, the utility of methylphenidate in adults with ADHD has also been tested in a number of placebo-controlled clinical trials (Dodson, 2005). In an early crossover trial, 37 adults with ADHD, verified using the Wenders–Utah Rating Scale, demonstrated significant improvement in a number of symptoms including attentional difficulty and impulsivity during methylphenidate maintenance relative to placebo maintenance (Wender et al., 1985). This finding has been confirmed in other crossover trials as well as in parallel trials (Spencer et al., 1995, 2005).

Abuse potential of methylphenidate

Despite its documented efficacy, there are concerns regarding the potential misuse and abuse of methylphenidate particularly when diverted to individuals without ADHD. The methods for determining the abuse potential of a drug include chemical, pharmacological, behavioural and epidemiological analysis. At the chemical level of analysis, inferences concerning the abuse potential of a drug can be drawn on the basis of its structural similarity to known drugs of abuse. Inferences concerning the abuse potential of a drug can also be drawn on the basis of its pharmacological effects in the central nervous system relative to known drugs of abuse. Methylphenidate is a piperidine derivative, structurally related to amphetamine. Abused stimulants including D-amphetamine, methamphetamine and cocaine increase synaptic levels of dopamine, albeit by different mechanisms. Methylphenidate also increases synaptic dopamine levels. Methylphenidate, like cocaine, blocks the dopamine transporter (DAT) (Ritz et al., 1987). Methylphenidate and cocaine are similar in terms of their actions at the DAT and produce comparable increases in synaptic dopamine levels in baboons (Gatley et al., 1999; Volkow et al., 1999a, 1999b). Moreover, the in vivo potency of methylphenidate at the DAT is comparable to that of cocaine in human brain (Volkow et al., 1999b). The regional distribution of [11C]-methylphenidate is almost exactly the same as that of [11C]-cocaine in humans (Volkow et al., 1995). Because of its structural and pharmacological similarity to drugs such as cocaine and D-amphetamine, there is reason to suspect that methylphenidate may have at least some abuse potential.

Consistent with these chemical and pharmacological data, the results of human laboratory experiments suggest that the behavioural effects of methylphenidate overlap extensively with those of cocaine, D-amphetamine and methamphetamine. Below we review the behavioural effects of methylphenidate compared to commonly abused stimulants with special emphasis on measures traditionally used to assess the relative abuse potential of drugs. Special emphasis is given to those studies that determined the relative abuse potential of methylphenidate in humans under controlled laboratory conditions. The behavioural effects of a drug, however, are not the sole determinant of its abuse potential. Biological factors, social variables and drug availability, for example, systematically influence the abuse potential of a drug (Altmann et al., 1996). We, therefore, review epidemiological data to determine the extent of methylphenidate misuse and abuse. Only through the comparison to epidemiological data can the predictive validity and public health relevance of laboratory-based research be ascertained.

Reinforcing effects

The reinforcing effects of a drug may be the single most important determinant of its abuse potential (Foltin and Fishcman, 1991). Human laboratory studies often assess the reinforcing effects of a drug by determining whether it maintains self-administration. In a typical self-administration experiment, volunteers receive administrations of a drug or placebo contingent upon some response (e.g. button pressing). Drugs that maintain rates of self-administration greater than those observed with placebo are deemed to be reinforcers. An alternative method for assessing the reinforcing effects of drugs involves a choice procedure wherein volunteers sample drug or placebo under double-blind conditions on separate days and are then given the opportunity to choose which drug they wish to take on subsequent days. The reliable selection of the drug-containing capsules demonstrates that the drug is a reinforcer (Johanson and Uhlenhuth, 1980a, 1980b).

We know of three published studies in which the reinforcing effects of orally administered methylphenidate were compared to D-amphetamine in humans (Chait, 1994; Rush et al., 2001; Stoops et al., 2004). In the first study, non-drug-abusing volunteers were allowed to choose between methylphenidate (20–40 mg, dose varied across volunteers) and placebo using a discrete-choice procedure. Methylphenidate was chosen on 28% of occasions, which was not statistically significant. While the results of this study suggest that methylphenidate does not function as a reinforcer and, by inference, does not have abuse potential, they must be viewed cautiously because of the methods used. Most notably, the discrete-choice procedure may not be sensitive to the reinforcing effects of commonly abused stimulants in non-drug-abusing volunteers. In support of this notion is the fact that this report included results from a methodologically similar experiment in which the reinforcing effects of D-amphetamine were assessed. In this experiment, volunteers were allowed to choose between D-amphetamine (7.5–20 mg, dose varied across individual volunteers) and placebo; D-amphetamine was chosen on 38% of occasions, which was not significant. Thus, D-amphetamine, a drug with documented abuse potential, also failed to function as a reinforcer.

In a series of studies conducted in our laboratory, we compared the reinforcing effects of methylphenidate and D-amphetamine using a progressive-ratio procedure (Rush et al., 2001; Stoops et al., 2004). Under a progressive-ratio schedule, the response requirement to obtain a reinforcer (e.g. a drug dose) systematically increases. The last ratio completed to obtain a reinforcer is referred to as the break point and is the dependent measure. Progressive-ratio schedules are thought to provide an index of reinforcing efficacy or 'strength' (Hodos, 1961). In the first experiment, we compared the reinforcing effects of methylphenidate (20 and 40 mg),

D-amphetamine (10 and 20 mg) and placebo in eight recreational drug users (Rush et al., 2001). A modified progressive-ratio schedule was used to assess drug reinforcement in which a sampling session always preceded a self-administration session. During sampling sessions, volunteers received a drug dose to acquaint them with the drug effects. Drug doses were administered in eight identical capsules (i.e. each capsule contained 12.5% of the total dose). During self-administration sessions, which generally were conducted the next day, volunteers were given eight opportunities to work on a computer and could earn all, or some, of the capsules that were administered the previous day. To earn the first capsule, volunteers had to click a computer mouse 50 times. The number of clicks required to earn each additional capsule doubled (i.e. 100, 200, 400, 800, 1600, 3200 and 6400 clicks). Both doses of D-amphetamine increased break point significantly above placebo levels, while only the high dose of methylphenidate did so (Figure 5.1a). Break-point values for the doses of methylphenidate and D-amphetamine that maintained the greatest responding did not differ significantly. In the second experiment, we compared the reinforcing effects of methylphenidate (16, 32 and 48 mg), D-amphetamine (8, 16 and 24 mg) and placebo in 10 drug-abusing volunteers (Stoops et al., 2004). The intermediate dose of methylphenidate and D-amphetamine increased, responding significantly above placebo levels (Figure 5.1b). The effects of the intermediate doses of methylphenidate and D-amphetamine did not differ significantly. These data suggest that methylphenidate, like D-amphetamine, functions as a reinforcer under a modified progressive-ratio schedule and, by inference, has at least some abuse potential.

Discriminative-stimulus effects

Drug-discrimination experiments determine whether novel drugs share similar interoceptive effects and, by inference, abuse potential with a known drug of abuse. In a typical drug-discrimination experiment, one response (e.g. right button press) is reinforced following the administration of a drug and a different response (e.g. left button press) is reinforced following the administration of placebo. Following training, novel drugs are administered to determine if they share discriminative-stimulus effects with the training drug (i.e. occasion similar response patterns). The human drug-discrimination procedure has several advantages: first, drug-discrimination is contingency-based in that correct identifications are usually reinforced with money; second, human drug discrimination involves extensive training; third, volunteers usually need to meet a predetermined accuracy criterion before progressing to a test phase in which novel drugs are administered to determine if they share discriminative-stimulus effects with the training drug. Volunteers, therefore, have similar recent pharmacological and behavioural histories. Collectively, these procedures may reduce variability within and across volunteers. Finally, drug-discrimination is pharmacologically specific in that drugs from the same class as the training drug generally increase drug-appropriate responding as a function of dose, while drugs from different classes generally produce placebo-appropriate

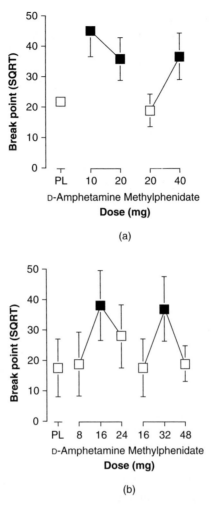

(a)

(b)

Figure 5.1 Dose–response functions for methylphenidate and D-amphetamine for break point on the progressive-ratio procedure in (a) stimulant users (redrawn from Rush et al. (2001)) and (b) abusers (redrawn from Rush et al. Stoops et al. (2004)). Data points above PL designate placebo values. Filled symbols denote a significant difference from placebo response. Brackets indicate one standard error of the mean (SEM).

responding (Lile et al., 2006; Rush and Baker, 2001; Rush et al., 1997, 1998, 2002; Sevak et al., 2009; Stoops et al., 2005).

We know of seven published reports in which the discriminative-stimulus effects of methylphenidate were compared to those of another abused stimulant (Heishman and Henningfield, 1991; Lile et al., 2006; Rush and Baker, 2001; Rush et al., 1998, 2002; Sevak et al., 2009; Stoops et al., 2005). The results of these studies are remarkably consistent in that the discriminative effects of methylphenidate overlapped extensively with those of cocaine, D-amphetamine and methamphetamine.

In three studies conducted in our laboratory, we compared the discriminative-stimulus effects of methylphenidate and D-amphetamine (Lile et al., 2006; Rush et al., 1998; Stoops et al., 2005). In the first study, the discriminative-stimulus effects of a range of doses of D-amphetamine (2.5–20 mg), methylphenidate (5–40 mg) and triazolam (0.0625–0.5 mg) were examined in five volunteers who had learned to discriminate oral D-amphetamine (20 mg) (Rush et al., 1998). D-Amphetamine and methylphenidate generally dose-dependently increased drug-appropriate responding (Figure 5.2, a). Triazolam on average occasioned low levels of drug-appropriate responding. In the other two studies, we examined the discriminative-stimulus effects of methylphenidate (5–30 mg), D-amphetamine (2.5–15 mg), triazolam (0.0625–0.375 mg) and placebo in volunteers (i.e. 6 per study) who had learned to discriminate 30-mg oral methylphenidate (Lile et al., 2006; Stoops et al., 2005). Methylphenidate and D-amphetamine dose-dependently increased methylphenidate-appropriate responding, while triazolam produced low levels of drug-appropriate responding (see Figure 5.2b for representative data).

In two other studies conducted in our laboratory, we compared the discriminative-stimulus effects of methylphenidate to those of the more widely abused stimulants, cocaine and methamphetamine (Rush and Baker, 2001; Sevak et al., 2009). In the first study, we examined the discriminative-stimulus effects of methylphenidate (15–90 mg), cocaine (50–300 mg), triazolam (0.125–0.75 mg) and placebo in six human volunteers with recent histories of cocaine use who had learned to discriminate 200-mg oral cocaine (Rush and Baker, 2001). Cocaine and methylphenidate dose-dependently increased cocaine-appropriate responding, while triazolam produced low levels of drug-appropriate responding (Figure 5.2c). In the other study, we examined the discriminative-stimulus effects of methamphetamine (2.5–15 mg), D-amphetamine (2.5–15 mg), methylphenidate (5–30 mg), triazolam (0.0625–0.375 mg) and placebo in seven volunteers with histories of illicit stimulant use who had learned to discriminate 10-mg oral methamphetamine (Sevak et al., 2009). Methamphetamine, D-amphetamine and methylphenidate dose-dependently increased methamphetamine-appropriate responding, while triazolam produced low levels of drug-appropriate responding.

In summary, the discriminative-stimulus effects of methylphenidate overlap extensively with those of cocaine, D-amphetamine and methamphetamine. By inference, then, methylphenidate has at least some abuse potential.

Subjective effects

Human laboratory studies often characterise the subjective effects of the drug of interest (e.g. methylphenidate) relative to those of a standard compound (e.g. D-amphetamine) (e.g. de Wit and Gritffiths, 1991). A range of acute doses are administered and volunteers complete a battery of subjective drug-effect questionnaires before drug administration and periodically afterwards for several hours. Standardised mood questionnaires such as the Addiction Research Center Inventory (ARCI) or Profile of Mood States (POMS) are often employed along with

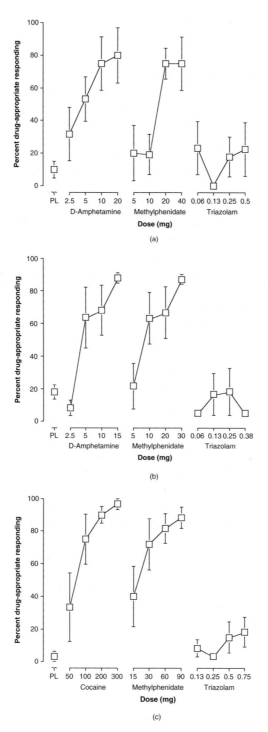

Figure 5.2 Dose effects for percentage of drug-appropriate responding. Data points above PL designate placebo values. Redrawn from Rush et al. (1998, (a)); Stoops et al. (2005, (b)); and Rush and Baker (2001, (c)).

investigator-constructed instruments. The investigator-constructed instruments usually consist of several items (e.g. like drug, stimulated, willing to take drug again) that are rated using a 5-point ordinal scale (i.e. 0 = Not at All, 4 = Extremely) or a 100-mm visual-analogue line (e.g. extreme left labelled 'Not at All' and extreme right labelled 'An Awful Lot'). Compounds that produce subjective ratings (e.g. euphoria or drug liking) similar to those of abused drugs are inferred to have abuse potential. Measures of drug liking are among the more sensitive subjective effects when assessing the abuse potential of drugs (Griffiths et al., 2003).

As part of the drug discrimination studies described above, volunteers also completed a battery of subjective-effects questionnaires before drug administration and periodically afterwards for several hours (Lile et al., 2006; Rush and Baker, 2001; Rush et al., 1998, 2002; Sevak et al., 2009; Stoops et al., 2005). In one study, for example, the subjective effects of methylphenidate (5–40 mg), D-amphetamine (2.5–20 mg), triazolam (0.06–0.5 mg) and placebo were assessed using an Adjective Rating Scale, the ARCI, the POMS, an investigator-developed Drug-Effect Questionnaire and an investigator-developed End-of-Day Questionnaire. Methylphenidate and D-amphetamine produced prototypical subjective effects (e.g. increased ratings of active, alert, energetic; drug liking; good effects; stimulated); these effects were an orderly function of dose. The effects of methylphenidate and D-amphetamine were qualitatively and quantifiably similar (see Figure 5.3 a for representative data). Triazolam, by contrast, produced sedative-like subjective effects (e.g. increased ratings of sluggish, lazy, fatigued). In another study, the subjective effects of methylphenidate (15–90 mg), cocaine (50–300 mg), triazolam (0.125–0.75 mg) and placebo were assessed in volunteers who reported recent cocaine use (Rush and Baker, 2001). Methylphenidate and cocaine produced prototypical subjective effects (e.g. increased ratings of drug liking; good effects; willing to take again; stimulated). These effects were an orderly function of dose. The dose-related effects of methylphenidate and cocaine did not differ significantly on these measures (see Figure 5.3 b for representative data). To the extent that the subjective effects of drugs might predict abuse potential, the results of these studies suggest that methylphenidate, like other stimulants, has at least some potential for abuse.

While the studies described above suggest that methylphenidate, like other stimulants, has at least some potential for abuse, it is worth noting that all of the drugs were administered orally. A number of case studies have described the abuse of intranasal methylphenidate (Coetzee et al., 2002; Garland, 1998; Jaffe, 1991, 2002; Massello and Carpenter, 1999). These reports suggest that adolescents pulverise two to five standard methylphenidate tablets and insufflate the powder. In another study conducted in our laboratory, we characterised the acute reinforcing and subjective effects of intranasal methylphenidate (0, 10, 20 and 30 mg) in eight volunteers with recent histories of recreational stimulant use (Stoops et al., 2003). Drug doses were administered in a double-blind fashion under medical supervision, but for safety purposes, they were administered in ascending order. The effects of intranasal methylphenidate were assessed before drug administration and periodically afterwards for 2 hours. Intranasal methylphenidate increased the crossover

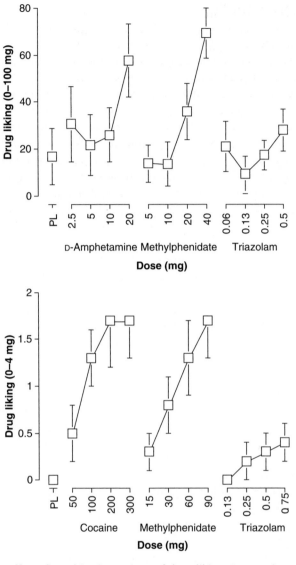

Figure 5.3 Dose effects for subjective ratings of drug liking. Data points above PL designate placebo values. Redrawn from Rush et al. (1998, (a)), Rush and Baker (2001, (b)).

point on the Multiple-Choice Questionnaire, a measure of drug reinforcement, in a linear fashion, which suggests that intranasal methylphenidate functioned as a reinforcer. Intranasal methylphenidate also produced linear dose-dependent prototypical stimulant-like subjective effects. The results of this study suggest that across a range of doses intranasal methylphenidate produces behavioural effects that are characteristic of abused stimulants.

Epidemiological findings

While the results of human laboratory studies suggest that the abuse potential of methylphenidate is comparable to that of licit and illicit stimulants (i.e. cocaine, D-amphetamine and methamphetamine), these findings need to be validated with data on relative rates of abuse in a naturalistic setting. The results of epidemiological studies suggest that the incidence of illicit methylphenidate use is comparable to, and in some instances exceeds, rates observed for cocaine and methamphetamine. A recent survey found that of 4580 college students 8.3% had used illicit prescription stimulants in their lifetime and 5.9% had used illicit prescription stimulants in the past year (Teter et al., 2006). Of the respondents that reported using illicit prescription stimulants in the past year, 25% reported using methylphenidate. In another sample of 2250 undergraduate students, 3% reported past-year illicit use of methylphenidate (Teter et al., 2003). Results from a third survey, which sampled 283 undergraduate students from a small north-eastern liberal arts college, showed that more than 16% of students had used methylphenidate recreationally and that almost 13% had used it intranasally (Babcock and Byrne, 2000).

Methylphenidate misuse and abuse is not limited to non-ADHD individuals. One survey study conducted with 334 college students found that 76 had been prescribed a stimulant for ADHD (Upadhyaya et al., 2005). Of the 76 that had been prescribed a stimulant, 29% reported selling or giving away their medication and 25% ($n = 19$) reported using their medication to get 'high'. Methylphenidate had been prescribed for 10 of the 19 individuals that reported using their medications to get 'high' (Upadhyaya et al., 2005).

Methylphenidate misuse and abuse is not limited to young adults or college students. The Indiana Prevention Resource Center (2006), for example, reported that approximately 4.2% of ninth-, tenth- and eleventh-grade students used illicit methylphenidate annually and more than 2% used it monthly. The results of another study that surveyed 12 990 students in seventh, ninth, tenth and twelfth grade revealed that 6.6% reported lifetime illicit methylphenidate use and 84% reported using illicit methylphenidate one to four times in the past year (Poulin, 2007). In addition, 57 students included in that sample reported both medical and non-medical use of methylphenidate.

At least 2% of children and young adults surveyed in the above-mentioned studies reported using methylphenidate illicitly (Babcock and Byrne, 2000; Poulin, 2007; Teter et al., 2003, 2006; Upadhyaya et al., 2005). Approximately 2% of individuals aged 18–25 years reported current cocaine use (SAMHSA, 2006). Amongst ninth, tenth and eleventh graders, annual rates of cocaine use are between 3.3 and 5.5% while monthly rates of cocaine use among these individuals are between 1.7 and 2.7% (Indiana Prevention Resource Center, 2006). Approximately 0.6% of individuals aged 18–25 years report current methamphetamine use (SAMHSA, 2006). Annual rates of methamphetamine use are between 2.2 and 2.7% amongst ninth, tenth and eleventh graders while monthly rates of methamphetamine use among these individuals are between 1.2 and 1.5% (Indiana Prevention Resource Center,

2006). Thus, the incidence of illicit methylphenidate use is comparable to, and in some instances exceeds, rates observed for cocaine and methamphetamine.

The illicit use of methylphenidate is also associated with a maladaptive behaviour pattern that could affect the health and well-being of the individual. Past-year illicit methylphenidate users are significantly more likely to smoke tobacco cigarettes, use other illicit substances and binge drink compared to non-users. Moreover, past-year illicit methylphenidate users reported experiencing greater consequences associated with their drug and alcohol use (Teter et al., 2003). In addition, methylphenidate misuse and abuse may lead to dependence. Results from epidemiological studies suggest that up to 38% of individuals using illicit methylphenidate snort the medication and some inject it (Babcock and Byrne, 2000; Teter et al., 2006). Snorting and injecting methylphenidate creates a quicker 'high' which may lead to the development of dependence on the medication. Consistent with this notion, approximately 10% of non-methamphetamine illicit prescription stimulant users between the ages of 12 and 25 meet the criteria for stimulant dependence (Kroutil et al., 2006).

Overall, then, the epidemiological studies reviewed above suggest that methylphenidate is misused and abused. The prevalence of methylphenidate abuse is comparable to that of other stimulants including cocaine and methamphetamine. The abuse of methylphenidate, like other stimulants, is associated with maladaptive behaviour and dependence. The results of epidemiological studies are concordant with those from human laboratory studies and suggest that laboratory models are valid for predicting the relative abuse potential of stimulant medications.

Summary

The results of controlled laboratory experiments and epidemiological studies suggest that methylphenidate, like other stimulants, has abuse potential. Clinicians, researchers and pharmaceutical manufacturers recognise this problem, and in recent years have begun to systematically examine ways to minimise the abuse potential of methylphenidate (Volkow, 2006). A number of novel formulations of methylphenidate have recently been introduced for clinical use. These novel formulations of methylphenidate, like traditional preparations, are effective in the management of ADHD (e.g. Coghill and Seth, 2006; Reimherr et al., 2007). In general, these formulations release methylphenidate slowly over an extended period of time. The premise behind reformulating methylphenidate is that reducing the rate of onset will minimise the abuse potential. Rate of onset is believed to be an important determinant of abuse potential (Farré and Cami, 1991). Users of illicit drugs often prefer substances that produce their behavioural effects rapidly (Jaffe, 1990). Furthermore, drug users tend to use routes of administration that produce effects quickly (e.g. insufflate, inhale or inject).

The results of two laboratory experiments support the notion that sustained-release formulations of methylphenidate have less abuse potential than immediate-release preparations (Kollins et al., 1998; Spencer et al., 2006). In the first experiment, the acute behavioural effects of orally administered sustained-release methylphenidate (20 and 40 mg), immediate-release methylphenidate (20 and 40 mg) and placebo were assessed in ten volunteers (Kollins et al., 1998). Drug effects were assessed before drug administration and periodically afterwards for 6 hours using a battery of subjective drug-effect questionnaires. As expected, immediate-release methylphenidate produced stimulant-like subjective effects (e.g. increased ratings of elated, good effects and high) that generally varied as a function of dose and time. Sustained-release methylphenidate, by contrast, produced very transient effects on these measures that were smaller in magnitude than those observed with the immediate-release doses. While the results of this experiment suggest that sustained-release methylphenidate has less abuse potential than similar immediate-release doses, blood plasma levels were not assessed; perhaps the immediate-release methylphenidate produced greater plasma concentrations than sustained-release drug. In the second experiment, the subjective effects of immediate-release (40 mg) and osmotic controlled-release (90 mg) methylphenidate were examined in 12 volunteers (i.e. 6 per condition) (Spencer et al., 2006). These doses produced comparable plasma concentrations. Volunteers who received immediate-release drug reported significantly greater subjective responses, including drug liking, relative to those who received controlled-release methylphenidate.

The results of these experiments suggest that sustained- or controlled-release formulations of methylphenidate have less abuse potential than immediate-release preparations. However, it is worth noting that the controlled- or sustained-release properties of many of the formulations are circumvented if the tablet is crushed or pulverised. The development of a sustained-release formulation of methylphenidate that is tamper resistant might obviate this problem.

Consequences of methylphenidate use

The widespread use of methylphenidate, and of other stimulants, has raised concerns regarding the consequences of treating ADHD patients. For example, ADHD patients are at increased risk to develop substance use disorders relative to their non-ADHD counterparts (e.g. Biederman et al., 1999; Tercyak et al., 2002). There is disagreement whether treating ADHD patients with stimulants decreases or increases their risk for substance use disorders (e.g. Barkley et al., 2003; Biederman et al., 1999; Faraone et al., 2007; Lambert and Hartsough, 1998; Molina et al., 2007; Wilens et al., 2003). Some trials reported that ADHD children treated with stimulants were more likely to try cocaine or develop cocaine problems relative to untreated patients (Barkley et al., 2003; Lambert and Hartsough, 1998). In another study, the effects of stimulant treatment on substance use were examined in stimulant-treated ($N = 56$) and untreated ADHD ($N = 19$) patients (Biederman et al., 1999). The stimulant-treated ADHD patients were significantly less likely to develop substance abuse disorders than their untreated counterparts. A recent trial failed to demonstrate either a deleterious or protective effect of stimulant treatment for the development of substance abuse disorders (Molina et al., 2007). Finally, the prevalence of substance use disorders was assessed in three groups of adult ADHD patients (i.e. no stimulant treatment, $N = 108$; past stimulant treatment, $N = 33$; current and past stimulant treatment, $N = 65$) (Faraone et al., 2007). There were no significant differences between these groups in terms of the prevalence of alcohol or drug abuse/dependence. Given the widespread use of stimulants such as methylphenidate to treat ADHD and the public health concerns associated with substance use disorders, more research is needed to elucidate the relationship between stimulant treatment and subsequent substance use disorders in ADHD children and adults.

Smoking or nicotine dependence, like other forms of substance use disorders, is more prevalent in ADHD patients than non-ADHD individuals (e.g. Lambert and Hartsough, 1998; Milberger et al., 1997a, 1997b; Pomerleau et al., 1995; Tercyak et al., 2002). In one survey, data were obtained from 218 ADHD and 182 non-ADHD adults (i.e. Lambert and Hartsough, 1998). By 17 years of age, 46% of the ADHD adults reported smoking daily compared to 24% of the non-ADHD controls. Because stimulants, including methylphenidate, are prescribed for the treatment of ADHD (Reeves and Schweitzer, 2004; Spencer et al., 2004), clinicians and researchers have been interested in determining whether these drugs increase the risk of smoking or nicotine dependence.

The results of laboratory experiments suggest that prescription stimulants, including methylphenidate, increase smoking (Chait and Griffiths, 1983; Cousins et al., 2001; Henningfield and Griffiths, 1981; Rush et al., 2005; Schuster et al., 1979; Tidey et al., 2000; Vansickel et al., 2007). Across a series of experiments, we have examined the acute effects of a range of doses of methylphenidate (10, 20 and 40 mg) and placebo in 22 non-ADHD cigarette smokers who were not attempting to quit. Each dose of methylphenidate was tested once while placebo was tested twice. One hour after ingesting drug, volunteers were allowed to smoke ad libitum for 4 hours. Methylphenidate dose-dependently increased the total number cigarettes smoked and carbon monoxide levels (Figure 5.4). While these results suggest that methylphenidate increases cigarette smoking, two caveats warrant mentioning. First, as noted above, non-ADHD volunteers were studied. Second, sustained-release formulations of methylphenidate are commonly used to manage the symptoms of ADHD, and, of course, drug is administered chronically (e.g. Lage and Hwang, 2004). Prospective laboratory research is needed to determine whether chronically treating ADHD patients with controlled-release methylphenidate increases smoking.

The results of clinical trials are mixed regarding the effects of stimulant treatment on smoking in ADHD patients (Barkley et al., 2003; Biederman et al., 1999; Lambert, 2002; Lambert and Hartsough, 1998). The results of at least two studies suggest that stimulant-treated ADHD patients may be at increased risk to smoke relative to their untreated counterparts (Lambert, 2002; Lambert and Hartsough, 1998). In one study, for example, the effects of stimulant pharmacotherapy on substance use were examined in stimulant-treated ($N = 131$) and untreated ADHD ($N = 268$) patients that had been part of a 22-year longitudinal study

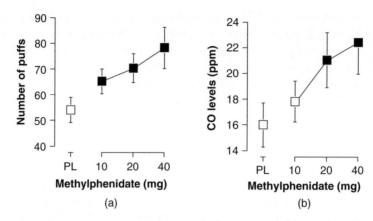

Figure 5.4 Dose–response functions for (a) number of cigarettes and (b) carbon monoxide (CO) levels. Data points above PL designate placebo values. Data points show means of 22 volunteers; brackets show ±1 SEM. Filled symbols indicate those values which are significantly different from the placebo value ($p \leq 0.05$, Fisher's protected least significant difference post hoc test).

(i.e. 6–28 years of age) (Lambert, 2002). A significantly greater percentage of stimulant-treated patients reported regular smoking relative to untreated controls. In another study, the effects of stimulant pharmacotherapy were examined in stimulant-treated ($N = 56$) and untreated ADHD ($N = 19$) patients (Biederman et al., 1999). A non-significant trend was observed that suggests stimulant-treated patients were at increased risk for tobacco use or dependence relative to untreated patients. In yet another study, the effects of stimulant pharmacotherapy were examined in stimulant-treated ($N = 98$) and untreated ADHD ($N = 21$) patients (Barkley et al., 2003). A greater percentage of stimulant-treated patients reported having tried cigarettes relative to untreated controls (i.e. 52 versus 30%). While this difference was not statistically significant, the trend was noteworthy ($\chi^2 = 3.82$, $p = 0.051$). Given the public-health implications of smoking and the mixed results described above, more research is clearly needed.

Concluding remarks

Methylphenidate and other stimulants are clearly effective for the treatment of ADHD in children and adults. As is the case with nearly every psychotherapeutic medication, there are problems associated with methylphenidate and other prescription stimulants. Methylphenidate is diverted and used illicitly. The results of human laboratory experiments and epidemiological studies suggest that methylphenidate has at least some abuse potential. The results of studies that examined the relationship between stimulant treatment and subsequent substance use disorders, including cigarette smoking, are mixed. This uncertainty along with the public-health implications of substance use disorders and smoking clearly suggest more research is needed.

We would like to emphasise that the review of the possible abuse of methylphenidate and the relationship between substance use disorders, including smoking, and stimulant treatment of ADHD is not intended to discourage the clinical use of methylphenidate or other stimulants for ADHD. Rather, the intention is to raise awareness regarding the potential abuse of methylphenidate as well as possible consequences of stimulant treatment. The prescribing physicians, patients and their families will then have a better understanding of the potential adverse effects of methylphenidate at all ages. Weighing the benefits and risks will lead to informed decision-making. Heightened awareness of these issues and more informed decision-making, along with the conduct of additional research, will eventually result in the safer treatment of ADHD patients.

Acknowledgements

The National Institute on Drug Abuse Grants R01 DA010325, R01 DA020429, R01 DA017711 and R01 DA021155 (Craig R. Rush) supported this research. The National Institute on Mental Health Grant K08 MH070840 supports Dr Glaser. The National Institute of Health National Research Service Award NIDA DA 07304 (Thomas F. Garrity) supported Ms Vansickel.

References

Altmann, J., Everitt, B. J., Glautier, S., Markou, A., Nutt, D., Oretti, R., Phillips, G. D. and Robbins, T. W. (1996) The biological, social and clinical bases of drug addiction: commentary and debate. *Psychopharmacology* 125: 285–345.

Anderson, E. E., Clement, P. W. and Oettinger, L. (1981) Methylphenidate compared with behavioral self-control in attention deficit disorder: preliminary report. *Journal of Developmental and Behavioral Pediatrics* 2: 137–141.

Babcock, Q. and Byrne, T. (2000) Student perceptions of methylphenidate abuse at a public liberal arts college. *Journal of American College Health* 49: 143–145.

Barbaresi, W. J., Katusic, S. K., Colligan, R. C., Weaver, A. L., Leibson, C. L. and Jacobsen, S. J. (2006) Long-term stimulant medication treatment of attention-deficit/hyperactivity disorder: results from a population-based study. *Journal of Developmental and Behavioral Pediatrics* 27: 1–10.

Barkley, R. A., Fischer, M., Smallish, L. and Fletcher, K. (2003.) Does the treatment of attention-deficit/hyperactivity disorder with stimulants contribute to drug use/abuse? A 13-year prospective study. *Pediatrics* 111: 97–109.

Biederman, J., Wilens, T., Mick, E., Spencer, T. and Faraone, S. V. (1999). Pharmacotherapy of attention-deficit/hyperactivity disorder reduces risk for substance use disorder. *Pediatrics* 104: e20.

Brown, R. T., Amler, R. W. and Freeman, W. S., Perrin, J. M., Stein, M. T., Feldman, H. M., Pierce, K. and Wolraich, M. (2005) Treatment of attention deficit/hyperactivity disorder: overview of the evidence. *Pediatrics* 115: e749–e757.

Chait, L. D. (1994) Reinforcing and subjective effects of methylphenidate in humans. *Behavioural Pharmacology* 5: 281–288.

Chait, L. D. and Griffiths, R. R. (1983) Effects of caffeine on cigarette smoking and subjective response. *Clinical Pharmacology and Therapeutics* 34: 612–622.

Coetzee, M., Kaminer, Y. and Morales, A. (2002) Megadose intranasal methylphenidate (ritalin) abuse in adult attention deficit hyperactivity disorder. *Substance Abuse* 23: 165–169.

Coghill, D. and Seth, S. (2006) Osmotic, controlled-release methylphenidate for the treatment of ADHD. *Expert Opinion on Pharmacotherapy* 7: 2119–2138.

Cousins, M. S., Stamat, H. M. and de Wit, H. (2001) Acute doses of D-amphetamine and bupropion increase cigarette smoking. *Psychopharmacology (Berlin)* 157: 243–253.

de Wit, H. and Gritffiths, R. R. (1991) Testing the abuse liability of anxiolytic and hypnotic drugs in humans. *Drug and Alcohol Dependence* 28: 83–111.

Dodson, W. W. (2005) Pharmacotherapy of adult ADHD. *Journal of Clinical Psychology* 61: 589–606.

Faraone, S. V., Biederman, J., Spencer, T. J. and Aleardi, M. (2006) Comparing the efficacy of medications for ADHD using meta-analysis. *Medscape General Medicine* 8: 4.

Faraone, S. V., Biederman, J., Wilens, T. E. and Adamson, J. (2007) A naturalistic study of the effects of pharmacotherapy on substance use disorders among ADHD adults. *Psychological Medicine* 12: 1–10.

Farré, M. and Cami, J. (1991) Pharmacokinetic considerations in abuse liability evaluations. *British Journal of Addictions* 86: 1601–1606.

Foltin, R. W. and Fishcman, M. W. (1991) Assessment of abuse liability of stimulant drugs in humans: a methodological survey. *Drug and Alcohol Dependence* 28: 3–48.

Garland, E. J. (1998) Intranasal abuse of prescribed methylphenidate. *Journal of American Academy of Child and Adolescent Psychiatry* 37: 573–574.

Gatley, S. J., Volkow, N. D., Gifford, A. N., Fowler, J. S., Dewey, S. L., Ding, Y. S. and Logan, J. (1999) Dopamine-transporter occupancy after intravenous doses of cocaine and methylphenidate in mice and humans. *Psychopharmacology* 146: 93–100.

Griffiths, R. R., Bigelow, G. E. and Ator, N. A. (2003) Principles of initial experimental drug abuse liability assessment in humans. *Drug and Alcohol Dependence* 70: S41–S54.

Heishman, S. J. and Henningfield, J. E. (1991) Discriminative stimulus effects of D-amphetamine, methylphenidate, and diazepam in humans. *Psychopharmacology* 103: 436–442.

Henningfield, J. E. and Griffiths, R. R. (1981) Cigarette smoking and subjective response: effects of D-amphetamine. *Clinical Pharmacology and Therapeutics* 30: 497–505.

Hodos, W. (1961) Progressive ratio as a measure of reward strength. *Science* 134: 943–944.

Horn, W. F., Ialongo, N. S., Pascoe, J. M., Greenberg, G., Packard, T., Lopez, M., Wagner, A. and Puttler, L. (1991) Additive effects of psychostimulants, parent training, and self-control therapy with ADHD children. *Journal of the American Academy of Child and Adolescent Psychiatry* 30: 233–240.

Indiana Prevention Resource Center (2006) The Indiana Prevention Resource Center 2006 prevalence statistics main findings. Available at www.drugs.indiana.edu. Accessed on 8 August 2007.

Jaffe, J. H. (1990). Drug addiction and drug abuse. In: Gilman, A. G., Rall, T. W., Nies, A. A. and Taylor, P. (eds), *The Pharmacological Basis of Therapeutics*, 8th edn. New York: MacMillan Publishing Co, pp. 522–573.

Jaffe, S. L. (1991) Intranasal abuse of prescribed methylphenidate by an alcohol and drug abusing adolescent with ADHD. *Journal of the American Academy of Child and Adolescent Psychiatry* 30: 773–775.

Jaffe, S. L. (2002) Failed attempts at intranasal abuse of concerta. *Journal of the American Academy of Child and Adolescent Psychiatry* 41: 5.

Johanson, C. E. and Uhlenhuth, E. H. (1980a) Drug preference and mood in humans: D-amphetamine. *Psychopharmacology (Berlin)* 71: 275–279.

Johanson, C. E. and Uhlenhuth, E. H. (1980b) Drug preference and mood in humans: diazepam. *Psychopharmacology (Berlin)* 71: 269–273.

Klein, R. G. and Abikoff, H. (1997) Behavior therapy and methylphenidate in the treatment of children with ADHD. *Journal of Attention Disorders* 2: 89–114.

Kollins, S. H., Rush, C. R., Pazzaglia, P. J. and Ali, J. A. (1998) Comparison of the acute behavioral effects of sustained-release and immediate-release methylphenidate. *Experimental and Clinical Psychopharmacology* 6: 367–374.

Kroutil, L. A., Van Brundt, D. L., Herman-Stahl, M. A., Heller, D. C., Bray, R. M. and Penne, M. A. (2006) Nonmedical use of prescription stimulants in the United States. *Drug and Alcohol Dependence* 84: 135–143.

Lage, L. and Hwang, P. (2004) Effect of methylphenidate formulation for attention deficit hyperactivity disorder on patterns and outcomes of treatment. *Journal of Child and Adolescent Psychopharmacology* 14: 575–581.

Lambert, N. M. (2002) Stimulant treatment as a risk factor for nicotine use and substance abuse. In: Jensen, P. S. and Cooper, J. R. (eds), *Attention Deficit Hyperactivity Disorder: State of Science, Best Practices*. Kingston, N. J.: Civic Research Institute (CRI), pp. 18-1–18-24.

Lambert, N. M. and Hartsough, C. S. (1998) Prospective study of tobacco smoking and substance dependencies among samples of ADHD and non-ADHD participants. *Journal of Learning Disabilities* 31: 533–544.

Lile, J. A., Stoops, W. W., Durell, T. M., Glaser, P. E. A. and Rush, C. R. (2006) Discriminative-stimulus, self-reported, performance, and cardiovascular effects of atomoxetine in methylphenidate-trained humans. *Experimental and Clinical Psychopharmacology* 14: 136–147.

Massello, W. III. and Carpenter, D. A. (1999) A fatality due to the intranasal abuse of methylphenidate. *Journal of Forensic Science* 44: 220–221.

Milberger, S., Biederman, J., Faraone, S. V., Chen, L. and Jones, J. (1997a) Further evidence of an association between attention-deficit/hyperactivity disorder and cigarette smoking. Findings from a high-risk sample of siblings. *American Journal of Addictions* 6: 205–217.

Milberger, S., Biederman, J., Faraone, S. V., Wilens, T. and Chu, M. P. (1997b) Associations between ADHD and psychoactive substance use disorders. Findings from a longitudinal study of high-risk siblings of ADHD children. *American Journal of Addictions* 6: 318–329.

Molina, B. S., Flory, K., Hinshaw, S. P., Greiner, A. R., Arnold, L. E., Swanson, J. M., Hechtman, L., Jensen, P. S., Vitiello, B., Hoza, B., Pelham, W. E., Elliott, G. R., Wells, K. C., Abikoff, H. B., Gibbons, R. D., Marcus, S., Conners, C. K., Epstein, J. N., Greenhill, L. L., March, J. S., Newcorn, J. H., Severe, J. B. and Wigal, T. (2007) Delinquent behavior and emerging substance use in the MTA at 36 months: prevalence, course, and treatment effects. *Journal of the American Academy of Child and Adolescent Psychiatry* 46: 1028–1040.

Pliszka, S. R., Browne, R. G., Olvera, R. L. and Wynne, S. K. (2000). A double-blind, placebo-controlled study of adderall and methylphenidate in the treatment of attention-deficit hyperactivity disorder. *Journal of the American Academy of Child and Adolescent Psychiatry* 39: 619–626.

Pomerleau, O. F., Downey, K. K., Stelson, F. W. and Pomerleau, C. S. (1995) Cigarette smoking in adult patients diagnosed with attention deficit hyperactivity disorder. *Journal of Substance Abuse* 7: 373–378.

Poulin, C. (2007) From attention-deficit/hyperactivity disorder to medical stimulant use to the diversion of prescribed stimulants to non-medical stimulant use: connecting the dots. *Addiction* 102: 740–751.

Reeves, G. and Schweitzer, J. (2004) Pharmacological management of attention-deficit hyperactivity disorder. *Expert Opinion on Pharmacotherapy* 5: 1313–1320.

Reimherr, F. W., Williams, E. D., Strong, R. E., Mestas, R., Soni, P. and Marchant, B. K. (2007) A double-blind, placebo-controlled, crossover study of osmotic release oral system methylphenidate in adults with ADHD with assessment of oppositional and emotional dimensions of the disorder. *Journal of Clinical Psychiatry* 68: 93–101.

Ritz, M. C., Lamb, R. J., Goldberg, S. R. and Kuhar, M. J. (1987) Cocaine receptors on dopamine transporters are related to self-administration of cocaine. *Science* 237: 1219–1223.

Robison, L. M., Sclar, D. A., Skaer, T. L. and Galin, R. S. (1999) National trends in the prevalence of attention-deficit/hyperactivity disorder and the prescribing of methylphenidate among school-age children: 1990–1995. *Clinical Pediatrics* 38: 209–217.

Rush, C. R. and Baker, R. W. (2001) Behavioral pharmacological similarities between methylphenidate and cocaine in cocaine abusers. *Experimental and Clinical Psychopharmacology* 9: 59–73.

Rush, C. R., Essman, W. D., Simpson, C. A. and Baker, R. W. (2001) Reinforcing and subject-rated effects of methylphenidate and D-amphetamine in non-drug-abusing volunteers. *Journal of Clinical Psychopharmacology* 21: 273–286.

Rush, C. R., Higgins, S. T., Vansickel, A. R., Stoops, W. W., Lile, J. A. and Glaser, P. E. A. (2005) Methylphenidate increases cigarette smoking. *Psychopharmacology* 181: 781–789.

Rush, C. R., Kelly, T. H., Hays, L. R. and Wooten, A. F. (2002) Discriminative-stimulus effects of modafinil in cocaine-trained humans. *Drug and Alcohol Dependence* 67: 311–322.

Rush, C. R., Kollins, S. H. and Pazzaglia, P. J. (1998) Discriminative-stimulus and participant-rated effects of methylphenidate, bupropion and triazolam in D-amphetamine-trained humans. *Experimental and Clinical Psychopharmacology* 6: 32–44.

Rush, C. R., Madakasira, S., Goldman, N. H., Woolverton, W. L. and Rowlett, J. K. (1997) Discriminative-stimulus effects of zolpidem in pentobarbital-trained subjects: II. Comparison with triazolam and caffeine in humans. *Journal of Pharmacology and Experimental Therapeutics* 280: 174–188.

Schuster, C. R., Lucchesi, B. R. and Emley, G. S. (1979) The effects of D-amphetamine, meprobamate, and lobeline on the cigarette smoking behavior of normal human subjects. In: Krasnegor, N. A. (ed.) *Cigarette Smoking as a Dependence Process*. National Institute on Drug Abuse Research Monograph 23. Department of Health, Education, and Welfare, Public Health Service, Alcohol, Drug Abuse, and Mental Health Administration, National Institute on Drug Abuse, Division of Research, Rockville, MD, pp. 91–99.

Sevak, R. J., Stoops, W. W., Hays, L.R. and Rush, C. R. (2009) Discriminative-stimulus and subject-rated effects of methamphetamine, D-amphetamine, methylphenidate and triazolam in methamphetamine-trained humans. *Journal of Pharmacology and Experimental Therapeutics* 328: 1007–1018.

Spencer, T., Biederman, J. and Wilens, T. (2004) Stimulant treatment of adult attention-deficit/hyperactivity disorder. *Psychiatric Clinics of North America* 27: 361–372.

Spencer, T., Biederman, J., Wilens, T., Doyle, R., Surman, C., Prince, J., Mick, E., Aleardi, M., Herzig, K. and Faraone, S. (2005) A large, double-blind, randomized clinical trial of methylphenidate in the treatment of adults with attention-deficit/hyperactivity disorder. *Biological Psychiatry* 57: 456–463.

Spencer, T., Wilens, T., Biederman, J., Faraone, S. V., Ablon, J. S. and Lapey, K. (1995) A double-blind, crossover comparison of methylphenidate and placebo in adults with childhood-onset attention-deficit hyperactivity disorder. *Archives of General Psychiatry* 52: 434–443.

Spencer, T. J., Biederman, J., Ciccone, P. E., Madras, B. K., Dougherty, D. D., Bonab, A. A., Livni, E., Parasrampuria, D. A. and Fischman, A. J. (2006) PET study examining pharmacokinetics, detection and likeability, and dopamine transporter receptor occupancy of short- and long-acting oral methylphenidate. *American Journal of Psychiatry* 163: 387–395.

Stoops, W. W., Fillmore, M. T., Glaser, P. E. A. and Rush, C. R. (2004) Reinforcing, subject-rated, performance and physiological effects of methylphenidate and D-amphetamine in stimulant abusing humans. *Journal of Psychopharmacology* 18: 534–543.

Stoops, W. W., Glaser, P. E. A. and Rush, C. R. (2003) Reinforcing, subject-rated and physiological effects of intranasal methylphenidate: a dose–response analysis. *Drug and Alcohol Dependence* 71: 179–186.

Stoops, W. W., Lile, J. A., Glaser, P. E. A., Rush, C. R. (2005) Discriminative-stimulus and self-reported effects of methylphenidate, D-amphetamine, and triazolam in methylphenidate-trained humans. *Experimental and Clinical Psychopharmacology* 13: 56–64.

Substance Abuse and Mental Health Services Administration (SAMHSA) (2006) *Results from the 2005 National Survey on Drug Use and Health: National Findings*. Office of Applied Studies, NSDUH Series H-30, DHHS Publ No. SMA 06–4194. Rockville, MD: Substance Abuse and Mental Health Services Administration.

Tercyak, K. P., Lerman, C. and Audrain, J. (2002) Association of attention-deficit/hyperactivity disorder symptoms with levels of cigarette smoking in a community sample of adolescents. *Journal of the American Academy of Child and Adolescent Psychiatry* 41: 799–805.

Teter, C. J., McCabe, S. E., Boyd, C. J. and Guthrie, S. K. (2003) Illicit methylphenidate use in an undergraduate student sample: prevalence and risk factors. *Pharmacotherapy* 23: 609–617.

Teter, C. J., McCabe, S. E., LaGrange, K., Cranford, J. A. and Boyd, C. J. (2006) Illicit use of specific prescription stimulants among college students: prevalence, motives, and routes of administration. *Pharmacotherapy* 26: 1501–1510.

Tidey, J. W., O'Neill, S. C. and Higgins, S. T. (2000) D-Amphetamine increases choice of cigarette smoking over monetary reinforcement. *Psychopharmacology (Berlin)* 153: 85–92.

Upadhyaya, H. P., Rose, K., Wang, W., O'Rourke, K., Sullivan, B., Deas, D. and Brady, K. T. (2005) Attention-deficit/hyperactivity disorder, medication treatment, and substance use patterns among adolescents and young adults. *Journal of Child and Adolescent Psychopharmacology* 15: 799–809.

Vansickel, A. R., Stoops, W. W., Glaser, P. E. A. and Rush, C. R. (2007) A pharmacological analysis of stimulant-induced increases in smoking. *Psychopharmacology* 193: 305–313.

Volkow, N. D. (2006) Stimulant medications: how to minimize their reinforcing effects? *American Journal of Psychiatry* 163: 359–361.

Volkow, N. D., Ding, Y. S., Fowler, J. S., Wang, G. J., Logan, J., Gatley, S. J., Dewey, S., Ashby, C., Liebermann, J., Hitzemann, R. and Wolf, A. P. (1995) Is methylphenidate like cocaine? Studies on their pharmacokinetics and distribution in the human brain. *Archives of General Psychiatry* 52: 456–463.

Volkow, N. D., Fowler, J. S., Gatley, J. S., Dewey, S. L., Wang, G. J., Logan, J., Ding, Y. S., Franceschi, D., Gifford, A., Morgan, A., Pappas, N. and King, P. (1999a) Comparable changes in synaptic dopamine induced by methylphenidate and cocaine in the baboon brain. *Synapse* 31: 59–66.

Volkow, N. D., Wang, G. J., Fowler, J. S., Fischman, M., Foltin, R., Abumrad, N. N., Gatley, S. J., Logan, J., Wong, C., Gifford, A., Ding, Y. S., Hitzemann, R. and Pappas, N. (1999b) Methylphenidate and cocaine have similar in vivo potency to block the dopamine transporters in the human brain. *Life Sciences* 65: 7–12.

Wender, P. H., Reimher, F. W., Wood, D. and Ward, M. (1985) A controlled study of methylphenidate in the treatment of attention deficit disorder, residual type, in adults. *American Journal of Psychiatry* 142: 547–552.

Wender, P. H., Wolf, L. E. and Wasserstein, J. (2001) Adults with ADHD: an overview. *Annals of the New York Academy of Science* 93: 1–16.

Wilens, T. E., Faraone, S. V., Biederman, J. and Gunawardene, S. (2003) Does stimulant therapy of attention-deficit/hyperactivity disorder beget later substance abuse? A meta-analytic review of the literature. *Pediatrics* 111: 179–185.

Chapter 6

AMPHETAMINE TREATMENT IN THE UK: THE ROLE OF SUBSTITUTE PRESCRIBING

Richard Pates

This chapter looks at the role of the prescription of dexamphetamine as a substitute for street amphetamine in the treatment of amphetamine dependence. In the UK dexamphetamine prescription has been a treatment intervention for two decades although the evidence for the efficacy of this intervention is scant. The chapter concentrates on the evidence that exists, including reports regarding problems with the intervention and a report on a randomised controlled trial.

Introduction

While the use of methadone (and more recently other opioid drugs) as replacement therapy in the treatment of opiate addiction has been commonplace for many years in many parts of the world, the use of substitute drugs for the treatment of amphetamine problems has remained controversial and, with the exception of some projects in the UK, has been rarely used. The arguments against substitute prescribing include the fact that there is no obvious long-acting drug similar to methadone that could be used, and that the same harm could potentially be caused by prescribing amphetamine as caused by street drugs. An experiment of substitute prescribing in the 1960s was found not to have been useful (see description below).

An 'epidemic' of injectable methylamphetamine use in London in the late 1960s (Hawks et al., 1969) led to a trial of prescribing of the drug. This was the result of the drug being diverted onto the black market after being prescribed in large quantities by a small number of doctors. The treatment trial was deemed appropriate because all of the group were injecting and using large doses of the drug and contact with the users was frequently lost when they were referred to treatment services. There was also a high level of amphetamine psychosis among this group. The treatment trial (Mitcheson et al., 1976) involved the prescription of methylamphetamine to a group of 12 patients, and although one patient showed improvement in social stability and two became abstinent the trial was thought to have been a failure. Mitcheson et al. (1976) commented that for the two patients who became abstinent 'something considerable was attained – although originally prescribed Methedrine they are now off all drugs' (p. 158). This is an interesting contrast to recent news from the BBC (30 October 2007) that reported that only 3% of clients currently leave treatment drug free.

In another paper, Gardner and Connell (1972) described their findings of 104 users of non-opioid drugs, who were mainly amphetamine users, attending a clinic in London between March 1968 and February 1969. Amphetamine psychosis occurred in 35% of the cases and was a more frequent complication of intravenous use. Garner and Connell concluded that 'except in rare circumstances amphetamines were not prescribed because of their widespread availability and of the dangers of toxic effects if the prescribed dose was supplemented by illicit use. The few exceptions who were maintained on amphetamine were usually older persons from "outside" the drug scene who had been receiving prescriptions from their General Practitioners'. The authors claimed that maintenance was not likely to be an effective treatment for young people despite the fact that 25% of them were receiving a prescription from their general practitioners. Their recommendation for treatment was a probation order with a condition of attendance at a drug clinic.

By the late twentieth century in Britain, amphetamine had become the second most widely used illicit drug after cannabis (Pickering and Stimson, 1994). Amphetamine was almost entirely amphetamine sulphate of poor quality and was often used recreationally. There was also considerable injecting of amphetamine, and thus it had the same risks of blood-borne virus transmission as any other injected drug. As well as the risks of disease transmission, users were often in poor health, often underweight and malnourished because of the anorectic qualities of the drug and often in difficult social circumstances, with some being involved in crime and prostitution. Treatment services in the UK were perceived as treatment services for opiate users, and many of the services did not feel they had much to offer stimulant users. This was reflected in comments by the clients who often felt little was offered to them. The Advisory Council on the Misuse of Drugs (ACMD), a committee that advises the British Government on drug policy, said in one of their reports that 'the prescription of stimulants is unlikely to lead to desirable changes in behaviour, and carries a number of risks. This is borne out by previous experience in this country of prescribing stimulants regularly to drug misusers, which is generally acknowledged to have been disastrous, resulting in an increase in chaotic behaviour' (ACMD, 1989, p. 46). This was the trial previously mentioned (Mitcheson et al., 1976) of 12 patients who were prescribed injectable methamphetamine. The Department of Health's *Guidelines on Clinical Management* of drug problems also warned against prescribing amphetamines as 'the risk of them being diverted is very high' (Department of Health, 1991).

A number of clinicians in the UK in the early 1990s who were concerned about lack of effective treatment services for amphetamine users began to prescribe dexamphetamine in oral form for amphetamine users in an attempt to help them to stop, improve their health, and wean them off the drug by using a reducing dose. In an article intending to challenge the orthodoxy of non-prescription and to stir debate, Pates (1994) wrote, 'Prescribing is no panacea. It should be part of a package including services such as counselling, and is not suitable for all amphetamine users, particularly those using small amounts and not injecting. That still leaves many heavy, chaotic users for whom prescribing might provide the opportunity for change' (p. 17).

A gradual cautious change was noted in attitudes towards amphetamine prescribing. In 1996 the government's Task Force to Review Services for Drug Misusers suggested, 'There may be a role for amphetamine substitution prescribing in some cases but further research is needed. Preliminary reports from small-scale open studies suggest that further study of this different form of substitute prescribing should be undertaken'. In 1998 the government's own ten-year strategy for tackling drug misuse highlighted the fact that the treatment of stimulant dependency is a priority research area (Department of Health, 1998). In 1999, the Department of Health's *Guidelines on the Clinical Management of Drug Dependence* advised that dexamphetamine substitution should be limited to experienced specialist practitioners and noted that there was currently 'no research to guide practitioners'. However in 2007 the Department of Health changed the advice and in the new version of the prescribing guidelines (Department of Health, 2007, page 62) stated that "there is no indication for the prescription of amphetamines in the treatment of stimulant withdrawal . . . . substitute stimulant prescribing does not have demonstrated effectiveness and accordingly should not ordinarily be provided." This reversal of opinion appears to go against the evidence of the advantages of prescribing as described in this chapter.

One of the problems in the late 1990s was that although a number of reports on amphetamine prescribing had been published (these are reviewed below) there had been no randomised controlled trial published on the efficacy of amphetamine prescribing for amphetamine-dependent individuals. Bradbeer et al. (1998) surveyed the practice in England and Wales and found that of 149 respondents, 46% were currently prescribing amphetamine and 60% saw the role of it in the treatment of amphetamine dependence. They concluded that amphetamine prescribing was widespread in England and Wales despite the fact that there was little evidence for its efficacy. Strang and Sheridan (1997) found that between 900 and 1000 individuals were being prescribed dexamphetamine for the treatment of amphetamine dependence in England and Wales.

The British experience of prescribing

The lack of presentation to treatment of amphetamine users has been a cause for concern for many agencies in the UK. The risks of the spread of blood-borne virus infection via injecting is similar to that of heroin users, who are more likely to access treatment. Fleming and Roberts (1994) reported on the first 3 years of the practice of prescribing dexamphetamine to amphetamine users in Portsmouth. They found that relatively few problematic amphetamine users presented to treatment agencies and commented that injecting amphetamine users are a high-risk group as far as HIV transmission is concerned. Fleming and Roberts found that more than half of their patients ceased injecting and that there was a considerable reduction by the remainder. Eighty five per cent had not used or shared injecting equipment during the programme. The use of street amphetamine was lower than previously but did not cease. Offending also reduced but there was little change in sexual practices.

Most importantly, there was an increase in primary amphetamine users presenting for treatment.

Pates et al. (1996) described a pilot programme in prescribing dexamphetamine for amphetamine users in Wales. Wales has had a high prevalence of amphetamine use for many years, but few of these users were presenting to services. The aims of the project were not necessarily to bring about abstinence in the patients but (a) to reduce the frequency of injecting, (b) to reduce the use of street amphetamine and (c) to stabilise lifestyle as measured by decrease in prostitution, crime and an improvement in general health. Inclusion criteria were (1) a history of injecting amphetamine for at least the previous 6 months, (2) urine positive for amphetamines and negative for opiates, (3) that amphetamine was being used dependently and not recreationally and (4) a stable psychiatric state and no evidence of a history of non-drug-induced psychosis.

Fourteen patients were originally recruited for the study; one failed to attend the initial assessment, two dropped out early in the programme and one had a transient psychotic episode as a result of still using street amphetamine heavily. This last one was excluded from the trial because of mental health problems. Clients were obliged to attend the clinic four times per week and on these occasions were required to take their prescription on the premises. Doses were commenced at 30 mg per day and increased to a maximum of 60 mg. At the end of the trial of 24 weeks the frequency of injecting had decrease from an average of 38 times per week to an average of 1.3 times per week and four clients had ceased injecting. The use of street amphetamine had reduced from an average of 40.45 g/week to an average of 1.6 g/week with four clients using no street amphetamine. Lifestyle changes were reported with five of the six patients who had been sex workers and had stopped working completely and the other worked only occasionally; all reported a reduction in crime and an improvement in general health.

This was not a randomised controlled trial, and the changes could have been confounded by the fact that they had to attend a group four times per week. However, the fact that they attended was probably due to the prescription; without this they may not have continued to attend. Most of the results were self-reports, but they did show improvements in skin condition consistent with reductions in injecting.

In another study from Wales, McBride et al. (1997) compared 63 patients who were receiving dexamphetamine substitution with 25 patients who received treatment before the service started prescribing dexamphetamine. They wanted to answer three important questions: (1) Are high-risk users attracted into a service prescribing dexamphetamine? (2) Will the prescribing of dexamphetamine retain patients in treatment? (3) Will the prescribing produce behaviour change? McBride et al. compared figures for 29 months before dexamphetamine prescribing began with 28 months after the prescribing began. The number of primary amphetamine users increased from 83 to 197, with the proportion of all patients who were primary amphetamine users from 24.3 to 42.7%. The patients being prescribed dexamphetamine were retained in treatment for an average of 11.7 months compared with an average of 1.4 months for the control group. Less than half the control group were seen more than twice, preventing a comparison of behaviour change. In the prescribed group those who reported injecting fell from 63 to 37 and those sharing injecting equipment fell from 16 to 2.

The evidence for reduction or cessation of injecting during dexamphetamine prescribing is quite strong. Charnaud and Griffiths (1998) compared the efficacy of dexamphetamine prescribing for injecting amphetamine users with methadone prescribing for injecting opiate users. One hundred and twenty primary opiate misusers were prescribed oral methadone, and 60 primary amphetamine misusers were prescribed dexamphetamine elixir. The level of injection drug misuse at the time of discharge for the two groups was similar, with 67% of the opiate misusers and 70% of the amphetamine misusers having stopped injecting.

In a study from the West of England, White (2000) surveyed retrospectively the records of 220 subjects who had been prescribed dexamphetamine for the treatment of amphetamine users. Cross-sectional socio-demographic data and longitudinal outcome data were available for 148 of them. All of them had received treatment from a community service in Cornwall during the period 1992–1996. They included both intravenous users and oral users. Outcomes were similar for both groups, but the intravenous group showed more overall gains in treatment than the oral group. Over 63% of the injectors stopped injecting and 57% of these stopped within 2 months of coming into treatment. Females were slower to change drug-using behaviour but stayed longer in treatment. Being male was a predictor of dropping out of treatment by 1 year, and failing to complete 1 year of treatment was associated with being younger, using only amphetamines and having a forensic history. Of the 220 users in the original sample, there were no reported cases of a first psychotic episode although seven individuals had a previous history of psychosis, four being diagnosed with schizophrenia and three with drug-induced psychosis.

White comments that dexamphetamine prescription was not a good means of retaining people in treatment, with 35% of injectors being discharged for non-attendance and 52% failing to complete or to stay in treatment. As time in treatment is often associated with changes in drug use, White considered this a very negative outcome; however as McBride et al. (1997) commented, without prescription the dropout rates approach nearly 100%. White remained optimistic in that he considered that the dangers of amphetamine have probably been overestimated. Of the 220 people in White's study who were monitored for 2640 person months and prescribed higher levels of dexamphetamine than in other services, there were only five episodes of psychosis recorded and these were all in people with a previous history of psychosis who had continued to inject street drugs.

Potential problems with dexamphetamine prescribing

Critics of substitute prescribing for amphetamine users have cited a number of problems. Firstly, the early experience of substitute prescribing in the 1960s was a failure. It should be noted that this was quite a different situation from more recent prescribing conditions. The people being studied had been prescribed Methedrine in ampoule form, a much stronger drug than the amphetamine sulphate commonly available in the UK. The prescribing treatment consisted of continuing to prescribe injectable Methedrine which gave no incentive to cease injecting. It was also a time when the fears of blood-borne infections via injecting were of less concern since at that time HIV and hepatitis C had not been identified; cessation of injecting is now an important aim of treatment. It is also interesting to note that the results may not have been as negative as they were then thought to be. We now look at treatment aims as being much more than cessation of drug use and the authors of the study (Mitcheson et al., 1976) were, perhaps, too hard on themselves.

Specific concerns have been expressed concerning possible harm associated with long-term prescribing, the effects on the unborn fetus when pregnant women are being prescribed, and the effects on mental health. Most of the projects where dexamphetamine is prescribed have strict inclusion and exclusion criteria. Inclusion criteria include a history of amphetamine injecting (some projects will only prescribe to injectors), evidence of dependence and not being dependent on alcohol or opiates. Exclusion criteria include a history of mental illness, being pregnant, being hypertensive or being anorexic (a BMI of less than 17.5).

In a study on the long-term effects of dexamphetamine prescribing (Myton et al., 2004) the notes of 20 patients treated with dexamphetamine between 1984 and 1998 were examined. Demographic features, drug use at initial contact, subsequent management and outcomes including health and social circumstances were assessed. Patients who had stopped attending for at least 6 months were compared with those in treatment. Myton and colleagues found that those retained in dexamphetamine treatment showed reduction in injecting and illicit drug use and an improvement in employment status. Retention in treatment was also associated with older age, longer history of drug use, a stable relationship and fewer prison sentences during treatment. It was noted that some illicit drug use continued as did criminal activity. Because there were no limits to the duration of treatment, some patients had been receiving dexamphetamine for 14 years without ill effect. Psychotic symptoms developed in 5 out of the 20 patients; one suffered a possible myocardial infarction. Myton et al. concluded that from a selected sample, the study provided some evidence of the benefits of the prescription of dexamphetamine in terms of improved outcome in amphetamine users and does not inevitably lead to physical or psychiatric complications. Mental illness is often a contraindication for prescription of dexamphetamine, but Myton et al. comment that those who have become psychotic through chaotic drug use may benefit if prescription stabilises substance use and lifestyle.

In a study specifically addressing dexamphetamine prescription and the effects on mental health, Carnwath et al. (2002) retrospectively examined case notes. They looked at the notes of eight schizophrenic patients who had been prescribed dexamphetamine for coexisting amphetamine dependence. They commented that patients with coexisting problems have been shown to have poorer treatment outcomes; they often do not comply with treatment plans and have frequent periods of hospitalisation. In four out of the eight cases, the prescription of dexamphetamine led to good progress in terms of both substance use and their mental health. In two cases the progress was more equivocal but there appeared to be some benefit. Two of the cases were judged to be treatment failures, but the condition and situation of the patients was no worse at the end of treatment than at the beginning. They found that adherence to neuroleptic regimes increased in most cases and none of the patients suffered an exacerbation of their psychosis as a result of treatment.

Carnwath et al. commented that patients with severe mental illness have significant rates of concurrent amphetamine use and that given the difficult nature of this patient group and previous failure to respond to intensive treatment the rate of success was satisfactory. They suggest that benefits may be gained from increased compliance with psychiatric treatment when dexamphetamine is prescribed and that this may outweigh possible risks. They acknowledge that their results are tentative given the nature of the study and recommend further prospective study be undertaken.

White et al. (2006) described the effects of prescribing dexamphetamine to pregnant women. In this study the antenatal care and birth outcomes of 47 amphetamine-using women who were prescribed dexamphetamine were compared with 41 who were not and with local population norms. Data was also collected for two equivalent samples of heroin users. The results showed that the prescribed amphetamine users and heroin users received adequate antenatal care. There was, however, a high incidence of low birth rate in both groups. The results were slightly better for both the prescribed group and the non-prescribed group as compared to the heroin users. The authors believe that these findings in the dexamphetamine-prescribed group were not due to the prescription of dexamphetamine as they were similar to those women with an amphetamine problem who did not receive a prescription. There was also no relationship between these results and maximum dose or duration of prescribing. The best predictor of adverse birth outcomes was the use of more drugs on top of their prescribed dose. White et al. point out that their sample of pregnant drug users was younger than the general population which may contribute to the low birth weight and that smoking among this group appeared to account for half the birth-weight reduction.

White et al. are cautious in interpreting these findings. They conclude that the risk–benefit ratio of prescribing dexamphetamine to pregnant women can only be calculated when definitive conclusions have been reached regarding the efficacy of dexamphetamine substitution for amphetamine users. Dexamphetamine appears effective at drawing users into treatment and appears to be reasonably safe, but it should be used as a treatment of last resort and pregnant amphetamine users should be encouraged to remain abstinent where possible. These findings are important in countries such as the UK where pregnant drug users are unwilling to access antenatal services because of discriminatory attitudes towards them by both health and social services: when women are at least presenting to and remaining in treatment, proper antenatal care may be provided.

Randomised controlled trials of the prescription of dexamphetamine

One of the major criticisms of the practice of prescribing dexamphetamine in the treatment of amphetamine dependence has been the paucity of the randomised controlled trial. Early studies in the UK were not randomised controlled trials, but they did produce useful evidence of the potential for demonstration of the efficacy of this intervention.

In an Australian study, Shearer et al. (2001) reported a pilot randomised controlled study of the prescription of dexamphetamine for amphetamine dependence. The study did not aim to definitively evaluate the effectiveness of amphetamine substitution. Forty-one treatment-seeking amphetamine users were recruited to the trial, the design of which was an open two-group pre–post randomised controlled trial. Twenty-one patients were randomised to the treatment arm of the project and 20 to the control arm. All subjects received weekly counselling sessions. The treatment arm received prescribed oral dexamphetamine up to a maximum dose of 60 mg; the dose was reduced to 40 mg at week 12.

In the treatment group, no adverse events were reported, and no psychotic symptoms were reported for any subjects. Two subjects ceased treatment during the induction phase, one reported agitation and aggressive behaviour and insomnia was reported in three of the subjects; all these complaints ceased before entry to the trial. Twelve of the treatment group reached the 12-week stage of the trial and nine dropped out. The dropout rate of the control group was not reported although it was reported that attrition rats were similar. Attendance at the counselling sessions differed with 57% of the treatment group attending an average of 2.6 sessions and 25% of the control group attending an average of 1.4 sessions. The proportion of methylamphetamine in the urine samples decreased in both groups between baseline and week 6, but there was no significant difference between the groups. In the treatment group, urine levels remained stable at 12 weeks, but these increased in the control group. Self-reported street drug use declined in both groups as did injecting. Improvements in psychological adjustment, health and a reduction in criminal behaviour were apparent in both groups; there was no significant difference between the groups. The authors conclude that substitution therapy deserves further consideration, as a range of interventions for problematic amphetamine use and rigorous controlled trials of amphetamine substitution with adequate sample sizes and follow-ups are needed.

One of the significant developments was the technology to differentiate street amphetamine from dexamphetamine in the urine. This enabled researchers to confirm whether subjects were still using street amphetamine. Tetlow and Merrill (1996) developed a method for determining whether those in dexamphetamine substitution treatment were supplementing prescribed dexamphetamine with street amphetamine by separating and quantifying stereoisomers, expressing results as ratios of L- to D-isomers.

The only published randomised controlled trial of substitute prescribing in the UK has been the study by Merrill et al. (2005). This study was funded by the Department of Health and took place across two sites: Manchester and Cardiff. The aims of the study were as follows: (a) to investigate the impact of dexamphetamine prescribing for the treatment of amphetamine dependence, (b) to assess the practicalities of a research methodology for studying dexamphetamine prescribing in UK clinical settings, (c) to asses the effectiveness of dexamphetamine substitution on recognised best available treatment of amphetamine dependence, (d) to describe the nature and extent of any benefits or harms on the mental or physical health of those receiving dexamphetamine and (e) to contribute to the development of guidelines for best practices in the management of amphetamine dependence.

The inclusion criteria for the trial were as follows:

- Primary drug used is amphetamine
- Fulfilling DSM IV criteria for dependence
- Using amphetamine on 4 or more days a week over a minimum period of 12 months
- Urinalysis confirms recent use of amphetamine
- Aged 18 years or older
- Informed written consent to enter the trial

Exclusion criteria were as follows:

- Pregnancy or lactation
- Blood pressure when seated over 150/100 mm Hg
- History of cardiovascular disease, glaucoma or epilepsy
- Diagnosis of schizophrenia or other serious mental illness
- Amphetamine psychosis within the previous 6 months
- Body mass index below 17.5
- Opiate dependence
- Alcohol dependence

The two arms of the trial were of, for the control group, best available treatment (BATA) which consisted of literature on the effects of amphetamine, motivational interviewing, recording of recent behaviour using a retrospective drug diary, discussions of cues, coping with lapses and advice on healthier lifestyles. Also included was harm minimisation advice, including advice on safer injecting, referral to appropriate non-drug agencies for health or social issues, symptomatic prescribing for depression, anxiety and insomnia and the possibility for inpatient detoxification if clinically indicated. The dexamphetamine arm of the trial (the DEX group) included all the BATA above plus the prescription of up to 100 mg. dexamphetamine per day dispensed on a daily basis through a community pharmacy.

After treatment, randomisation subjects were seen weekly for 4 weeks and then fortnightly until 7 months at which point the treatment study of the phase finished. During the first 4 months participants in the DEX group received a maintenance dose of dexamphetamine from which they were gradually withdrawn over the next 3 months according to a pre-defined schedule. Independent research assessments took place at entry to treatment, 1 month, 4 months, seven 7 and 9 months.

Appointments were sent to 165 subjects. Ninety-six (58%) subjects attended for the initial assessment appointment and 69 (42%) subjects failed to attend (DNA ['did not attend']). Of the 96 subjects who attended 59 (61%) entered the trial and 37 (39%) were ineligible. Thirty-two subjects were randomised to the DEX arm and 27 to the BATA arm.

There was a reported reduction of an illicit amphetamine use in both groups although this did not differ significantly between groups. There was also evidence of reduced polydrug use in the DEX group during the maintenance phase. There was no evidence of reduced injecting behaviour in the DEX group compared with the BATA group. The DEX group also showed improvements in physical health outcomes during the maintenance phase with some evidence that this was maintained over the later outcome period. There was a statistical trend showing improvements in psychological health in the DEX group compared to the BATA group in both early and late outcome periods. Blood pressure increased in the DEX group but remained within normal range. Both groups showed an overall weight gain. Prescribing dexamphetamine did not have any adverse physical or psychological effects on the participants. One DEX subject did have a brief psychotic episode, but this was in the context of severe emotional stress.

The main conclusions of the study were as follows:

1. This pilot study demonstrated the feasibility of conducting a randomised controlled trial comparing the treatment of amphetamine dependence with BATA and BATA supplemented by amphetamine substitution using dexamphetamine tablets (DEX).
2. Both treatments resulted in substantial falls in self-reported amphetamine use during the first month of treatment, which were maintained after the end of the treatment phase.
3. Treatment with dexamphetamine resulted in better physical health early in treatment, and trends towards improvements in other problem areas. Although there was a tendency towards better outcomes for treatment with DEX over BATA, the difference was less marked than suggested by previous uncontrolled studies.
4. The study did not support concerns raised by some that treatment with dexamphetamine confers significant risks to the physical and mental health of patients.
5. The evidence to date supports the Department of Health's current clinical guidelines that dexamphetamine substitution should remain a specialist treatment intervention carried out by experienced practitioners. When offered, dexamphetamine should be part of a complete treatment package incorporating psycho-social interventions employed in BATA and clinical monitoring procedures including urine drug screening with the ability to differentiate prescribed from illicit amphetamine, blood pressure checks and mental state reviews.
6. Future studies must involve higher numbers of subjects that are based on power calculations that assume more limited benefits to dexamphetamine prescribing than previously assumed and that anticipate difficulties in recruitment and retention.

Conclusions

As clinicians we have noticed some remarkable changes in clients who were prescribed dexamphetamine, with much improved health reduction in street drug use and injecting, and with a few others it would be seen as an opportunity to supplement street amphetamine use. As the McBride et al. (1997) study showed, prescribing it did make for a much better retention in treatment. The Merrill et al. (2005) study participants were paid for attendance at the regular research interviews and, although this was a small amount, this may have influenced the BATA group's retention.

The prescription of dexamphetamine for the treatment of amphetamine-dependent persons is now quite common in the UK despite the lack of a full randomised controlled trial. The evidence suggests that it does attract this group of clients into services and that fears over the potential harm are generally unfounded. One advantage of prescribing is that if clients are attending a clinic and become unwell they can be treated. There is evidence that prescribing will reduce the use of street drugs and some evidence (although not from the British pilot randomised controlled trial) that it may lead to a reduction in injecting. As with other forms of substitute prescribing (e.g. methadone) it should not stand alone, but be used in conjunction with some form of motivational therapy.

References

Advisory Council on the Misuse of Drugs (1989) *AIDS and Drug Misuse Part 2*. London: HMSO.

Bradbeer, T. M., Fleming, P. M., Charlton, P. and Crichton, J. S. (1998) Survey of amphetamine prescribing in England and Wales. *Drug and Alcohol Review* 17(3): 299–304.

Carnwath, T. Garvey, T. and Holland, M. (2002) The prescription of dexamphetamine to patients with schizophrenia and amphetamine dependence. *Journal of Psychopharmacology* 16(4): 373–377.

Charnaud, B. and Griffiths, V. (1998) Levels of intravenous drug misuse among clients prescribed oral dexamphetamine or oral methadone: a comparison. *Drug and Alcohol Dependence* 52: 79–84.

Department of Health (1991) *Drug Misuse and Dependence: Guidelines on Clinical Management*. London: HMSO.

Department of Health (1998) *Tackling Drugs to Build a Better Britain: the Government's Ten-Year Strategy for Tackling Drug Misuse*. London: HMSO.

Department of Health (1999) *Drug Misuse and Dependence: Guidelines on Clinical Management*. London: HMSO.

Department of Health (2007) *Drug Use and Dependence: UK guidelines on Clinical Management*. London: HMSO.

Fleming, P and Roberts, D. (1994) Is the prescription of amphetamine justified as a harm reduction measure? *Journal of the Royal Society of Health* 114(3): 127–131.

Gardner, R. and Connell, P. H. (1972) Amphetamine and other non-opioid drug users attending a special drug dependence clinic. *British Medical Journal* 2(5809): 322–326.

Hawks, D., Mitcheson, M., Ogborne, A. and Edwards, G. (1969) Abuse of methylamphetamine. *British Medical Journal* 2: 715–721.

McBride, A. J., Sullivan, G., Blewett, A. E. and Morgan, S. (1997) Amphetamine prescribing as a harm reduction measure: a preliminary study. *Addiction Research* 5: 95–112.

Merrill, J., McBride, A. J., Pates, R., Peters, L., Tetlow, A., Roberts, C., Arnold, K., Crean, J., Lomax, S. and Deakin, B. (2005) Dexamphetamine substitution as a treatment of amphetamine dependence: a two-centre randomised controlled trial. *Drugs: Education, Prevention and Policy* 12(Suppl 1): 94–97.

Mitcheson, M., Edwards, G., Hawks, D. and Ogborne, A. (1976) Treatment of methylam-phetamine users during the 1968 epidemic. In: Edwards G., Russell, M. A. H., Hawks, D. and Maccafferty, M. (eds), *Drugs and Drug Dependence*. London: Saxon House Publishers.

Myton, T., Carnwath, T. and Crome, I. (2004) Health and psychosocial consequences associated with long-term prescription of dexamphetamine to amphetamine misusers in Wolverhampton 1985–1998. *Drugs: Education, Prevention and Policy* 11(2), 157–166.

Pates, R. (1994) Speed on prescription. *Druglink* 9(3): 16–17.

Pates, R., Coombes, N., Ford, N. (1996) A pilot programme in prescribing dexamphetamine for amphetamine users part I. *Journal of Substance Misuse* 1: 80–84.

Pickering, H., and Stimson, G. (1994) Prevalence and demographic function of stimulant use. *Addiction* 89: 1385–1390.

Shearer, J., Wodak, A., Mattick, R. P., van Beek, I., Lewis, J., Hall, W. and Dolan, K. (2001) Pilot randomized controlled study of dexamphetamine substitution for amphetamine dependence. *Addiction* 96(9): 289–1296.

Strang, J. and Sheridan, J. (1997) Prescribing amphetamines to drug misusers: data from the 1995 national survey of community pharmacies. *Addiction* 92: 833–838.

Task Force to Review Services for Drug Misusers (1996) *Report of an Independent Review of Drug Treatment Services in England*. London: Department of Health.

Tetlow, V. A. and Merrill, J. (1996) Rapid determination of amphetamine stereoisomer ratios is urine by gas chromatography–mass spectroscopy. *Annals of Clinical Biochemistry* 33: 50–54.

White, R. (2000) Dexamphetamine substitution in the treatment of amphetamine abuse: an initial investigation. *Addiction* 95(2): 229–238.

White, R., Thompson, M., Windsor, D., Walsh, M., Cox, D. and Charnaud, B. (2006) Dex-amphetamine substitute-prescribing in pregnancy: a 10-year retrospective audit. *Journal of Substance Use* 11(3): 205–216.

Chapter 7

TREATMENTS FOR METHAMPHETAMINE DEPENDENCE: CONTINGENCY MANAGEMENT AND THE MATRIX MODEL

Richard A. Rawson

As methamphetamine (MA) use and dependence has spread through North America, Southeast Asia, Australia, South Africa and some parts of Europe since the mid-1990s, efforts to develop effective treatments have increased. As of 2009, an effective pharmacotherapy has not been identified, although bupropion (Elkashef et al., 2007) methylphenidate (Tiihonen et al., 2007) and vigabatrin (Brodie et al., 2003, 2005) have shown promise. Consequently, there is considerable interest in the status of behavioural/psychosocial treatment development and evaluation. Despite this interest, there is relatively modest research literature on empirically supported treatments for MA dependence.

At present, only two specific psychosocial treatment protocols (contingency management and the Matrix Model) have been evaluated in adequately powered, randomised, controlled clinical trials with MA-dependent participant samples. However, it should be noted that comparisons of treatment responses by MA users and cocaine users to specific behavioural protocols and to community treatments have indicated that psychosocial treatments with demonstrated efficacy for cocaine dependence appear equally useful for individuals for MA dependence. (Copeland and Sorensen, 2001; Huber et al., 1997; Luchansky et al., 2007; Rawson et al., 2006). Consequently, treatments including cognitive behavioural therapy (CBT) (Carroll et al., 1991, 1994a, b; Morgenstern et al., 2001; Rawson et al., 2006), community reinforcement approach (Higgins et al., 2003), 12-step facilitation (Nowinski et al., 1992) and the National Institute on Drug Abuse (NIDA) drug counselling approach (Daley and Mercer, 1999) should be considered for treating MA-dependent individuals.

Contingency management

Contingency management (CM) applies the principles of positive reinforcement for performance of desired behaviours consistent with MA abstinence. Typically, CM involves the contingent delivery of a voucher (which can be traded for desired items or privileges) or other incentives for behaviours such as attendance at treatment sessions or production of a drug-negative urine specimen. CM has been widely applied to other drug-dependence disorders, and a meta-analysis of research findings has documented strong evidence of efficacy across many studies, types of disorders and populations (Prendergast et al., 2006). Petry (2000) has written on how this technique can be used efficiently and cost-effectively.

The validity of CM for the treatment of MA dependence has been confirmed in a study conducted within the NIDA Clinical Trials Network in which a CM procedure was combined with counselling for a group of 113 MA-dependent individuals (Roll et al., 2006). Study participants were randomly assigned to receive a structured counselling programme (Matrix Model, see below; $n = 62$) or structured counselling plus a CM condition ($n = 51$). In the CM condition, individuals could earn small incentives for providing MA-free urine samples on a variable ratio schedule of reinforcement. Study results indicated that participants who received the CM intervention had more drug-free urine test results, longer periods of abstinence and were more likely to be abstinent during the study period compared to those who only received counselling. At 12-month post-treatment, both CM and standard counselling participants had comparable outcomes.

Another study compared the effectiveness of CM and CBT for treating cocaine- and MA-dependent individuals (Rawson et al., 2006) over a 16-week outpatient trial. Stimulant-dependent individuals ($n = 177$) were randomly assigned to receive either a (1) group-based, three-times-per-week CBT programme ($n = 58$), (2) CM programme for provision of stimulant-free urine samples, with no counselling ($n = 60$) or (3) combination of CM and CBT conditions ($n = 59$). Study results demonstrated that all groups had a significant reduction in MA use during treatment, when compared to pretreatment levels. Participants receiving CM were retained in treatment significantly longer than those receiving only CBT, and they provided more drug-free urine samples during treatment. The gains from CM and CBT were sustained at 6- and 12-month follow-ups, although there were no between group differences at follow-up. Clearly, the CM approach is a validated, powerful tool for the treatment of MA dependence.

The Matrix Model of intensive outpatient treatment

The approach for treating MA-dependent individuals that has received the most systematic study is the Matrix Model of intensive outpatient treatment. The model is presented in some detail in this chapter, as it has been the subject of considerable investment by the US federal government. The initial Matrix Manual was produced with funds from NIDA (Rawson et al., 1989) and evaluated in a major multi-site trial by the Substance Abuse and Mental Health Services Administration (SAMHSA; Rawson et al., 2004). This multi-element model was developed as a package of complementary therapeutic strategies that were combined in a manner to produce an integrated outpatient treatment experience (The Matrix Intensive Outpatient Treatment for People with Stimulant Abuse Disorders manuals are available at www.ncadi.samhsa.gov; Matrix Model manuals are also available from Hazelden Publishing at www.hazelden.com). Research reports describing clinical experiences with the model, plus the results of the major multi-site trial, have provided information on the application of the entire package of techniques (Huber et al., 1997; Rawson et al., 1995, 2004). However, many of the treatment strategies, including CBT, relapse prevention techniques, motivational interviewing strategies, psycho-educational information and 12-step programme involvement, are derived from the clinical research literature. One purpose of this chapter is to deconstruct the Matrix Model into its essential elements and treatments.

Matrix Model background

The Matrix Model of outpatient treatment was developed at the height of the stimulant epidemic in Southern California in the 1980s (Obert et al., 2000). In the urban areas of Los Angeles, cocaine (including crack cocaine) was the major drug affecting communities, but 50 miles to the east of downtown Los Angeles, in San Bernardino County, large numbers of MA users began to present at the Matrix Institute clinic in Rancho Cucamonga (one of three clinics in the Southern California area) for assistance. At the time, there was no established approach for structuring outpatient services to meet the needs of these two groups of psycho-stimulant users. Therefore, with funding from NIDA, the authors of the Matrix approach attempted to integrate existing knowledge and empirically supported techniques into a single, multi-element manual that could serve as an outpatient 'protocol' for the treatment of cocaine and MA users (Rawson et al., 1989, 1995). It was hoped that by creating a single protocol that could be delivered at all Matrix Institute sites in a standardised manner, it would be possible to systematically collect information on how well the approach worked with these populations.

The development of the Matrix Model was influenced by an ongoing interaction between clinicians working with patients and researchers collecting clinical research data. As clinical experience with stimulant-dependent individuals was amassed, clinical impressions frequently generated questions that were answered by using relevant research findings. For example, stimulant users in outpatient treatment frequently gave the impression of being unmotivated or uncooperative because they failed to understand information and follow through on counsellors' directions. These patients might have been considered resistant or not ready for treatment and, therefore, discharged or referred to a higher level of care. New information on stimulants and the brain provided an alternate view of these patients for Matrix clinicians. They began to understand that it was not a psychological issue, but rather a physiologic issue involving brain chemistry changes that contributed to patients' inability to recognise and deal rationally with their self-destructive behaviour.

Once the Matrix clinical staff understood this concept, a decision was made to share this information with patients and their families as part of the therapeutic process. In order to do this, materials had to be developed that captured the essence of how MA changes the brain, yet were simple enough to be readily understood by clinical staff patients and their families. Manuals were written to guide clinical staff in how to work collaboratively with patients and their families and effectively teach them basic brain research concepts and findings.

Similarly, as Matrix staff worked with these stimulant users, they identified specific clinical issues (e.g. conditioned cues, drug craving, anhedonia) which created challenges for patients. Materials were adopted from the cognitive behavioural and relapse prevention literature to provide patients with an understanding of these phenomena and 'tools' to deal with them. Matrix staff also identified a set of clinical issues in working with the family members of these patients (e.g. anger, blaming, poor understanding of addiction), and therefore, materials were adapted from the family therapy literature to aid in work with family members. In order to standardise the delivery of a common set of materials across patients, therapists and clinics, a treatment manual was created which consisted of a session-by-session set of clinical exercises and information (Rawson et al., 1989, 1995).

Several variations of the Matrix treatment model have been developed. The original model, referred to as the Neurobehavioural Model, was a 12-month version that relied heavily on a series of 52 structured, 45-minute individual counselling sessions. These were conducted by a trained master's level therapist during the first 6 months of intensive treatment. This was supplemented by an educational group for patients and their families that met for 12 weekly sessions; a stabilisation group session that met on Friday nights during the first month to help patients stay sober through the weekend; relapse prevention group sessions to provide specific information about relapse and ways to avoid it; family group sessions to help relatives cope with the stimulant user's addiction; random, weekly urine testing; on-site Alcoholics Anonymous (AA) meetings to encourage patients' ongoing participation as part of recovery plans; and ongoing social support group sessions in which more stable patients could interact with programme graduates, serving as role models for the resocialisation of those newly abstinent (Rawson et al., 1989).

In the 16-week version of the Matrix-intensive outpatient treatment for stimulant abuse and dependence disorders (used in all research and dissemination efforts), the individual/conjoint sessions have been reduced to three – scheduled at the beginning, middle and end of the active treatment phase – and group interactions and learning are stressed in a total of 40 structured sessions targeted at the skills needed in early recovery and for relapse prevention (Obert et al., 2000). A primary therapist conducts both the individual and group sessions for a particular patient and is responsible for coordinating that patient's entire treatment experience. Materials are also available for 12 weekly family and patient education sessions and for weekly social support group sessions for patients that are conducted through Week 52. Regular urine testing continues to be a part of the programme; patients are encouraged to participate in 12-step meetings as an important supplement to intensive treatment and as a continuing source of positive emotional and social support.

Programme components

- *Individual counselling* is limited to three 45-minute sessions at the beginning, middle and end of the active therapy effort and can include a significant other. Additional sessions may be scheduled to handle crises or conduct the optional conjoint sessions.

- *Early recovery groups* meet for eight skill-building sessions that impart the cognitive-behavioural and behavioural tools for identifying and controlling the triggers for drug use, understanding withdrawal symptoms, reducing craving, scheduling time, committing to the discontinuation of all psychoactive substances, and connecting with 12-step activities and other community resources for successful recovery.
- *Relapse prevention groups* are the critical mechanism for providing information about relapse in 32 structured sessions that focus on behaviour change, alteration of participants' cognitive/affective orientation, understanding conditioning principles, managing emotions and other practical issues, repairing relationships and connecting with 12-step support groups. The sessions are very directive and combine didactic information with discussion and homework assignments. They are not emotional exploration-experiential groups.
- *Family education groups* that include patients and their relatives use PowerPoint presentations, videos and discussions in a 12-week series focused on topics such as the biology of addiction (e.g. neurotransmitters, brain structure, drug tolerance), conditioning (e.g. cues that lead to drug use, extinction, conditioned abstinence), the medical effects of stimulants on organ systems and how addiction impacts family relationships.
- *12-step meetings* are optimally held on-site one night a week to introduce patients to AA concepts and philosophy. Patients are strongly encouraged to participate in outside groups for ongoing support.
- *Urine and breath tests* are conducted randomly on a weekly basis, and the results are used to review and improve the treatment plan, not to be punitive.
- *Relapse analysis* is a standardised, structured exercise that closely examines the issues and events preceding unexpected or repeated drug use to find clues for preventing future relapses.
- *Social support group sessions* are provided from Weeks 13 to 52; these groups help patients establish new drug-free friendships and activities and transition to long-term continuing care that supports recovery.

Schedule of treatment

The original Matrix protocol called for 6 months of active treatment requiring attendance at treatment sessions up to 3 days a week during three stages of tapering intensity. Weekly support was provided for another 6 months of continuing care. The 16-week version of Matrix that is usually scheduled during evening hours entails the following:

Stage I: Weeks 1–4 include $6\frac{1}{2}$ hours of group meetings on three evenings a week, including:
- 1-hour early recovery group sessions on Monday and Friday
- $1\frac{1}{2}$-hour relapse prevention group sessions on Monday and Friday
- $1\frac{1}{2}$-hour family education group sessions on Wednesday
- Weekly urine and breath testing

- Weekend AA meetings
- One 45-minute individual sessions during this month

Stage II: Weeks 5–16 require $4\frac{1}{2}$ hours of group meetings on three evenings a week, including:

- $1\frac{1}{2}$-hour relapse prevention group sessions on Monday and Friday
- $1\frac{1}{2}$-hour family education group sessions on Wednesday for 12 weeks
- Social support group sessions for patients in the final 4 weeks of this stage
- Weekly urine and breath testing
- AA meetings on Tuesday, Thursday and weekends
- Bimonthly 45-minute individual sessions

Stage III: Weeks 17–52 require $1\frac{1}{2}$ hours of group meeting weekly, including:

- $1\frac{1}{2}$-hour social support group sessions
- Continuing urine and breath testing
- Weekend or more frequent AA meetings

Primary clinical constructs

The Matrix Model has a number of central therapeutic constructs. These include:

(1) Establishing a positive and collaborative relationship with the patient
(2) Creating explicit structure and expectations
(3) Teaching psycho-educational information (including information on brain chemistry and other research-derived clinically relevant knowledge)
(4) Introducing and applying cognitive-behavioural concepts
(5) Positively reinforcing desired behavioural change
(6) Educating family members regarding the expected course of recovery
(7) Introducing and encouraging self-help participation
(8) Monitoring drug use through the use of urinalyses

Positive and collaborative therapeutic relationship

The Matrix Model is characterised by a positive and collaborative relationship between the patient and the therapist. Within this model, the therapist is required to be directive but to maintain a patient-centred therapeutic stance. As cited in much psychotherapy research, it is essential to deliver accurate empathy, positive regard, warmth and genuineness. This means treating patients with dignity, respect and listening attentively and reflectively to their unique experience without imposing judgments. Use of confrontation and the therapist imposition of treatment goals are contraindicated. This collaborative climate increases patients' readiness to learn new skills and practice more adaptive coping strategies and establishes an environment where the successes and failures of using these new strategies can be shared.

The motivational interviewing techniques developed by Miller and Rollnick (1991, 2002) are extremely useful in building a successful therapeutic relationship with MA users in the Matrix outpatient treatment approach. Motivational interviewing skills are of tremendous value throughout the treatment course, but they are especially valuable during the early weeks of treatment.

Potential problems in the early stages of treatment

Clinicians may face several challenges when providing treatment for MA-dependent patients, especially in the initial stages of treatment, including the following:

- MA users frequently enter treatment with many of the pharmacological effects of MA still limiting their functioning. It is very common for MA users in the early stage of treatment to be paranoid and suspicious. This paranoia can make the rapid establishment of trust and cooperation very difficult. Therapist mannerisms and style are important elements in working with patients during this period. It is important to speak slowly and clearly and to maintain a calming demeanour. Use of humour can sometimes be misinterpreted by the patient, as impaired MA users are not always able to understand humorous references. Steady and consistent expressions of support and encouragement are essential to the establishment of a positive relationship with MA users in early treatment. Sarcasm and confrontation are counterproductive.
- A therapist's attitude strongly influences patient's behaviours and expectations. It is important for therapists to establish and maintain the role of a positive re-inforcer throughout the treatment episode. However, patient non-compliance, resistance and continued drug/alcohol use can result in frustration for the therapist. These behaviours may signal that the treatment goals are unattainable and should be adjusted to more realistic levels. Once the patient experiences success, more ambitious goals can be set.
- Early in treatment, many MA-dependent patients have cognitive difficulties or memory problems. Cognitive impairment can be misconstrued as resistance or deliberate non-compliance. To deal with this issue, the topic material and behavioural goals of patients need to be very clear and reviewed repeatedly with patients during the early stages of treatment. Use of reminder cards and written schedules are important aids in giving patients needed support to enhance their compliance and promote successful behaviour change.
- MA users experience substantial mood fluctuations during treatment. Anxiety and depression coupled with lethargy and apathy are common struggles throughout the first months of MA abstinence. These symptoms are signals for the therapist to educate or remind the patient that this is a predictable part of the recovery from MA, that it is a temporary condition and that it will improve with time away from the drug.

Structure and expectations

Structure is a critical element in any effective outpatient programme. In outpatient settings, structure is created by defining the activities that are required parts of a patient's treatment involvement. These activities include attendance at the individual and group sessions of the programme, participation in community self-help groups and the scheduling of daily activities in such a manner as to minimise contact with drugs and avoid high-risk situations that can trigger drug use. The structure provided by treatment helps to define what is expected of patients in treatment and gives them a 'roadmap' for their recovery. The 'routine' that is created by these structure-creating activities decreases stress and provides consistency and predictability, as opposed to the spontaneous, unplanned and chaotic lifestyle that is characteristic of people who are addicted to substances.

The primary tool in building a structure during outpatient treatment is a daily, hour-by-hour schedule for their activities. The act of planning and committing to a predetermined set of activities is frequently a new or forgotten skill for many stimulant addicts. Proactively planning future activities and following through on this plan is typically not part of an active addict's repertoire. Mastering this skill of purposely determining behaviours, as opposed to acting with no plan, is an important step towards creating a drug-free lifestyle.

The term 'scheduling' can be misleading. The purpose of this exercise is not to create a list of one activity after another. The intent of the exercise is to impart (a) the concept of proactive planning on a daily basis, (b) tools for making these plans and (c) reinforcement for successfully following the schedule. For example, a realistic time plan incorporates a collection of activities that include work activities, treatment and recovery activities, family and recreational activities, and relaxation activities such as television watching, taking naps and so forth. Within the context of this scheduling exercise, it is possible to teach a patient how to avoid high-risk settings and people as well as to promote engagement in new, non-drug-related alternative behaviours.

Scheduling is important in that it is a way to identify upcoming high-risk situations, thus giving clinicians and patients the opportunity to discuss responses to potential risky circumstances. An added benefit of scheduling is that it gives the therapist an opportunity to review the patient's daily living activities in detail and identify potential problem areas. It also keeps patients accountable for their time, thereby reducing the chance of them having free time to acquire and use alcohol and drugs. Creating a 24-hour schedule with patients can help them operationalise how to stay abstinent 'one day at a time'. The schedule is written out with the patient during treatment sessions to promote compliance.

It is helpful for the patient take the schedule with them so that they can refer to it during day-to-day activities. Patients can change their plan if necessary, but they should take the time to actually change the written schedule and write in the new activity.

It is generally advised that scheduling skills be taught in an individual session, if possible. The individual sessions provide an opportunity to learn much about a patient's day-to-day life, and they present occasions for rapport building and education regarding treatment issues. In cases in which it is necessary to conduct the initial scheduling sessions in group sessions, the basic principles discussed above are the same.

Possible scheduling pitfalls

Therapists should be aware of potential problems that may arise in the scheduling process, including the following:

- Patients (and therapists) may forget to schedule in leisure activities, time to rest, time to relax and so forth. The schedule can become a marathon of productive activities. This type of unrealistic scheduling will lead to non-compliance and quickly make the scheduling activity pointless. One helpful way to make sure that the schedule is realistic is to review the events of typical drug-free days for the patient and see what a normal routine for them would be. If the schedule created is too different from normal habits, it will be difficult for the patient to incorporate it into their routine.
- Many patients have difficulty making an hour-by-hour schedule. If this is the case, the process should be simplified. One way to do that is to simply use a small, pocket-sized card with the day divided into four sections: morning, midday, afternoon and evening. Initial scheduling is easier if the patient can just plan activities for these four times of the day.
- Some families want to help 'plan' (or dictate) a patient's schedule. Spouses and parents, especially, have lots of ideas for things that have been neglected or things that the patient should do. Since many patients are trying to win back the support of their families, they can be easily convinced that they should do whatever family members want rather than what they need to do sustain a plan for their recovery. If someone else's wishes and desires are the basis for the schedule regularly, sooner or later the recovering person will become resentful and will not find the scheduling useful or helpful. It will be viewed as a 'sentence' imposed by the family member, and the therapist will be viewed as a colluding compatriot. It is important for the patient to be the person who is responsible for constructing the schedule with input from the therapist.

Psycho-education

A key component of the Matrix Model is educating patients about conditioning and neurobiology in relation to MA dependence (Obert et al., 2002). Accurate, understandable information helps patients gain an understanding of predictable changes that will occur in their thinking, mood and relationships over the course of several months of abstinence from MA. This educational process identifies and normalises symptoms, thereby empowering patients to draw upon resources and techniques to help manage their symptoms.

The use of patient education as a treatment component is a not a new treatment concept, nor unique to the Matrix Model. However, teaching patients and their families about how cocaine and MA produce changes in brain functioning in a manner that has direct application to patients' behaviour is a relatively new strategy. It is very helpful for patients and their families to know that cocaine and MA use changes brain functioning. Two very basic lectures on 'brain chemistry made simple' were developed to be delivered to patients and their families by a senior clinical staff person. New therapists are coached on how to explain the essence of this brain chemistry change process, along with the concept of classical conditioning. One of the lectures covers the changes in brain chemistry as the healing brain attempts to regain normal functioning. This knowledge reinforces the value of continuing relapse prevention activities for patients and supports vigilant treatment participation far beyond the initial withdrawal phase.

Other lectures present information derived from research about the role of classical conditioning in the development of drug craving and why craving is stimulated by specific cues and emotional states. The research on the relationship of alcohol and marijuana use to stimulant relapse is presented to support the clinical recommendation for abstinence from these drugs as important in preventing relapse to stimulants. Information on the relationship between MA use, route of administration, sexual behaviour and HCV and HIV transmission is also discussed as part of the psycho-educational curriculum.

In the Matrix Model, the science-made-simple lectures are delivered midweek during the education group sessions for patients and their families. They are part of a series of 12 educational group sessions that the senior clinical person in each clinic conducts.

Potential problems in delivering psycho-education

Clinicians should keep the following potential problems in mind when delivering psycho-education to MA-dependent patients and their families:

- The presentation of psycho-educational information based on science can be dull and tedious for patients and families if presented improperly. The material from the research literature has to be 'translated' into non-technical language and presented at eighth- to tenth-grade levels. Visual aids including clear and understandable pictures and videos can be very useful in conveying this information. It is important that the material be presented in a context of clinical issues so that patients and their family members understand the relevance of the information and how it applies to their recovery from addiction.
- The individual who presents this material as part of the Matrix programme has to be well versed in the neurobiological concepts and related research information. For the material to be understood and used by patients, the presenter must have credibility, be able to expand on the material and make the material relevant to patients' clinical challenges.

Teaching cognitive behavioural skills

Knowledge and skills that have been developed within the field of CBT play a large role in the Matrix Model. The work of Marlatt and Gordon (1985), Carroll and colleagues (1991, 1994a, b) and others have contributed greatly to the content and group treatment activities of the Matrix Model. While this form of cognitive behavioural outpatient therapy is structured and focused on relapse prevention, it can be individualised to the patient's unique experiences, thoughts and behaviours. The educational aspect of CBT teaches patients how to self-monitor and utilise the information gained in preventing relapse. The goal of self-monitoring is to bring into the patient's awareness any dysphoric or uncomfortable symptoms, thoughts, warning signs, high-risk situations and subtle precipitating events. The patient is given skills training in identifying triggers, developing coping skills and managing immediate problems. They are encouraged to practice and experiment with new behaviours outside the clinic setting. In the group, they are asked to report on what worked and what did not work, what obstacles were encountered and what changes need to be made to make the interventions successful in the future.

Each of the Matrix group sessions is anchored by a specific CBT topic, for example, 'Internal and External Triggers'. At the initiation of the group sessions, each patient receives a handout/worksheet that explains the concept and includes questions that can be used by patients to personalise the concept and make it relevant to their lives. The topics are usually introduced by the therapist, and a brief explanation is given about how this topic relates to the achievement of a successful recovery. Each patient in the group discusses how the topic is a factor in their life and how the skills being introduced could (or could not) help them with specific challenges they face in recovery. The discussion is not confrontational, and while the primary exchange is typically between the patient and the therapist/group leader, frequently other patients make observations about similarities and differences between their experiences and those of other patients. Frequently, the therapist will suggest that one or more of the group members apply the skill in the following days as a homework assignment.

Potential problems in teaching cognitive behavioural skills

The following are problems that therapists may face in teaching cognitive behaviour strategies:

- Therapists may find that they have difficulty simultaneously delivering the topic material and paying attention to the group dynamics. For example, a therapist may be reviewing a topic where one patient has discussed a high-risk situation they were in, while another patient is becoming agitated and triggered as a result of the discussion. This is not an uncommon occurrence in the Matrix groups. It is sometimes necessary for a patient to step outside the group with the therapist or a senior group member to get through this craving experience.
- A cognitive behavioural orientation involves an engaging and non-judgmental stance by the therapist and communicates positive regard for the patient. If the topic is not accompanied with useful real-world examples of how the topic can actually relate to patient challenges and benefits, the sessions can feel excessively

didactic and academic, or, in short, boring. The skill of the therapist in this kind of CBT group is to keep the topic interesting and relevant and find ways to apply it to patients in the group.

- When CBT-oriented groups are employed, there are challenges in maintaining a stimulating pace, staying on topic and managing the time of the group. Speaking calmly and redirecting patients is an effective way to keep the group focused and on task. (As noted previously, with MA use there may be some cognitive impairment, which should not be confused with 'resistance' or 'non-compliance'.)
- Mandated patients who have not decided they need or want treatment may present a problem within a CBT group. These patients have not yet recognised a need to change their behaviour and are therefore not ready to hear suggestions regarding how to become drug free. Often, the cohesiveness and positive momentum of the group can move them in this direction.
- It is not unusual for an intoxicated patient to attend a group session. If another counsellor is available on-site, he or she can work with the client to ensure safe transportation home. Any discussion regarding the patient's drug or alcohol use should be avoided until the next appointment. If possible, an individual session should be scheduled to address the particular issues surrounding the relapse.

Positive reinforcement

Rigorous research and empirical evidence support positive outcomes when CM techniques are used to shape and maintain drug recovery behaviours (Petry, 2000; Roll et al., 2006). As reviewed earlier in this chapter, CM techniques are, at their core, the systematic application of positive reinforcement principles to the modification of behaviour. As the research evidence has accumulated on the effectiveness of CM for stimulant dependence (Rawson et al., 2006; Roll et al., 2006), the clinics of the Matrix Institute have added CM strategies as a standard component of the standard Matrix Model treatment.

Positive reinforcement to promote behaviour change can be accomplished in ways other than CM. Simple ways of administering positive reinforcement include verbal praise for attendance at sessions, for using newly learned skills, for giving clean urine tests and for active participation in group sessions. Encouragement and praise decreases negative attitudes and negative expectations about therapy.

Another technique for reinforcing positive behaviour is the recording of sober days on a calendar. To implement this exercise, patients are asked at the beginning of each session to place coloured stickers, or 'dots', on a calendar for each drug-free day. This public recording of data provides an excellent opportunity to explicitly reinforce patients' achievements.

Family education

The Matrix Model involves family members in the treatment programme. 'Family' includes all those people who are part of patients' everyday existence and are close to them. This includes biological family members as well as partners, close friends, associates and extended family members. Family involvement in the Matrix Model of treatment leads to better retention of patients in the treatment. One of the reasons it is important for significant others to be involved is to help patients be better prepared for the changes they may experience during the recovery process. This allows family members to better understand what normally occurs for a recovering person and some of the difficulties they may encounter. It is not uncommon for some patients to not want family members involved, especially those who may be critical or overly controlling.

It is often necessary for therapists using the Matrix Model to schedule a session with family members to explain the ways in which they can be helpful in the treatment process and strongly encourage them to attend scheduled sessions. By presenting their role as providing supportive and positive assistance, as opposed to entering 'therapy' for their family systems pathology, family members are often more willing to help support the recovery process and attend treatment.

Not all family members will want to be a part of the recovery process, despite the urging by the therapist or patient. There are many reasons for this. One may be that family members feel they have been through tremendous stress and disappointment and that they cannot put themselves through any more emotional turmoil. Another reason for family members being unwilling to participate may be that they are very angry. They may be tired of all the family resources being expended fruitlessly on battling the addiction. Other family members say they are just tired of all the deception and turmoil that is part of the addiction and they are not willing to invest more energy into helping the patient recover. These family members might say something such as 'This is your problem, not mine. Go get fixed and when you are all better we can continue leading our lives together'.

Despite all these scenarios, it is often possible to find at least one family member who is willing to participate. Just because a family member does not choose to be actively involved at the outset of treatment, it should not be assumed they are forever unwilling to participate. The counsellor should, with the consent of the patient, continue to maintain contact (by telephone if necessary) and issue open invitations for involvement to family members.

Potential pitfall of family involvement

Involving families in the treatment of MA-dependent individuals can be very helpful; however:

- Since patients and family members are both present in the family education group sessions, there is the potential for discussions to erupt into disagreements about current or past problems between family members. The group leader has to be skilled in defusing the situation, reminding participants that this is not a 'therapy' session and that conjoint sessions can be scheduled with the therapist to address these issues. Family therapy referrals can also be useful to provide a more appropriate venue for these clinical issues.

Self-help groups

Because AA meetings have occurred since the 1930s, they are familiar to much of the public and are frequently an available resource. Recently, there have been well-designed studies that have demonstrated empirically the usefulness of participation in 12-step programmes (e.g. Humphreys et al., 2004).

Not everyone responds favourably to the concepts of the 12 steps or to the groups themselves. Many patients are not willing to attend 12-step meetings, or sample one or two meetings and find them unhelpful or aversive. However, there is a substantial effort within the Matrix approach to promote the use of this free, widely available support system.

Much of the resistance to participation in 12-step programmes often concerns the 'spiritual' dimension of AA. This resistance can be reduced by urging patients to focus on other benefits of the 12-step programme that they find useful. For example, one basic principle of the Matrix approach is the creation of structure and development of non-drug-related activities. Attendance at 12-step group sessions can be presented as part of constructing a schedule with drug-free activities during high-risk time periods. Often motivational interviewing strategies can be helpful in addressing resistance to participation in 12-step programme involvement.

Potential pitfall of encouraging 12-step involvement

- A substantial number of individuals will be resistant to attending 12-step programme meetings. It is important that this issue does not turn into a power struggle between the patient and the therapist. As with all Matrix treatment activities, participation is voluntary and patients should not be penalised or criticised for their unwillingness to attend these meetings. Often other group members who are benefiting from 12-step programme participation can be helpful in promoting attendance.

Urine and breath tests

The Matrix approach requires accurate information on the drug use of patients as they progress through treatment. The most accurate means of monitoring patients for drug and alcohol use during treatment is through the use of urine and breath alcohol testing. Urine testing should not be presented to the patient primarily as a monitoring measure. Instead of being used as a policing device, testing should be seen as a way to help a person not use drugs. Urine and breath alcohol testing done in a clinical setting for clinical purposes is quite different from urine testing that is done for legal monitoring.

Potential pitfalls of urine and breath testing

- Some patients may resist the necessity of urine testing. They may view the procedure as coercive or indicative of mistrust by the treatment programme staff.

It is possible to mitigate this resistance by describing the purpose of the testing as offering objective evidence of the patient's abstinence if family members or others make accusations of drug use. Patients will often say things such as 'You don't need to test me. Why would I come in here and lie about using? I will tell you if I use'. It is important to let new patients know that the testing procedure is a standard part of the programme and that urine testing is not a way of 'catching' misbehaviour.

Applications of the Matrix Model

Since the mid-1980s, the Matrix Model has been used with over 10 000 stimulant-dependent individuals. It is currently being used throughout the USA, typically in areas of heavy MA use. It has been translated into seven languages, and there are substantial clinical efforts using the approach in Thailand, Spain and Lebanon. In addition to the manuals published by SAMHSA and Hazelden, the Matrix organisation has produced a full set of manuals in Spanish, as well as manuals for the treatment of male gay and bisexual MA users (Shoptaw et al., 1998, www.uclaisap.org) and adolescent MA users (www.hazelden.org), and a special manual for Native Americans (www.matrixinstitute.org). Current efforts are underway to evaluate these specialty manuals.

Summary and conclusions

At the present time, the main treatment approaches for individuals who are dependent upon MA are behavioural and psychosocial. Treatments with demonstrated efficacy for cocaine dependence are appropriate for the treatment of MA users. The research supporting the use of CM is quite robust, and it is clear that this technique can be of great value in improving treatment retention and reducing drug use when individuals are in treatment.

The Matrix Model is a different treatment approach in that it is a collection of strategies, integrated into a single protocol. Although the research on the Matrix approach (Huber et al., 1997; Rawson et al., 1995, 2004) supports its value as a standardised package, the treatment elements can be disaggregated into individual elements and applied in a variety of treatment settings. The content of the individual elements and specific clinical constructs are founded in many of the seminal research-based clinical techniques supported by empirical evidence over the past 20 years (e.g. motivational interviewing, CBT, relapse prevention, 12-step programme participation, family therapy).

The international problem of MA use and its consequences appears to be expanding. It is imperative that new treatments and new specific strategies be developed to augment the existing treatment methods. As new methods are developed and alternative approaches are established, treatment efforts with MA-dependent individuals will continue to improve.

References

Brodie, J. D., Figueroa, E. and Dewey, S. L. (2003) Treating cocaine addiction: from pre-clinical to clinical trial experience with gamma-vinyl GABA. *Synapse* 50: 261–265.

Brodie, J. D., Figueroa, E., Laska, E. M. and Dewey, S. L. (2005) Safety and efficacy of gamma-vinyl GABA (GVG) for the treatment of methamphetamine and/or cocaine addiction. *Synapse* 55: 122–125.

Carroll, K. M., Rounsaville, B. J. and Gawin, F. H. (1991) A comparative trial of psychotherapies for ambulatory cocaine abusers: relapse prevention and interpersonal psychotherapy. *American Journal of Drug and Alcohol Abuse* 17: 229–247.

Carroll, K. M., Rounsaville, B. J., Gordon, L. T., Nich, C., Jatlow, P. M., Bisighini, R. M. and Gawin, F. H. (1994a) Psychotherapy and pharmacotherapy for ambulatory cocaine abusers. *Archives of General Psychiatry* 51: 177–197.

Carroll, K. M., Rounsaville, B. J., Nich, C., Gordon, L. T., Wirtz, P. W. and Gawin, F. H. (1994b) One year follow-up of psychotherapy and pharmacotherapy for cocaine dependence: delayed emergence of psychotherapy effects. *Archives of General Psychiatry* 51: 989–997.

Copeland, A. L. and Sorensen J. L. (2001) Differences between methamphetamine users and cocaine users in treatment. *Drug and Alcohol Dependence* 62(1): 91–95.

Daley, D. C. and Mercer, D. E. (1999) *Counseling for Cocaine Addiction: The Collaborative Cocaine Treatment Study Model*. Therapy Manuals for Drug Abuse: Manual 4, NIH Publ No 99–4380. Bethesda, MD: National Institute on Drug Abuse. Available at http://www.drugabuse.gov/TXManuals/DCCA/DCCA1.html. Accessed 31 March 2009.

Elkashef, A. M., Rawson, R. A., Anderson, A. L., Li, S.-H., Holmes, T., Smith, E. V., Chiang, N., Kahn, R., Vocci, F., Ling, W., Pearce, V. J., McCann, M., Campbell, J., Gorodetzky, C., Haning, W., Carlton, B., Mawhinney, J. and Weis, D. (2007) Bupropion for the treatment of methamphetamine dependence. *Neuropsychopharmcology* 33(5): 1162–1170.

Higgins, S. T., Sigmon, S. C., Wong, C. J., Heil, S. H., Badger, G. J., Donham, R., Dantona, R. L. and Anthony, S. (2003) Community reinforcement therapy for cocaine-dependent outpatients. *Archives of General Psychiatry* 60(10): 1043–1052.

Huber, A., Ling, W., Shoptaw, S., Gulati, V., Brethen, P. and Rawson, R. (1997) Integrating treatments for methamphetamine abuse: a psychosocial perspective. *Journal of Addictive Diseases* 16(4): 41–50.

Humphreys, K., Wing, S., McCarty, D., Chappel, J., Gallant, L., Haberle, B., Horvath, A. T., Kaskutas, L. A., Kirk, T., Kivlahan, D., Laudet, A., McCrady, B. S., McLellan, A. T., Morgenstern, J., Townsend, M. and Weiss, R. (2004) Self-help organizations for alcohol and drug problems: toward evidence based practice and policy. *Journal of Substance Abuse Treatment* 26(3): 151–158.

Luchansky, B., Krupski, A. and Stark, K. (2007) Treatment response by primary drug of abuse: does methamphetamine make a difference? *Journal of Substance Abuse Treatment* 32(1): 89–96.

Marlatt, G. A. and Gordon, J. R. (eds). (1985) *Relapse Prevention: Maintenance Strategies in the Treatment of Addictive Behaviors*. New York: Guilford Press.

Miller, W. R. and Rollnick, S. (1991) *Motivational Interviewing: Preparing People for Change*. New York: Guilford Press.

Miller, W. R. and Rollnick, S. (2002) *Motivational Interviewing: Preparing People for Change*, 2nd edn. New York: Guilford Press.

Morgenstern, J., Morgan, T. J., McCrady, B. S., Keller, D. S. and Carroll, K. M. (2001) Manual-guided cognitive-behavioral therapy training: a promising method for disseminating empirically supported substance abuse treatments to the practice community. *Psychology of Addictive Behaviors* 15(2): 83–88.

Nowinski, J., Baker, S. and Carroll, K. (1992) *Twelve Step Facilitation Therapy Manual: A Clinical Research Guide for Therapists Treating Individuals with Alcohol Abuse and Dependence*. Rockville, MD: National Institute on Alcohol Abuse and Alcoholism.

Obert, J. L., London, E. D. and Rawson, R. A. (2002) Incorporating brain research findings into standard treatment: an example using the Matrix Model. *Journal of Substance Abuse Treatment* 23: 107–114.

Obert, J. L., McCann, M. J., Brethen, P., Marinelli-Casey, P. and Rawson, R. A. (2000) The Matrix Model of outpatient substance abuse treatment: history and description. *Journal of Psychoactive Drugs* 32: 157–165.

Petry, N. M. (2000) A comprehensive guide to the application of contingency management procedures in clinical settings. *Drug and Alcohol Dependence* 58: 9–25.

Prendergast, M., Podus, D., Finney, J., Greenwell, L. and Roll, J. (2006) Contingency management for treatment of substance use disorders: a meta-analysis. *Addiction* 101(11): 1546–1560.

Rawson, R. A., Marinelli-Casey, P., Anglin, M. D., Dickow, A., Frazier, Y., Gallagher, C., Galloway, G. P., Herrell, J., Huber, A., McCann, M. J., Obert, J., Pennell, S., Reiber, C., Vandersloot, D., Zweben, J. and Methamphetamine Treatment Project Corporate Authors (2004) A mutli-site comparison of psychosocial approaches for the treatment of methamphetamine dependence. *Addiction* 99(6): 708–717.

Rawson, R. A., McCann, M. J., Flammino, F., Shoptaw, S., Miotto, K., Reiber, C. and Ling, W. (2006) A comparison of contingency management and cognitive-behavioral approaches for stimulant-dependent individuals. *Addiction* 101(2): 267–274.

Rawson, R. A., Obert, J. L., McCann, M. J., Smith, D. P. and Scheffey, E. H. (1989) *The Neurobehavioral Treatment Manual*. Beverly Hills, CA: Matrix.

Rawson, R. A., Shoptaw, S. J., Obert, J. L., McCann, M. J., Hasson, A. L., Marinelli-Casey, P., Brethen, P. R. and Ling, W. (1995) An intensive outpatient approach for cocaine abuse treatment: the Matrix Model. *Journal of Substance Abuse Treatment* 12(2): 117–127.

Roll, J. M., Petry, N. M., Stitzer, M. L., Brecht, M. L., Peirce, J. M., McCann, M. J., Blaine, J., MacDonald, M., DiMaria, J., Lucero, L. and Kellogg, S. (2006) Contingency management for the treatment of methamphetamine use disorders. *American Journal of Psychiatry* 163(11): 1993–1999.

Shoptaw, S., Reback, C. J., Freese, T. E. and Rawson, R. A. (1998) *Behavioral Interventions for Methamphetamine Abusing Gay and Bisexual Men: A Treatment Manual Combining Relapse Prevention and HIV Risk-Reduction Interventions*. Los Angeles, CA: Friends Research Institute, Inc.

Tiihonen, J., Kuoppasalmi, K., Föhr, J., Tuomola, P., Kuikanmäki, O., Vorma, H., Sokero, P., Haukka, J. and Meririnne, E. (2007) A comparison of aripiprazole, methylphenidate, and placebo for amphetamine dependence. *American Journal of Psychiatry* 164(1): 160–162.

Chapter 8
AMPHETAMINE USE IN CANADA

Diane Riley

Introduction

In their review of the history of psychostimulant use, Hando and Hall point out that since the medical introduction of cocaine in the 1880s, several 'epidemics' of stimulant use have been described (Hando and Hall, 1997). Such extensive use was probably due to a belief in the relative safety of the use of stimulants in conjunction with wide availability. Cocaine was also promoted by persons of standing, such as the psychoanalyst Sigmund Freud, as a cure for heroin addiction. A second wave of widespread cocaine use occurred in the USA during the mid-1980s and included the newly introduced 'crack cocaine'. This wave was followed by an increase in amphetamine use in the USA and Canada, which continues to the present time.

Experimentation with amphetamine in North America began in the late 1920s, when it was used for everything from depression to congestion. In the 1930s, it began to be sold as Benzedrine in an over-the-counter inhaler and its misuse rose. Methamphetamine (MA) first became popular for recreational use in the 1960s. In the 1980s, illegal street forms in a powder form that could be injected, inhaled or taken orally appeared. In the late 1980s, a smokable form known as ice or glass was being sold on the streets of West Coast mainland cities in the USA and Canada (Vancouver Coastal Health, 2004). Since the late 1990s, MA has shown up in very large quantities in Canada as well as in the USA, partly because of the ease and cost-efficiency of manufacturing this form of the drug.

Like Australia, Canada has a long history of amphetamine use in many sections of society, including recreational use by young adults, functional use among workers such as long distance transport drivers, performance enhancement in athletes and students, and heavy, chronic use by dependent drug users (see Chapter 9 in this volume). As in Australia, amphetamine is available throughout the country – in rural and urban areas and on native reserves. This is likely due to the availability of precursors from agriculture, mining, and long distance transport (Rawson et al., 2002) and due to off-reserve Aboriginal persons taking drugs to the reserves.

MA is currently the most popular illicit form of amphetamine in Canada, using pseudoephedrine as the main precursor. In the 1930s, MA was marketed as a decongestant in Canada, but currently it is not legally available. The increase in recreational use and availability of illegal forms of the drug mirrored that in the USA, especially on the West Coast. During the 1990s, the range of psychos-timulants available on illicit markets became wider, and levels of use increased. Worldwide, police and customs seizures of amphetamine-type stimulants reached record levels (see UNODC World Drug Report 2008 for details, which is available at http://www.unodc.org/unodc/en/data-and-analysis/WDR-2008.html. Accessed 19 November 2008).

Illicit MA is now readily available in Canada and elsewhere and can be produced easily and inexpensively. There are literally thousands of websites offering recipes and information about making MA. Typically, MA is produced in clandestine laboratories using over-the-counter medication ingredients such as ephedrine, pseudoephedrine, phenylpropanolamine and iodine, as well as commonly available chemicals such as red phosphorous, hydrochloric acid, ether, hydriodic acid and anhydrous ammonia. A small laboratory can produce an ounce per production cycle, or 'cook' (1 oz equals about 110 MA 'hits'); super-laboratories can produce kilograms per cycle (Vancouver Coastal Health, 2004).

In August 2005, the federal government attempted to address the increase in availability by increasing penalties for the producers and distributors of MA, putting it in the same category as cocaine and heroin (Canada Gazette, 2005; Gordon, 2006; Mills, 2005). Restrictions on the purchase of precursor ingredients have also been put in place (Canada Gazette, 2005; Mills, 2005). In 2007, the federal government introduced changes to the drug laws that increase penalties and impose mandatory minimum sentences for production and distribution of all drugs.

Patterns and prevalence

MA use, especially in the crystal form, has been reported to be the cause of an increasing number of harms across Canada in the past few years, especially in the West (Lee, 2005; Mills, 2005). Patterns of use include chronic and dependent use by the socially marginalized groups, use by young, often socially well-integrated people in recreational settings and by certain occupational groups or in particular work settings. Rates of crystal MA use are highest among street youth, gay and bisexual youth, and people who attend raves (Barrett et al., 2005; Gross et al., 2002; Lampinen et al., 2006; Martin et al., 2006). Despite the extensive media attention and legal changes that have been made to address the growing problem of crystal MA use in Canada, little research has been conducted to assess the purported increase in use of the drug.

The 2004 Canadian Addictions Survey (CAS) was the first national survey conducted in Canada since 1994 and is the most comprehensive overview available of alcohol and other drug use among Canadians 15 years and older (Adlaf et al., 2005). For the general population of Canadians, the use of illicit drugs is usually limited to cannabis only. About 29% of Canadians (63.4% of lifetime users) report using only cannabis during their lifetime, and 11.5% (79.1% of past-year users) used only cannabis during the past year. The survey equated amphetamine-type substances (ATS) with speed and found that 6.4% of Canadians reported use at least once in their lifetime, with less than 1% reporting use in the 12 months preceding the survey. Although the survey did not measure MA use specifically, the results suggest a low level of use of this type of substance by the general population. By comparison, lifetime use of hallucinogens was 11.4%, cocaine 10.4% and ecstasy 4.1%. The lifetime use of inhalants, heroin, steroids and drugs by injection was about 1% or less. Most current rates of drug use – those occurring during the past 12 months – are generally 1% or less, with the exception of cocaine use (1.9%). The national rate of lifetime and past-year illicit drug use, other than cannabis (16.5 and 3.0%), is highest among men (21.1 and 4.3%, respectively): 18- to 19-year-olds (30.6 and 17.8%, respectively) and 20- to 24-year-olds (28.1 and 11.5%, respectively); and single (24.0 and 8.9%, respectively) and previously married respondents (13.7% lifetime only). Men are more likely than women to report lifetime use of cocaine (14.1 vs. 7.3%), speed (8.7 vs. 4.1%) and ecstasy (5.2 vs. 3.0%) and are more likely to report use of any of these drugs. Analysis of ATS use in the western provinces showed that reports of more than one ATS use in the past year were the same for rural (4%) and non-rural (4.1%) areas. British Columbia had reported rates of 5.1% (190 000 users), followed by Alberta (4% or 108 000 users), Manitoba (3% or 33 400 users) and Saskatchewan (2.8% or 27 700 users). These figures pertain to all ATS users, but anecdotal reports from addiction treatment providers suggest that the drug of choice is MA.

Provincial student surveys give a good indication of overall incidence rates of drug use since initial drug use often occurs during adolescence. Several provinces conduct such surveys, but only Manitoba (AFM, 2001) and Ontario (Centre for Addiction and Mental Health, 2003) have specifically asked about the use of amphetamine. According to these surveys, past-year use of amphetamine (in the form of MA) was 2.7% in Manitoba and 3.3% in Ontario, a decline from 5% in 1999.

For several reasons, it is unlikely that studies such as CAS and student surveys reflect the full extent of amphetamine use in Canada. The CAS was conducted through a telephone survey, and the student surveys were conducted in schools. These studies do not include data on hard-to-reach populations such as street-involved youth, Aboriginal communities in remote and rural settings, and people without a telephone.

Piran and Gadalla (2007) examined the comorbidity between eating disorders and substance use in a large nationally representative sample of Canadian women and men. The research was based on secondary analyses of data collected by Statistics Canada in the Mental Health and Well-being cycle 1.2 of the Canadian Community Health Survey (CCHS). Data included the Eating Attitude Test (EAT-26) and modules of the short form of the Composite International Diagnostic Interview (CIDI-SF) to assess alcohol and drug use, dependence and interference. Problematic alcohol use and amphetamine use were associated with the risk for an eating disorder in both women and men. In the women sample only, risk for an eating disorder was associated with illicit drug use, dependence and problematic use, as well as with the number of substance classes used.

Young people

After a peak in 1979, the use of most substances among high school students declined steadily until the early 1990s. In the following decade, substance use by students tended to increase, and has now stabilised at levels close to those of the late 1970s (AADAC, 2003; Adlaf et al., 2000; Adlaf and Paglia, 2004). On average, one-quarter to one-third of Canadian high school students (aged 12–19 years) used no drugs in the past year. The most commonly used drugs among youth remain alcohol, cannabis and tobacco. There is little reliable information on club or dance drugs such as ATS. Rates of ecstasy use (or drugs called by that name) apparently increased more than any other substance in the 1990s (3.2–6% of students reporting use in the last year).

Along with increases in stimulant use by young people in Canada and the USA in recent years, major increases in the prescribing of methylphenidate have been observed (Miller et al., 1998; Safer et al., 1996; Zito et al., 2000). Patterns of use are related to gender, with several studies reporting a preponderance of females taking diet pills and males taking methylphenidate; the amount of methylphenidate prescribed increased about fivefold from the early to the mid-1990s (Johnson et al., 1999; LeFever et al., 1999; Miller et al., 1998; Safer et al., 1996; Zito et al., 2000). One study conducted in the Province of Nova Scotia found that the annual prevalence of non-medical stimulant use among adolescents increased from 5% in 1991 to 11% in 1998 (Poulin, 2001). In 1998, a self-reported anonymous questionnaire was administered to a random sample of students in grades 7, 9, 10 and 12 in New Brunswick, Nova Scotia, Prince Edward Island, and Newfoundland and Labrador about their medical and non-medical use of stimulants (Benzedrine, Dexedrine, Ritalin, Cylert, diet pills, 'speed', 'uppers', 'bennies' and 'pep pills'). A total of 13 549 students completed the questionnaire, representing a 99% participation rate among the students present at school on the day of the survey. Of the 5.3% of students who reported medical use of stimulants in the 12 months before the survey, 14.7% reported having given away some of their medication, 7.3% having sold some of their medication, 4.3% having experienced theft and 3.0% having been forced to give up some of their medication. Non-medical stimulant use by students who did not have a prescription for stimulants was significantly related to increased numbers of students who gave or sold some of their prescribed stimulants.

Street youth are youth (aged 12–25 years) who are absent from home without their parents' permission for 24 hours or more. Data on substance use among street youth in Canada are limited; prevalence and patterns vary by city, but are always much higher than student use. Several studies report that at least one in five street youth, including Aboriginal youth, have injected drugs (Roy et al., 1998). It is estimated that as many as 200 000 street youths move through Canadian cities every year (Covenant House, Canada, 2007). The lifestyles of street youth involve many high-risk behaviours including licit and illicit drug use and needle sharing (Haley et al., 2003; McKenzie et al., 1997). The most popular drugs are alcohol, tobacco, cannabis and stimulants. A survey of a sample of street youth (aged 14–30 years) conducted in Vancouver in 2000 found that 71% had tried ATS and 57% had used them more than ten times (Vancouver Coastal Health, 2004).

In British Columbia, as elsewhere in Canada, amphetamine is used more frequently by younger people. In 2002, a study of 1900 lower mainland youth (average age 17 years) found that 18.7% had tried crystal MA, with an average first use at 14.5 years of age (Pacific Community Resources, 2002, Accessed 19 Novemember 2008 http://www.pcrs.ca/content/home.asp). Among homeless youth in Vancouver, more young (aged <19 years) used amphetamines than older youth (Between the Cracks, McCreary Centre, British Columbia, 2002). The specialised youth centre in Victoria has seen admissions for detoxification from crystal MA increase from 17 to 117 over the past 4 years. More than 70% of all admissions are now for crystal MA, and average age of admission is 16 years (Victoria Youth Empowerment Society, 2002). In 2003, a survey of youth in Vancouver and Victoria comparing high school youth and vulnerable youth showed that 10% of Victoria high school students and 70% of street-involved Vancouver youth had used crystal MA, and there is evidence that this level of use by street youth in Vancouver has continued or increased over recent years (Fairbairn et al., in press).

Injection

The number of Canadians reporting use of an injectable drug at some point in their life increased from 1.7 million in 1994 (7.4% overall: 10% of males, 4.9% of females) to a little more than 4.1 million in 2004 (16.1% overall: 20.8% males, 11.7% females) (Adlaf et al., 2005). Of those who used an injectable drug at least once in their lifetime, 7.7% (132 000) reported past-year use by injection in 1994 compared with 6.5% (269 000) in 2004. The percentage of those who are injecting amphetamine is not known; anecdotal reports from syringe exchanges and other services suggest that it is still relatively small, but increasing.

A recent study directly addresses the issue of rates of MA injection. Fairbairn and colleagues evaluated the trends in crystal MA injection and factors associated with injection of the drug among a cohort of injection drug users (IDU) in Vancouver (Fairbairn et al., in press). The researchers conducted a prospective analysis of factors associated with crystal MA injection among participants enrolled in the Vancouver Injection Drug Users Study (VIDUS); variables potentially associated with crystal MA injection were evaluated. Overall, 1587 IDU were enrolled into the VIDUS cohort between May 1996 and December 2004. The proportion of IDU who reported injecting crystal MA during the last 6 months increased significantly during the study, from 2.5% in 1997 to 6.7% in 2004. Crystal MA injection was independently associated with younger age, Caucasian ethnicity, syringe borrowing and syringe lending. The association of MA injection with younger age and syringe sharing is of particular concern, given the increased risks of HIV and hepatitis C infection in younger, inexperienced injectors (cf. Urbina and Jones, 2004).

Gay community

According to media and anecdotal reports, the use of psychostimulants, including MA, among members of the gay community in Canada is widespread, as it is in a number of other countries (Boddiger, 2005; Mansergh, 2005). As in Australia, the use of drugs in combination with music, dancing and sexual contact has been identified as a means to celebrate gay identity, with psychostimulants, in particular, being used to enhance energy for dancing and partying (Jenner and McKetin, 2004). There are a number of factors that contribute to patterns of drug use among the gay community, such as the nature of sexual relationships, misunderstanding of risks, impulsivity, the situational context of sexual activity, stress responses and age. MA use during sex is relatively prevalent in some men who have sex with men. One of the main reasons that MA is popular is that it enhances and/or prolongs intensity and frequency of sexual encounters and keeps a person active for long parties (McVinney, 2005; Siever, 2005). The Sex Now Survey conducted in 2004 reported that 25.4% of gay men in British Columbia had used MA, and anecdotal reports from the gay community around Canada suggested a similar pattern of use (Vancouver Coastal Health, 2004).

Police data

An increased prevalence of MA use is reflected in a significant and steady expansion in police contacts in Canada; greater numbers of clandestine laboratory seizures in western Canada indicate that the MA industry is expanding (Vancouver Coastal Health, 2004; RCMP data). Multiple sources such as law enforcement data, production rates and prevalence rates also suggest a gradual migration in MA use from the West Coast towards Manitoba and further to the east of the country. These indicators also suggest that MA use remains relatively low in the general population but seems to be on the rise, most notably among street-involved youth, gay men and young adults in the party scene. Law enforcement agencies in Canada believe that criminal organisations such as biker gangs are involved in the production and distribution of MA.

Emergency, hospital and treatment settings

An increased prevalence of MA use is reflected in a significant and steady expansion in hospital admissions and in the number of clients seeking treatment in community treatment centres; as in most countries, young persons represent a disproportionate share of MA treatment admissions in Canada (Vancouver Coastal Health, 2004). In British Columbia, crystal MA-related deaths increased from 3 in 2000 to 33 in 2004, most commonly as a result of overdose or motor vehicle accidents (BC Coroners Service, 2005).

In summary, an increased prevalence of MA use is reflected in the increase in hospital admissions, police contacts and in the number of clients seeking treatment in community treatment centres. There has also been an increase in the number of MA-related deaths. MA is being used increasingly as a substitute for other drugs, such as ecstasy, or in a mixture with these drugs. The increase in the number of clandestine laboratory seizures in western Canada indicates that the MA industry is expanding.

Interventions

There have been a wide variety of responses to increasing amphetamine use in Canada, ranging from detention and coerced treatment to harm reduction services and proposals for stimulant maintenance programmes.

Psychosocial interventions

As in most countries, systematic counselling forms the basis of most community-based treatments for amphetamine users in Canada. Approaches and programmes used include:

- Motivational interviewing
- Behavioural therapy and cognitive behavioural therapy
- Contingency management
- Residential rehabilitation
- Therapeutic communities
- Self-help groups
- Family and multi-systemic interventions
- Residential treatment
- 12-step programmes

The increase in stimulant-related problems and the specific needs of stimulant users has led to calls for tailored interventions and more intensive approaches, especially for young people.

One response to increased stimulant use by youth has been an increase in mandatory and coerced treatment in several provinces (Canadian Centre on Substance Abuse, 2006). Alberta's Protection of Children Abusing Drugs Act, which came into effect in 2006, requires persons under 18 with an apparent alcohol or other drug problem to participate, with or without their agreement, in an assessment and subsequent outpatient treatment or in a programme within a 'protective safe house'. The Youth Drug Detoxification and Stabilization Act passed in Saskatchewan in 2005 allows for the apprehension and detainment against the will of persons under 18 for assessment, detoxification and stabilisation of substance misuse problems. In Manitoba, the Youth Drug Stabilization (Support for Parents) Act came into effect in November 2006. The act provides a way to access involuntary detention and short-term stabilisation for young Manitobans under 18 years of age. The act is stated to be intended as a last resort, when other measures have been unsuccessful and where a youth is causing serious self-harm through severe, persistent substance misuse. The purpose of the stabilisation period is to provide a safe, secure environment to engage the youth and develop a treatment plan that he or she will follow after discharge.

Mandatory treatment is contrary to the harm reduction model, which is a human rights-based approach, determined by clients' choices, life circumstances and stages of change. There are also a number of ethical and legal issues. Forced treatment may be a violation of civil liberties and could result in legal challenges under the Canadian Charter of Rights and Freedoms. There are issues of professional ethics for treatment providers who deal with clients mandated to attend. For example, Canadian psychologists are required by Code of Ethics to recognise the self-determination and liberty of the clients they serve. Other ethical issues regarding mandatory treatment include potential breaches of client confidentiality when legal and court-appointed case management authorities enter into the treatment process.

Harm reduction services

In the knowledge that much psychostimulant use by the younger population is experimental or social in nature, the emphasis of many interventions has been aimed at reducing the harm caused by this time-limited or lower-level use (Weir, 2000). This has included the dissemination of information on the effects and risks of taking psychostimulants or being in a place where psychostimulants are freely available. Harm reduction strategies include teaching early signs of problematic use, how to assist peers with problems and where help is available for individuals with problems (Dennis and Ballard, 2002). The provision of sterile injection equipment is also part of any such harm reduction strategy.

Peer education on psychostimulant use usually involves the use of peers who are credible, influential and have received training to help them to support and educate users to reduce the potential harms of stimulants use to themselves and others. There is limited information that specifically addresses the effectiveness of peer education in regard to stimulant use. Users who take psychostimulants at dance events are the targets of organisations such as Ravesafe, an international initiative based in South Africa with a number of groups operating in Canada (www.Ravesafe.org). It is an organisation of volunteers that generally provides basic first aid, distributes information about street/dance drugs and safer raving, and provides a place at parties where people can feel safe and secure, often referred to as a 'chill out' area.

Crystal Clear, a peer-led harm reduction programme for young MA users in Vancouver, BC, which focuses on street-involved youth, is a well-designed and effective service in an area of high amphetamine and other drug use. Another innovative harm reduction service located in Vancouver is Insite, a safe injection site opened in 2004 under an exemption to the Federal drug laws to help deal with the many problems related to the high levels of public drug use in the Downtown Eastside area. Insite is a clean, safe environment where users can inject their own drugs under the supervision of clinical staff. Nurses and counsellors provide on-site access and referral to addiction treatment services, primary health care, and mental health providers, as well as first aid and wound care. The service has been extensively and thoroughly evaluated and found to be very effective in reducing risks and harms related to injecting such as syringe sharing and HIV infection and in connecting users of the facility with other health services (see, for example, Kerr et al., 2005a, b; Wood et al., 2003, 2004a, b, c). Drug use data were collected from 7278 unique individuals registered at Insite for the 2-year period from 1 April 2004 to 31 March 2006 (Tyndall et al., 2006). Heroin was used in 40.0% of all visits, morphine in 13.2%, and speedballs, a combination of heroin and cocaine, were used in 6.3% of all injections. There was a significant amount of powder cocaine being injected (28.2%), as well as a smaller amount of cocaine that was brought into the supervised injection facility (SIF) as crack cocaine (3.0%) and crushed. Crystal MA was injected at the SIF in only 1.5% of all visits. The authors speculate that there may be a population of MA injectors who are not using the SIF, but it is also likely that the injection of MA is not as common in this community.

Increased stimulant use has led to calls for stimulant maintenance programmes along the lines of those in the UK and Australian pilot programmes. Vancouver's last Mayor, Sam Sullivan, put forward a proposal to provide cocaine and MA users with prescription stimulants; under CAST (Chronic Addiction Substitution Treatment), up to 700 chronic cocaine and MA users would be provided with maintenance doses of stimulants (Mulla and MacPherson, 2007). The results of a poll showed strong support for the notion among Vancouver residents; the survey released showed that 61% of respondents would support such a program to deal with the numerous drug-related problems in the city's Downtown Eastside area. To introduce such a program, the city would need an exemption from Canada's drug laws from the federal government. Given attempts by the present Conservative government to shut down the city's safe injection site which operates on an exemption to drug laws it is highly unlikely that such a program will be put in place in the near future.

Conclusions

Amphetamine in the form of MA has been the focus of considerable discussion in Canada over the past few years, as it has been in Australia, the USA and other countries. Just as in these others countries part of this reaction may well be a moral panic, but health indicators do suggest an increase in amphetamine-related harms, rising from a low baseline to a level of concern. Crystalline MA is cheap, fairly pure and readily available in many parts of Canada, especially the west.

Since changing the penalties for MA production and the banning of precursor chemicals are likely to have a negligible impact on the use of this drug (Cunningham and Liu, 2003, 2005; Reuter, 2003), evidence-based, cost-effective interventions are needed to address the risks and harms of MA misuse. Given the rise in injection of MA among young users in Vancouver, the need for such interventions is clear (Kerr et al., 2005c; Reuter, 2003).

In prevention and harm reduction strategies, emphasis has been placed on information conveyed at raves and dance parties. These harm reduction initiatives need to better target possibly more 'at-risk' groups (e.g. street-involved youth and those involved with the criminal justice system) and other settings like parties where young people are likely to use psychostimulants. Since amphetamine users come from all sectors of society and a variety of backgrounds, there is a need for a range of prevention and harm reduction strategies that target both the traditional drug user networks and users who take pills occasionally and who do not see themselves as 'drug users'. This includes the need for harm reduction in schools. In addition, little is known about how best to attract youth to services such as drop-ins and needle exchanges. Barriers and facilitators to service access for use should be documented for different youth subgroups. This should include an analysis of the unique legal and ethical issues posed by dealing with minors. Lack of relevant services and treatment is particularly marked with respect to MA and crack cocaine. Studies also support the importance of developing assessment instruments and treatment strategies that address the co-occurrence of eating disorders and stimulant use for both women and men.

There is growing recognition that we need to maintain credibility with stimulant users through the provision of accurate, culturally appropriate and useful information. This includes acknowledging the relatively low risk associated with the infrequent use of low doses of amphetamine, while at the same time emphasising the well-established risks associated with the frequent use of high doses, particularly through injecting or smoking.

There is a pressing need to study and adopt new approaches to stimulants. As is the case with other chapters in this book, the interventions described here are far from uniform and no standard of treatment has yet been suggested to serve as 'best' practice.

References

Addiction Foundation of Manitoba (2001) *Substance Use Among Manitoba High School Students*. Winnipeg, Manitoba, Canada: Addiction Foundation of Manitoba.

Adlaf, E. M., Begin, P. and Sawka, E. (eds) (2005) *Canadian Addiction Survey (CAS): A National Survey of Canadians' Use of Alcohol and Other Drugs, Prevalence of Use and Related Harms: Detailed Report*. Ottawa: Canadian Centre on Substance Abuse.

Adlaf, E. M. and Paglia, A. (2004) Drug use among Ontario students. Document 14, Toronto, Ontario: Centre for Addiction and Mental Health Research.

Adlaf, E. M., Paglia, A., Ivis, F. J. and Ialomiteanu A. (2000) Nonmedical drug use among adolescent students: highlights from the 1999 Ontario Student Drug Use Survey. *Canadian Medical Association Journal* 162(12): 1677–1680.

Alberta Alcohol and Drug Addiction Commission (2003) *Alberta Youth Experience Survey 2002*. Edmonton: Alberta Alcohol and Drug Addiction Commission.

Barrett, S. P., Gross, S. R., Garand, I. and Pihl, R. O. (2005) Patterns of simultaneous polysubstance use in Canadian rave attendees. *Substance Use and Misuse* 40: 1525–1537.

BC Coroners Service (2005) *Deaths with Methamphetamine Present, 2000–2004*. Vancouver: BC Coroners Service.

Boddiger, D. (2005) Methamphetamine use linked to rising HIV transmission. *Lancet* 365: 1217–1218.

Canada Gazette (2005) *Order Amending Schedule I to the Controlled Drugs and Substances Act*, 15 November 2005, Vol. 139, No. 24.

Canadian Centre on Substance Abuse (2006) *Fact Sheet on Mandatory and Coerced Treatment*. Ottawa, Ontario: Canadian Centre on Substance Abuse.

Centre for Addiction and Mental Health (2003) *Ontario Addiction Survey*. Toronto: Centre for Addiction and Mental Health.

Covenant House, Canada (2007) Information Pamphlet. Available at www.covenanthouse.ca. Accessed 7 July 2008.

Cunningham, J. K. and Liu, L. (2003) Impacts of federal ephedrine and pseudoephedrine regulations on methamphetamine-related hospital admissions. *Addiction* 98: 1129–1137.

Cunningham, J. K. and Liu, L. (2005) Impacts of federal precursor chemical regulations on methamphetamine arrests. *Addiction* 100: 479–488.

Dennis, D. and Ballard, M. (2002) Ecstasy: it's the rave. *The High School Journal* 85(4): 64–70.

Fairbairn, N., Kerr, T., Buxton, J. A., et al. (in press) Increasing use and associated harms of crystal methamphetamine injection in a Canadian setting. *Drug and Alcohol Dependence* 88, 313.

Gordon, J. (2006) Crystal meth use soars to new high: seizure of synthetic drugs on rise. *The Gazette, British Columbia*, 11 July, p. A10.

Gross, S. R., Barrett, S. P., Shestowsky, J. S. and Pihl, R. O. (2002) Ecstasy and drug consumption patterns: a Canadian rave population study. *Canadian Journal of Psychiatry* 47: 546–551.

Haley, N., Leclerc, P. and Sochanski, B. (2003) Substance misuse and homelessness among youth. Paper presented at *the 14th International Conference on the Reduction of Drug Related Harm*, Chiang Mai, April.

Hando, J. and Hall, W. (1997) Patterns of amphetamine use in Australia. In: Klee, H. (ed), *Amphetamine Misuse: International Perspectives on Current Trends*. Amsterdam: Harwood Academic Publishers.

Jenner, L. and McKetin, R. (2004) Prevalence and patterns of psychostimulant use. In: Baker, A., Lee, N. and Jenner, L. (eds), *Models of Intervention and Care for Psychostimulant Users*, 2nd edn. Monograph Series No. 51. Australia: Commonwealth of Australia, pp. 13–34.

Johnson, L. D., O'Malley, P. M. and Bachman, J. G. (1999) Secondary School Students. *Volume 1 of National Survey Results on Drug Use from the Monitoring the Future Study, 1975–1998*. Washington, DC: US Department of Health and Human Services, NIH Publ No 99-4660.

Kerr, T., Oleson, M., Tyndall, M. W., Montagner, J. and Wood, E. (2005a) A description of a peer-run supervised injection site for injection drug users. *Journal of Urban Health* 82: 267–275.

Kerr, T., Tyndall, M., Li, K., Montagner, J. and Wood, E. (2005b) Safer injection facility use and syringe sharing in injection drug users. *Lancet* 366: 316–318.

Kerr, T., Wood, E., Grafstein, E., Ishida, T., Shannon, K., Lai, C., Montagner, J. and Tyndall, M. W. (2005c) High rates of primary care and emergency department use among injection drug users in Vancouver. *Journal of Public Health (Oxford)* 27: 62–66.

Lampinen, T. M., McGhee, D. and Martin, I. (2006) Increased use of 'club' drug use among gay and bisexual high school students in British Columbia. Journal of Adolescent Health 38(4): 458–461.

Lee, J. (2005). Crystal meth 'a massive problem'. *The Vancouver Sun*, 29 September, p. A4.

LeFever, G. B., Dawson, K. V. and Morrow, A. D. (1999) The extent of drug therapy for attention deficit-hyperactivity disorder among children in public schools. *American Journal of Public Health* 89: 1359–1354.

Mansergh, G. (2005) MSM methamphetamine use and sexual risk behavior for STD/HIV infection. Paper presented at *Science and Response Conference*, Salt Lake City, Utah.

Martin, I., Lampinen, T. M. and McGhee, D. (2006) Methamphetamine use among marginalized youth in British Columbia. *Canadian Journal of Public Health* 7(4): 320–324.

McKenzie, D. (1997) Street youth. In: McKenzie, D., Williams, B. and Single, E. (eds), *Canadian Profile: Alcohol, Tobacco and Other Drugs, 1997*. Ottawa: Canadian Centre on Substance Abuse.

McVinney, L. (2005) The pharmacology of crystal methamphetamine. Paper presented at *Science and Response Conference*, Salt Lake City, Utah.

Miller, A., Lee, S. K., Raina, P., Klassen, A., Zupancic, J. and Olsen, L. (1998) *A Review of Therapies for Attention-Deficit/Hyperactivity Disorder*. Ottawa: Canadian Coordinating Office for Health Technology Assessment.

Mills, A. (2005) Ottawa toughens laws on crystal meth; sentences lengthened for possession, trafficking of drug substance abuse experts warn that move won't deter use. *Toronto Star*, 12 August, p. A.06.

Mulla, Z. and MacPherson, D. (21 September 2007) Drug substitution and maintenance treatment. City of Vancouver Administrative Report, City of Vancouver, British Columbia, Canada.

Piran, N. and Gadalla, T. (2007) Eating disorders and substance abuse in Canadian women: a national study. *Addiction* 102(1): 105–113.

Poulin, C. (2001) Medical and nonmedical stimulant use among adolescents: from sanctioned to unsanctioned use. *Canadian Medical Association Journal* 165(8): 1039–1044.

Rawson, R., Anglin, M. D. and Ling, W. (2002) Will the methamphetamine problem go a away? *Journal of Addictive Diseases* 21: 5–19.

Reuter, P. (2003). Does precursor regulation make a difference? *Addiction* 98: 1177–1179.

Roy, E., Lemire, N. and Haley, N. (1998) Injection drug use among street youth: a dynamic process. *Canadian Journal of Public Health* 89(4): 239–240.

Safer, D. J., Zito, J. M. and Fine, E. M. (1996) Increased methylphenidate usage for attention deficit disorder in the 1990s. *Pediatrics* 98: 1084–1088.

Siever, M. D. (2005) Crystal methamphetamine. Paper presented at *Science and Response Conference*, Salt Lake City, Utah.

Tyndall, M., Kerr, T., Zhang, R., King, E., Montagner, J. and Wood, E. (2006) Attendance, drug use patterns, and referrals made from North America's first supervised injection facility. *Drug and Alcohol Dependence* 83: 193–198.

Urbina, A. and Jones, K. (2004) Crystal methamphetamine, its analogues, and HIV infection: medical and psychiatric aspects of a new epidemic. *Clinical and Infectious Diseases* 38: 890–894.

Vancouver Coastal Health (2004) Western Canadian Summit on Methamphetamine, Vancouver Coastal Health, Vancouver, British Columbia.

Victoria Youth Empowerment Society (2002) Annual Report, Victoria, British Columbia.

Weir, E. (2000) Raves: a review of the culture, the drugs and the prevention of harms. *Canadian Medical Association Journal* 162(13): 1843–1848.

Wood, E., Kerr, T., Lloyd-Smith, E., Buchner, C., Marsh, D. C., Montagner, J. S. and Tyndall, M. W. (2004a) Methodology for evaluating Insite: Canada's first medically supervised safer injection facility for injection drug users. *Harm Reduction Journal* 1: 9.

Wood, E., Kerr, T., Montagner, J. S., Strathdee, S. A., Wodak, A., Hankins, C. A., Schechter, M. T. and Tyndall, M. W. (2004b) Rationale for evaluating North America's first medically supervised safer-injecting facility. *Lancet Infectious Disease* 4: 301–306.

Wood, E., Kerr, T., Small, W., Li, K., Marsh, D. C., Montagner, J. S. and Tyndall, M. W. (2004c) Changes in public order after the opening of a medically supervised safer injecting facility for illicit injection drug users. *Canadian Medical Association Journal* 171: 731–734.

Wood, E., Kerr, T., Spittal, P. M., Small, W., Tyndall, M. W., O'Shaughnessy, M. V. and Schechter, M. T. (2003). An external evaluation of a peer-run 'unsanctioned' syringe exchange program. *Journal of Urban Health* 80: 455–464.

Zito, J. M., Safer, D. J., dosReis, S., Gardner, J. F., Boles, M. and Lynch, F. (2000) Trends in the prescribing of psychotropic medications to preschoolers. *Journal of American Medical Association* 283: 1025–1030.

Chapter 9

TREATMENT RESPONSES TO PROBLEMATIC METHAMPHETAMINE USE: THE AUSTRALIAN EXPERIENCE

James Shearer

Introduction

Australia has a long history of amphetamine use (cf. Hando and Hall, 1997) extending through many sections of society from recreational use among young adults, functional use in industries such as long-distance transport, performance enhancement among students and sports players, through to dependent use patterns among injecting drug users. Unlike some illicit drugs such as heroin, usually only readily available in major cities, amphetamine is available throughout the country; indeed amphetamine-related problems may be more prevalent on a per capita basis in regional areas of the country (McKetin et al., 2005b). This situation is similar to that in the western parts of Canada and the USA, where there is high incidence of amphetamine use in regional and rural areas possibly due to the availability of precursors from agricultural, mining and long-distance transport (Rawson et al., 2002).

The nature of amphetamine use in Australia has been highly fluid, mainly as a result of drug supply control efforts directed towards illicit manufacturing and chemical precursors. In 1994, the most common precursor used in the illicit manufacture of amphetamine was phenyl-2-propanone (P-2-P). The Australian chemical industry is highly concentrated, and it was relatively simple to identify and control this precursor (Caldicott et al., 2005). Illicit amphetamine manufacture shifted to a method which used pseudoephedrine as the main chemical precursor. Pseudoephedrine is a common ingredient in many cold and flu remedies and is readily available from pharmacy retailers and wholesalers. The pseudoephedrine method produces methamphetamine, an arguably more potent form than the racemic amphetamine produced using the P-2-P method. The pseudoephedrine technique was also much more efficient than other methods and required less material and expertise (Cho, 1990).

The shift from amphetamine sulphate to methamphetamine was rapid and complete. In 1998, we wanted to test a urinalysis technique developed in the UK that could distinguish dexamphetamine used in substitution therapy programmes from the racemic amphetamine used illicitly (Tetlow and Merrill, 1996). Such a technique could be used as an objective test of the effectiveness of dexamphetamine substitution in reducing hazardous illicit amphetamine use in dependent patients. All subjects recruited in that study tested positive to methamphetamine, which is not pharmaceutically available in Australia, and so the urinary isomer test was redundant for our purposes (Shearer et al., 2001). By 1999, nearly all illicit amphetamine seized in Australia were of the methamphetamine form (National Drug and Alcohol Research Centre, 2001). Drug supply control efforts refocused on regulating the availability of pseudoephedrine and the detection of the increasing number of smaller drug laboratories. Nevertheless, locally produced Australian methamphetamine was of low purity (5–15%) and presentations to treatment services recorded small but consistent year-on-year increases (Topp et al., 2002).

The importation of crystalline methamphetamine from Southeast Asia and North America, and latterly local illicit production, has added a new dynamic to the use of amphetamine in Australia and related harms. Crystalline methamphetamine (known locally as 'ice' or 'crystal') is highly pure (80% or more) and may be smoked as well as injected or ingested (McKetin et al., 2005a; Topp et al., 2002). Crystalline methamphetamine has been the subject of intense community, media and political interest in Australia, as it has been in North America. Emerging health, law enforcement and drug market data point to an increase in amphetamine-related harms, coinciding with the advent of crystalline methamphetamine (McKetin et al., 2006a). In particular, hospital and emergency department admissions for psychostimulant-induced psychosis have increased (Degenhardt et al., 2007). Crystalline methamphetamine use does appear to be associated with elevated levels of harm including dependence, and psychiatric sequelae including psychosis, compared to the less pure powder and base forms of the drug (McKetin et al., 2006a). While purity is one factor in the spread of crystalline methamphetamine, the fact that it can be smoked potentially introduces a wider range of otherwise irregular or recreational users of the drug. In inner city Sydney, we recently concluded recruitment into a trial of modafinil (200 mg/day) for amphetamine dependence. Every single subject recruited into the trial either injected or smoked crystalline methamphetamine (Shearer et al., 2007), illustrating again the adaptability of this market.

Prevalence of amphetamine use disorders

Lifetime-reported non-medical use of amphetamine in Australian adults has been estimated at 9.1% of the population or 1.5 million people (AIHW, 2005b), which places the prevalence of amphetamine use in the Australian population among the highest in the World (UNODC, 2006). Various Australian studies have found that the dependent amphetamine users are predominantly male, unemployed, young and likely to inject the drug (Baker et al., 2001; Hando et al., 1997; Vincent et al., 1998). There are an estimated 70 000 dependent methamphetamine users in Australia – a number greater than recent estimates of heroin users (McKetin et al., 2005b). Adverse consequences of regular amphetamine use include psychological morbidity (Dawe and McKetin, 2004), dependence (Topp and Darke, 1997), medical complications, blood-borne viral infections associated with unsafe sex and injecting (Hando and Hall, 1994, Vincent et al., 1999). Increased prevalence of amphetamine use in the Australian community has been accompanied by increased presentations for amphetamine-related problems to treatment services. National hospital admissions where amphetamines were the principal diagnosis have increased fourfold over the past decade to 2000 (Stafford et al., 2005), and stimulant-induced psychosis admissions increased sixfold to 1252 between 1998/1999 and 2000/2001 (McKetin et al., 2005a). The proportion of people presenting to drug and alcohol services with primary amphetamine problems in Australia increased between 1995 and 2005 from 6.5% (Shand and Mattick, 2001) to 11% (AIHW, 2006).

Treatment settings

Most treatment in Australia for amphetamine users is provided on an outpatient basis (65%) with inpatient services accounting for 24% of episodes and 4% occurring in outreach settings (AIHW, 2005a). In 2004–2005, there were 14 780 recorded drug treatment episodes for methamphetamine or amphetamine use in Australia through government and non-government organisations (NGOs) (AIHW, 2006). These treatment episodes consisted primarily of outpatient counselling (42%), information and assessment (16%), residential rehabilitation (15%) and withdrawal management (detoxification) (13%). People with psychostimulant problems present for treatment across a range of settings including hospital inpatient, emergency and outpatient departments, general medical practices, drug and alcohol specialist services, therapeutic communities, community health services, pharmacies and mental health/psychiatric care units. Unlike North America and Europe, psychiatrists have played a smaller role in the delivery and development of drug and alcohol treatment. General practitioners have for long had a role in the provision of pharmacotherapy for heroin addiction, and this has evolved into its own specialisation of addiction medicine with comparable specialisation for drug and alcohol nurses. Psychologists, counsellors, welfare and social workers have also played an important role, through establishing harm minimisation services such as Needle and Syringe Programs (NSPs) where Australia was a world leader and providing counselling and advisory services to the community. The setting of services has been an issue for amphetamine users, who in the past have perceived services as offering little amphetamine-specific help and more geared towards alcohol and opioid problems (Vincent et al., 1998; Wright et al., 1999). In turn, many health care professionals have limited training and little experience with psychostimulant disorders (Kamieniecki et al., 1998). Services with regular contact with psychostimulant users commonly manage acute presentations associated with psychosis (such as mental health services and hospital emergency departments) or provide harm reduction services such as methadone or NSPs. Psychostimulant dependence, arguably the underlying maladaptive pattern of drug use causing many of these problems, is often not specifically addressed.

Treatment presentations

Methamphetamine users present for treatment with either the acute effects of methamphetamine intoxication or the chronic effects of methamphetamine abuse or dependence. These may be two quite distinct treatment populations each with their own particular characteristics and treatment needs.

Emergency departments

The advent of crystalline methamphetamine has been accompanied by increased presentations to Australian hospital emergency departments. Patients typically present with acute features of amphetamine intoxication including agitation, aggression, delirium and stimulant-induced psychosis. A recent study in a large inner-city emergency department in Perth, Western Australia, found that amphetamine-related presentations accounted for 1.2% of attendances and represented a significant burden on the ED (Gray et al., 2007). These were high-acuity patients who were difficult to manage. Almost half were repeat attendees. Acute care systems are generally well equipped to deal with amphetamine-related emergencies (Dean and Whyte, 2004). There are a number of protocols and medications available although approaches are often not consistent or evidence based. Investigators in Adelaide, South Australia, attempted to examine the relative efficacy of either clonazepam (a benzodiazepine) or a combination of clonazepam and the atypical antipsychotic, olanzapine, for the treatment of amphetamine-induced psychosis. This trial was abandoned, however, after only three subjects could be recruited into the protocol (McIver et al., 2006). Apart from the usual difficulties of conducting clinical trials in ED settings (time pressures, the mental state of patients), it appeared that most potential patients were excluded due to prior diagnoses of schizophrenia or schizoaffective disorders. Given this experience, future trials should consider randomisation by treatment site and inclusion of subjects pre-existing psychiatric disorders including psychotic, anxiety and affective disorders. The very high rates of repeat presentations to EDs emphasise the need to engage patients in after-care drug treatment.

Detoxification and residential rehabilitation services

Detoxification and residential rehabilitation services represent around 28% of methamphetamine treatment episodes in Australia and the bulk of these are delivered by NGOs. NGOs are not-for-profit institutions that receive direct funding from governments but are run by charitable, religious and other welfare groups. These types of organisations have historically played a central role in the provision of welfare services, youth services, shelters for the homeless and drug rehabilitation services. These organisations recently attracted substantial additional funding as part of Australia's national response to the 'ice epidemic' (Stapleton, 2007). The specific effectiveness of these types of services for methamphetamine users is one focus of a current treatment cohort study (Mattick et al., 2007). Amphetamine withdrawal is not considered to be medically complicated (Jenner and Saunders, 2004), and many amphetamine-dependent persons have binge patterns of use with extended periods of abstinence due to physical exhaustion, or exhaustion of money or drugs. Thus, detoxification alone is not a treatment, although withdrawal programmes offer essential help for users in crisis and induct them into treatment. The Australian Treatment Outcome Study found residential rehabilitation was significantly more effective than either methadone or detoxification in reducing cocaine use in heroin-dependent individuals (Williamson et al., 2006). Taken with cohort studies conducted in the USA and UK, this may suggest a particular benefit for dual opioid–methamphetamine-dependent patients and those with welfare problems.

Counselling

Most treatment offered to methamphetamine users in Australia consists of supportive counselling. The specific efficacy of brief cognitive behavioural therapy (CBT) in the treatment of amphetamine dependence has been demonstrated in a multi-centre, randomised controlled trial (Baker et al., 2005). This evidence forms the basis of the recommendation of CBT as best practice in the treatment of methamphetamine dependence in Australia (Baker and Lee, 2003; Lee et al., 2007). In this pivotal study, 214 methamphetamine users were randomised to three conditions: a self-help booklet, two CBT sessions or four CBT sessions. The CBT sessions consisted of a motivational interview, two sessions introducing cognitive-behavioural techniques to help subjects cope with cravings and controlling thoughts about amphetamine, and a relapse prevention session. The most conservative data analysis approach, based on intention to treat, with missing data imputed as non-abstinent and a significance level set at $p < 0.01$, found that subjects in the intervention groups were significantly more likely to report abstinence at 6-month follow-up (33.8% two sessions, 37.9% four sessions) than those in the control condition (17.6%). Subjects in the intervention groups were three times more likely to report abstinence than control subjects after adjusting for duration of regular amphetamine use. The authors recommended a stepped-care approach varying in intensity between non-treatment and treatment settings, and response to treatment.

An important secondary finding was that the number of CBT sessions attended had a significant effect on levels of post-treatment depression. A subsequent trial of CBT for substance use in patients with psychotic disorders found a large effect size for reduced amphetamine use, although this was not statistically significant due the small number of amphetamine users in the sample (Baker et al., 2006). Common comorbid mental illnesses found in psychostimulant users include affective and mood disorders, such as depression and anxiety, and psychotic disorders such as schizophrenia and bipolar disorder (Baker and Dawe, 2005; Bartu et al., 2003; Dyer and Cruikshank, 2005; McKetin et al., 2006b). Clinical recommendations have been made to integrate psychosocial approaches to comorbid disorders (Dawe and McKetin, 2004) rather than treat them sequentially or separately. A stepped-care approach would also be relevant based on the severity of the co-occurring psychiatric problem (Baker and Dawe, 2005).

Evidence for the effectiveness of cognitive behavioural techniques, however, is not evidence for superiority over any other counselling and psychotherapeutic approaches. Indeed head-to-head comparisons of psychosocial approaches are probably inappropriate since they are *not necessarily mutually exclusive techniques* in the hands of skilled therapists. For this reason, the best experimental model remains that used by Baker and colleagues (2005), where the counselling approach was compared to a brief advice or self-help condition. Cognitive impairment is a feature of chronic amphetamine use and amphetamine withdrawal (Dyer and Cruikshank, 2005; Nordahl et al., 2003); accordingly CBT may have limited effectiveness for some amphetamine users.

One alternative is narrative therapy, which has won a following in many Australian drug and alcohol services including the Stimulant Treatment Program at Sydney's St Vincent's Hospital (Tarra Adam, Clinical Program Manager, personal communication). This approach is based on a shared examination of a person's life history and subsequent reconstruction or rewriting of their dependency story. Narrative therapy is derived from a post-modernist theoretical perspective, which seeks to empower the individual to escape from potentially negative social narratives (Campbell, 1997). Contingency management is another approach which includes community reinforcement and incentive-based programmes. These seek to reinforce a drug-free lifestyle through relationship counselling, vocational guidance, drug refusal skills, social skills and recreational opportunities, targeted vouchers and other rewards (Roll, 2007). In the USA, contingency management is recommended as the best treatment practice for psychostimulant problems (Rawson, 1999); however, it is not well understood in Australia where it is often misconceived as bribery or paying for good behaviour (Cameron and Ritter, 2007). Neither of these promising approaches has been adequately tested in Australian amphetamine users.

Overall, the effectiveness of existing treatment interventions is limited by poor rates of induction and retention (Shearer, 2007). In Australia, it has been estimated that only 10% of regular amphetamine users receive formal treatment in any given year, compared to over half of regular opiate users (Kelly et al., 2005). Data from the Australian national minimum dataset have shown that treatment for amphetamine use in Australia is significantly less successful than for other drugs. In cases where amphetamines were the principal drug of concern, fewer treatment episodes were closed due to completion of treatment and more amphetamine users ceased treatment without notice (AIHW, 2005a).

Pharmacological interventions

Safe and effective medication would be a valuable adjunct to most psychosocial programmes as an incentive to participation, and to facilitate retention through providing symptomatic relief in more severely dependent patients.

Dexamphetamine substitution, analogous to methadone maintenance for heroin users or nicotine replacement therapy for tobacco smokers, has been proposed for more severely dependent amphetamine users (Shearer et al., 2002). The earliest Australian observational report was a letter published by a general practitioner concerning the progress of 13 long-term intravenous amphetamine users in Melbourne who were prescribed 20–90 mg dexamphetamine supervised daily (Sherman, 1990). Half of these patients responded positively to the therapy reporting reduced craving, withdrawal symptoms and cessation of illicit amphetamine. The first prospective controlled trial of dexamphetamine (60 mg/day supervised doses) was conducted in Sydney (Shearer et al., 2001). Modest gains in favour of dexamphetamine treatment were observed and larger, more definitive trials were recommended. Interim data has been presented from a randomised placebo-controlled trial of sustained release dexamphetamine (20–110 mg daily supervised for 3 months) conducted in Adelaide (White et al., 2006). The interim analysis based on 30 subjects (20 received placebo, 10 received active) found trends towards superior retention and decreased methamphetamine use in the dexamphetamine group, but these were not significant due to the small sample size. Consistent with earlier observational reports, no adverse events were associated with dexamphetamine.

The very slow recruitment experienced in these trials suggests that dexamphetamine may only be effective in selected groups of highly dependent individuals. Such patients are likely to require higher sustained doses than offered in current programmes (usually up to 60 mg/day) and are also likely to have more severe personal and physical problems requiring careful supervision of doses and monitoring of progress. Apart from these reports, the prescription of dexamphetamine for amphetamine dependence is uncommon in Australia and closely regulated. Unsupervised doses as occur in the UK are not permitted in any state jurisdiction.

Modafinil is a novel non-amphetamine-type stimulant used in narcolepsy which has shown promise in the treatment of cocaine and amphetamine dependence in the USA (Comacho and Stein, 2002; Dackis et al., 2005; Malcolm et al., 2002). The precise pharmacological action of modafinil is unknown. It has specific glutamatergic and GABAergic activity that may account for its wakefulness and attention-enhancing effects. The reversal of glutamate depletion in the nucleus accumbens and prefrontal cortex may underpin its anti-craving effect. Modafinil is not water soluble and destroyed at high temperature, and thus cannot be injected or smoked. Together with its low direct affinity for dopamine receptors, modafinil appears to be safe with a low abuse liability (Jasinski and Kovacevic-Ristanovic, 2000). Modafinil 400 mg/day was examined in an open-label study in 14 amphetamine users undergoing a 10-day inpatient withdrawal programme (McGregor et al., 2004). The investigators from the University of Adelaide reported that modafinil was safe and well tolerated in amphetamine withdrawal and appeared to have no discernable reinforcing effects. Compared to open label studies of other compounds, modafinil appeared to be more effective in suppressing craving and withdrawal symptoms. Further studies in modafinil were recommended. We have completed recruitment in a randomised placebo-controlled trial of modafinil (200 mg/day for 10 weeks) in 87 methamphetamine-dependent subjects (Shearer et al., 2007) (see case studies in the following section).

Two case studies from a randomised placebo-controlled trial of modafinil

Case A

Pre-treatment history

Subject A was a 32-year-old single male, self-employed as a cleaner. He formerly dealt crystalline methamphetamine to other consumers but had recently abandoned that activity after being caught in an undercover police sting. He had no prison history or any other criminal record. He started smoking crystalline methamphetamine at the age of 26 and graduated to injection by age 27. Prior to joining the modafinil trial, he smoked around 2 'points' (0.2 g) of crystalline methamphetamine daily. He had reverted to smoking in an attempt to reduce his drug use. He had no other illicit drug use and was a non-smoker and non-drinker. He was under the care of a psychiatrist for an anxiety condition.

Treatment history

Subject A received 200 mg modafinil daily on waking under double-blind conditions. He was retained in treatment for the entire 10-week study period (70 days). He reported a positive response to modafinil including the almost complete abolition of methamphetamine craving (Figure 9.1). This subject did not attend any of the four CBT sessions as he was already attending a psychiatrist monthly for other mental issues and was apparently satisfied with effectiveness of modafinil.

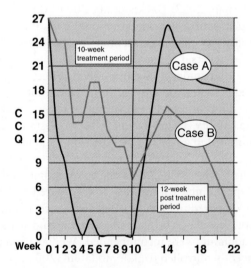

Figure 9.1 Craving questionnaire (CCQ) scores over study period. *Note:* Missing results imputed from last observation carried forward.

Post-treatment history

Subject A achieved an abstinence period of 65 days. He relapsed to baseline daily use patterns after accepting an offer of methamphetamine from a friend with whom he had a long history of shared drug use (see Table 1).

Case B

Pre-treatment history

Subject B was a university educated 36-year-old single male, self-employed as an IT consultant. He started smoking crystalline methamphetamine at age 28. Prior to joining the modafinil trial he had a relatively heavy habit, smoking in the order of 1 g/day. He also smoked cannabis and tobacco on a daily basis and used GHB most weekends. He had no other criminal or psychiatric history.

Treatment history

Subject B received 200 mg placebo daily on waking under double-blind conditions. He was retained in treatment for 26 days. He reported a positive response to the study medication although his craving and drug use did not decline as rapidly or completely as Case A. He attended two CBT sessions (a motivational interview and a coping with cravings and lapses session).

Post-treatment history

Subject B achieved an abstinence period of 119 days with one lapse. His craving for methamphetamine as measured by the CCQ (Weiss et al., 2003) continued to decline post-treatment (see Figure 9.1 and Table 9.1).

Comment

These cases are not strictly clinical case reports since both subjects believed they received active medication. While the modafinil-treated Case A had better outcomes in terms of methamphetamine craving and methamphetamine use during treatment, he rapidly deteriorated post-treatment, while placebo-treated Case B enjoyed

Table 9.1 Urinalysis results for methamphetamine use over study period.

Week	00	01	02	03	04	05	06	07	08	09	10	14	18	22
Case A	+	(+)	(+)	+	+	0	0	0	0	0	0	+	0	+
Case B	+	+	(+)	0	(+)	+	(+)	+	(+)	(+)	0	+	0	0

Notes: 0, methamphetamine negative samples; +, methamphetamine positive samples; (+), missing samples imputed as positive.

sustained reductions in these critical outcomes post-treatment. Case A preferred to rely on the medication effects to control his methamphetamine cravings and use and did not attend the CBT-based counselling offered as part of the study or make any other lifestyle changes. He was, arguably, less well prepared to deal with high-risk relapse situations post-treatment. Alternatively, a longer maintenance period of modafinil may have been beneficial. Case B not only attended CBT-based counselling but also made consequent lifestyle changes, including moving away from other methamphetamine using friends and taking a job that required more fixed working hours than his freelance consulting. Naturally, there were more complex psychosocial factors at play; however, these cases perhaps show that effective medications will almost always require effective psychosocial treatment.

Conclusion

Amphetamine, or more specifically methamphetamine, has been the subject of intense public interest in Australia in recent years. While some may view this as a moral panic or overreaction, health indicators do suggest a serious increase in amphetamine-related harms although from a low base. Crystalline methamphetamine is cheap, pure and plentiful in most Australian towns and cities. If the maxim that drug markets are driven by price, purity and availability holds, then Australia will require comprehensive, diverse and sophisticated programmes to minimise methamphetamine-related problems over the coming years. Australia has a strong drug and alcohol treatment and research infrastructure tempered by the heroin epidemic of the 1990s. Continued investment in this infrastructure will be required to deal with current and future methamphetamine presentations. The direct involvement of the brain's reward system adds a powerful, complex and enduring element to methamphetamine dependence. For this reason, psychosocial interventions play an especially important role in the effective long-term treatment of methamphetamine-related problems. New medications and rehabilitation also play an important part in bringing dependent users into treatment. Psychosocial interventions need to be more formally integrated into medication and rehabilitation regimens for methamphetamine dependence to achieve optimal results.

References

AIHW (2005a) Alcohol and other drug treatment services in Australia 2003–2004. Report on the National Minimum Data Set. Drug Treatment Series 4. AIHW Cat. No. HSE 100. Canberra: Australian Institute of Health and Welfare.

AIHW (2005b) National Drug Strategy Household Survey: Detailed Findings. AIHW Cat. No. PHE 66. Canberra: Australian Institute of Health and Welfare.

AIHW (2006) Alcohol and other drug treatment services in Australia 2004–05. Report on the National Minimum Data Set. Drug Treatment Series 5. Catalogue No. HSE 43. Canberra: Australian Institute of Health and Welfare.

Baker, A., Boggs, T. and Lewin, T. (2001) Characteristics of regular amphetamine users and implications for treatment. *Drug and Alcohol Review* 20: 49–56.

Baker, A., Bucci, S., Lewin, T., Kay-Lambkin, F., Constable, P. and Carr, V. (2006) Cognitive-behavioural therapy for substance use disorders in people with psychotic disorders: Randomised controlled trial. *British Journal of Psychiatry* 188: 439–448.

Baker, A. and Dawe, S. (2005) Amphetamine use and co-occurring psychological problems: Review of the literature and implications for treatment. *Australian Psychologist* 40: 88–95.

Baker, A. and Lee, N. (2003) A review of psychosocial interventions for amphetamine use. *Drug and Alcohol Review* 22: 323–335.

Baker, A., Lee, N., Claire, M., Lewin, T., Grant, T., Pohlman, S., Saunders, J., Kay-Lambkin, F., Constable, P., Jenner, L. and Carr, V. (2005) Brief cognitive behavioural interventions for regular amphetamine users: a step in the right direction. *Addiction* 100: 367–378.

Bartu, A., Freeman, N., Gawthorne, G., Codde, J. and Holman, C. (2003) Psychiatric comorbidity in a cohort of heroin and amphetamine users in Perth, Western Australia. *Journal of Substance Use* 8: 150–154.

Caldicott, D., Pigou, P., Beattie, R. and Edwards, J. (2005) Clandestine drug laboratories in Australia and the potential for harm. *Australian and New Zealand Journal of Public Health* 29: 155–162.

Cameron, J. and Ritter, A. (2007) Contingency management: perspectives of Australian service providers. *Drug and Alcohol Review* 26: 183–189.

Campbell, A. (1997) *Narrative Therapy in the Drug and Alcohol Field: An introduction. VAADA Vine* Melbourne: Victorian Alcohol and Drug Association.

Cho, A. (1990) Ice: a new dosage form of an old drug. *Science* 24: 631–634.

Comacho, A. and Stein, M. (2002) Modafinil for social phobia and amphetamine dependence (letter). *American Journal of Psychiatry* 159: 1947–1948.

Dackis, C., Kampman, K., Lynch, K., Pettinati, H. and O'Brien, C. (2005) A double-blind, placebo-controlled trial of modafinil for cocaine dependence. *Neuropsychopharmacology* 30: 205–211.

Dawe, S. and McKetin, R. (2004) The psychiatric comorbidity of psychostimulant use. In: Baker, A., Lee, N. and Jenner, L. (eds), *Models of Intervention and Care for Psychostimulant Users.* Canberra: Australian Government Department of Health and Ageing, pp. 154–168.

Dean, A. and Whyte, I. (2004) Management of acute psychostimulant toxicity, Chapter 6. In: Baker, A., Lee, N. and Jenner, L. (eds), *Models of Intervention and Care for Psychostimulant Users.* Canberra: Australian Government Department of Health and Ageing, pp. 85–101.

Degenhardt, L., Roxburgh, A. and McKetin, R. (2007) Hospital separations for cannabis- and methamphetamine-related psychotic episodes in Australia. *Medical Journal of Australia* 186: 342–345.

Dyer, K. and Cruikshank, C. (2005) Depression and other psychological health problems among methamphetamine dependent patients in treatment: implications for assessment and treatment outcome. *Australian Psychologist* 40: 96–108.

Gray, S., Fatovich, D., McCoubrie, D. and Daly, F. (2007) Amphetamine-related presentations to an inner-city tertiary emergency department: a prospective evaluation. *Medical Journal of Australia* 186: 336–339.

Hando, J. and Hall, W. (1994) HIV risk-taking behaviour among amphetamine users in Sydney, Australia. *Addiction* 89: 79–85.

Hando, J. and Hall, W. (1997) Patterns of amphetamine use in Australia. In: Klee, H. (ed.), *Amphetamine Misuse: International Perspectives on Current Trends*. Amsterdam: Harwood Academic Publishers.

Hando, J., Topp, L. and Hall, W. (1997) Amphetamine-related harms and treatment preferences of regular amphetamine users in Sydney, Australia. *Drug and Alcohol Dependence* 46: 105–113.

Jasinski, D. and Kovacevic-Ristanovic, R. (2000) Evaluation of the abuse liability of modafinil and other drugs for excessive daytime sleepiness associated with narcolepsy. *Clinical Neuropharmacology* 23: 149–156.

Jenner, L. and Saunders, J. (2004) Psychostimulant withdrawal and detoxification. In: Baker, A., Lee, N. and Jenner, L. (eds), *Models of Intervention and Care for Psychostimulant Users*, 2nd edn. Canberra: Australian Government Department of Health and Ageing, pp. 13–34.

Kamieniecki, G., Vincent, N., Allsop, S. and Lintzeris, N. (1998) *Models of Intervention and Care for Psychostimulant Users*. National Drug Strategy. Canberra: Commonwealth of Australia.

Kelly, E., McKetin, R. and McLaren, J. (2005) *Health Service Utilisation Among Regular Methamphetamine Users*. Sydney: National Drug and Alcohol Research Centre.

Lee, N., Johns, L., Jenkinson, R., Johnston, J., Connolly, K., Hall, K. and Cash, R. (2007) *Methamphetamine Dependence and Treatment. Clinical Treatment Guidelines for Alcohol and Drug Clinicians No.14*. Melbourne: Turning Point Alcohol and Drug Centre Inc.

Malcolm, R., Brook, S., Moak, D., Devane, L. and Czepowicz, V. (2002) Clinical applications of modafinil in stimulant abusers: low abuse potential. *The American Journal on Addictions* 11: 247–249.

Mattick, R., McKetin, R., Ross, J. and Kelly, E. (2007) *Methamphetamine Treatment Cohort Study*. Sydney: National Drug and Alcohol Research Centre.

McGregor, C., White, J., Srisurapanont, M., Mitchell, A. and Wickes, W. (2004) *Investigation of Potential Pharmacotherapies for Acute Amphetamine Withdrawal: Open-Label Pilot Studies of Mirtazapine and Modafinil*. Fremantle, Australia: Australian Professional Society on Alcohol and Other Drugs (APSAD).

McIver, C., Flynn, J., Baigent, M., Vial, R., Newcombe, D., White, J. and Ali, R. (2006) *Management of Methamphetamine Psychosis*. DASSA Research Monograph No.21. Adelaide: Drug and Alcohol Services South Australia.

McKetin, R., Kelly, E. and McLaren, J. (2006a) The relationship between crystalline methamphetamine use and methamphetamine dependence. *Drug and Alcohol Dependence* 85: 198–204.

McKetin, R., McLaren, J. and Kelly, E. (2005a) *The Sydney Methamphetamine Market: Patterns of Supply, Use, Personal Harms and Social Consequences*. NDLERF Monograph Series No.13. Adelaide: National Drug Law Enforcement Research Fund.

McKetin, R., McLaren, J., Kelly, E., Hall, W. and Hickman, M. (2005b) *Estimating the Number of Regular and Dependent Methamphetamine Users in Australia*. Technical Report No. 230. Sydney: National Drug and Alcohol Research Centre.

McKetin, R., McLaren, J., Lubman, D. and Hides, L. (2006b) The prevalence of psychotic symptoms among methamphetamine users. *Addiction* 101: 1473–1478.

National Drug and Alcohol Research Centre (2001) *Drug Trends Bulletin. Illicit Drug Reporting System*. Sydney: National Drug and Alcohol Research Centre.

Nordhal, T., Salo, R. and Leamon, M. (2003) Neuropsychological effects of chronic methamphetamine use on neurotransmitters and cognition: a review. *The Journal of Neuropsychiatry and Clinical Neurosciences* 15: 137–325.

Rawson, R. (1999) *Treatment for Stimulant Use Disorders. Treatment Improvement Protocol (TIP) Series*. Rockville, MD: Center for Substance Abuse Treatment.

Rawson, R., Anglin, M. D. and Ling, W. (2002) Will the methamphetamine problem go away? *Journal of Addictive Diseases* 21: 5–19.

Roll, J. (2007) Contingency management: an evidence-based component of methamphetamine use disorder treatments. *Addiction* 102: 114–120.

Shand, F. and Mattick, R. (2001) *Clients of Treatment Service Agencies: May 2001 Census Findings*. Canberra: AGPS.

Shearer, J. (2007) Psychosocial approaches to psychostimulant dependence: a systematic review. *Journal of Substance Abuse Treatment* 32: 41–52.

Shearer, J., Rodgers, C., Brady, D., Van Beek, I., Lewis, J., McKetin, R., Mattick, R., Darke, S. and Wodak, A. (2007) *Randomised Placebo Controlled Trial of Modafinil (200 mg/day) in Methamphetamine Dependence*. Sydney: National Drug and Alcohol Research Centre.

Shearer, J., Sherman, J., Wodak, A. and Van Beek, I. (2002) Substitution therapy for amphetamine users. *Drug and Alcohol Review* 21: 179–185.

Shearer, J., Wodak, A., Mattick, R., Van Beek, I., Lewis, J., Hall, W. and Dolan, K. (2001) Pilot randomised controlled study of dexamphetamine for amphetamine dependence. *Addiction* 96: 1289–1296.

Sherman, J. (1990) Dexamphetamine for 'speed' addiction. *Medical Journal of Australia* 153: 306.

Stafford, J., Degenhardt, L., Black, E., Bruno, R., Buckingham, K., Fetherston, J., Jenkinson, R., Kinner, S., Moon, C. and Weekley, J. (2005) *Australian Drug Trends 2004: Findings from the Illicit Drug Reporting System (IDRS)*. Monograph Series No.55. Sydney: National Drug and Alcohol Research Centre.

Stapleton, J. (2007) PM praised for $150m ice rehabilitation focus. *The Australian*, 23 April 2007.

Tetlow, V. and Merrill, J. (1996) Rapid determination of amphetamine steroisomer ratios in urine by gas chromatography-mass spectroscopy. *Annals of Clinical Biochemistry* 33: 50–54.

Topp, L. and Darke, S. (1997) The applicability of the dependence syndrome to amphetamine. *Drug and Alcohol Dependence* 48: 113–118.

Topp, L., Degenhardt, L., Kaye, S. and Darke, S. (2002) The emergence of potent forms of methamphetamine in Sydney, Australia. *Drug and Alcohol Review* 21: 341–348.

UNODC (2006) *World Drug Report 2006*. Vienna: United Nations Office on Drugs and Crime.

Vincent, N., Shoobridge, J., Ask, A., Allsop, S. and Ali, R. (1998) Physical and mental health problems in amphetamine users from metropolitan Adelaide. *Drug and Alcohol Review* 17: 187–195.

Vincent, N., Shoobridge, J., Ask, A., Allsop, S. and Ali, R. (1999) Characteristics of amphetamine users seeking information, help and treatment in Adelaide, South Australia. *Drug and Alcohol Review* 18: 63–73.

Weiss, R., Griffin, M., Mazurick, C., Berkman, B., Gastfriend, D., Frank, A., Barber, J., Blaine, J., Salloum, I. and Moras, K. (2003) The relationship between cocaine craving, psychosocial treatment, and subsequent cocaine use. *American Journal of Psychiatry* 160, 1320–1325.

White, J., Wickes, W. and Longo, M. (2006) *Randomised Controlled Trial of D-Amphetamine Maintenance for Treatment of Methamphetamine Dependence*. Cairns, Queensland: Australasian Professional Society in Alcohol and Other Drugs (APSAD).

Williamson, A., Darke, S., Ross, J. and Teeson, M. (2006) The association between cocaine use and short-term outcomes for the treatment of heroin dependence: findings from the Australian Treatment Outcome Study (ATOS). *Drug and Alcohol Review* 25: 141–148.

Wright, S., Klee, H. and Reid, P. (1999) Attitudes of amphetamine users towards treatment services. *Drugs: Education, Prevention and Policy* 6: 71–86.

Chapter 10

THE 'P' PROBLEM IN NEW ZEALAND

Chris Wilkins and Janie Sheridan

Introduction

Methamphetamine in New Zealand, commonly known as 'P' or 'pure', emerged in the late 1990s, creating the country's first new serious drug problem since the short-lived popularity of heroin in the mid-1970s. A United Nations report published in 2003 on the global trends in ecstasy and amphetamines ranked New Zealand as having the third highest population prevalence of methamphetamine in the world after Thailand and Australia (United Nations Office on Drugs and Crime, 2003). The use of methamphetamine has been linked to a range of social problems in New Zealand including drug addiction, mental illness, violent crime, domestic violence and property crime (Expert Advisory Committee on Drugs, 2002; Wilkins et al., 2004a).

As is often the case with so-called new drug trends, the use of methamphetamine was occurring within a small subculture in New Zealand for many decades preceding its more widespread popular emergence in the late 1990s. A small number of local outlaw motorcycle gangs (OMG) with international affiliations to gangs in other countries are believed to have used and manufactured methamphetamine on a small scale in New Zealand since the 1980s (Australian Bureau of Criminal Intelligence, 2002; Newbold, 2000; New Zealand Police, 2002). Methamphetamine use began to spread beyond the OMG subculture in the mid-1990s in New Zealand when the use of the drug became popular within the dance party culture (Horne, 1997; New Zealand Police, 2002; Schmidt, 2001; Zander, 2002). By 2001 amphetamines were New Zealand's second most popular illegal drug after cannabis (Wilkins et al., 2002b). This chapter traces the rise of P in New Zealand and the subsequent response by a range of agencies to its emergence. The final section of the chapter attempts to set out some policy lessons learned from the recent history of methamphetamine in New Zealand.

The terminology used to describe amphetamine-type drugs varies internationally, so for clarity in this chapter, the term 'amphetamine' will be used to denote any amphetamine such as amphetamine sulphate and methamphetamine.

Drug use in New Zealand before methamphetamine

The impact of methamphetamine use in New Zealand can only be fully appreciated if one understands the nature of the 'drug problem' in New Zealand before its emergence. The regular international supply of heroin to New Zealand had been effectively ended in the late 1970s by the arrest of the 'Mr Asia' drug ring, which had been smuggling heroin into the country since the early 1970s (Newbold, 2000; New Zealand Customs Service, 2002). The remaining opiate users responded by drawing on three local sources of opiates: morphine sulphate tablets (MST), codeine-based tablets which are made into a heroin/morphine mix known as 'homebake' and opium extracted from opium poppies (Adamson and Sellman, 1998).

The first household survey of drug use was conducted in New Zealand in 1990, which surveyed people aged 15–45 years in a major metropolitan and provincial region (Black and Casswell, 1993). This regional drug survey indicated that cannabis was by far New Zealand's most commonly used illegal drug, with 18% of the subjects having used cannabis at least once in the past year. The use of illegal drug types other than cannabis was much less common with only 2% reporting use of LSD (lysergic acid diethylamide), 2% having used hallucinogenic mushrooms, 1% having used a stimulant, 0.4% having used cocaine and 0.7% having used any opiate in the past year (Black and Casswell, 1993). The term 'stimulant' was used in the survey to refer to a broad range of amphetamines, which the interviewer described to the respondent as 'uppers, speed, amphetamine or methamphetamine'.

The availability of cannabis had become easier in New Zealand during the 1980s through the rise in large-scale clandestine cultivation of cannabis in several of the country's economically depressed rural regions (Australian Bureau of Criminal Intelligence, 2002; Newbold, 2000; Yska, 1990). The emergence of a domestic supply of high-potency cannabis replaced the previous international smuggling of cannabis from Thailand (Newbold, 2000; Yska, 1990).

The use of cocaine and 'crack' cocaine never became established in New Zealand (Australian Bureau of Criminal Intelligence, 2002; Black and Casswell, 1993; Field and Casswell, 1999b; New Zealand Customs Service, 2002). The low levels of heroin and cocaine in New Zealand are commonly explained through reference to New Zealand's geographical isolation, small population and effective border controls (New Zealand Customs Service, 2002).

Illegal drug use in New Zealand in the early 1990s was, therefore, dominated by the use of cannabis, with small-scale use of hallucinogens, low-potency stimulants, and opiates diverted from the medical system. While cannabis was considered a serious problem in New Zealand, in particular because of the link with ethnic gangs involved it its large-scale commercial cultivation and sale, there was very little experience of what the rest of world commonly described as a 'serious drug problem' (Australian Bureau of Criminal Intelligence, 2002; Newbold, 2000; Wilkins and Casswell, 2003). This situation began to change sometime in the mid-1990s.

The rise of methamphetamine

Tracking the rise in the use of methamphetamine in New Zealand during the 1990s is made difficult by the absence of any population drug survey during most of this decade. As described in the previous section, a regional household survey of drug use had been completed in New Zealand in 1990. Funding to complete a follow-up regional survey, and the first national survey, was not secured until 1998. Comparison of the regional findings of the 1990 and 1998 surveys suggested there had been some increase in amphetamine use in New Zealand during the 8-year gap in surveying (Field and Casswell, 1999a). Past-year prevalence of use of a stimulant had increased from 1% in 1990 to 4% in 1998 in the two regions surveyed (Field and Casswell, 1999a).

The increase in stimulant use detected in the 1990 and 1998 regional household drug survey comparison does not appear to have attracted much popular attention, or to have been linked to an increase in any 'new' type of amphetamine. There are a number of reasons why this may have been the case. Firstly, as discussed earlier, the broad category used in the household surveys to measure amphetamine use (i.e. stimulants) did not allow for the identification of any specific type of amphetamine. The increase in the general 'stimulant' category provided no indication that the traditional amphetamine sulphate (i.e. 'speed') was being supplanted by a more powerful stimulant, methamphetamine. Refining or expanding the stimulant category in future waves of the household drug survey was problematic for methodological reasons, as any change to the questionnaire could affect respondents' answers in unknown ways and hence impact on the validity of comparisons with previous survey waves. Secondly, the 1990 and 1998 regional household drug survey comparison also found large increases in the use of a range of other drug types, including LSD (2% in 1990 to 5% in 1998), hallucinogenic mushrooms (2% in 1990 to 3% in 1998) and ecstasy (MDMA) (0.4% in 1990 to 2% in 1998) (Field and Casswell, 1999a). LSD had been a popular drug in New Zealand for a number of decades, and hence any increase in its use was likely to be considered important. Ecstasy was a new drug at this time with a worldwide reputation, and hence any increase in its use was likely to attract more attention than it otherwise might have (see Australian Bureau of Criminal Intelligence, 2002; New Zealand Customs Service, 2002). Thirdly, a specialised knowledge of illegal drug use was required to link the increase in stimulant use in the New Zealand household surveys to the growing use of methamphetamine in neighbouring countries, and this research capacity had yet to be developed in New Zealand.

The rising use of methamphetamine in New Zealand during the 1990s was, however, clearly identified by New Zealand Police. A New Zealand Police report written in 1997 states that the police had noted a rising use of amphetamines, in particular methamphetamine and ecstasy 'since the early 1990s' (Horne, 1997, p. 9). The police report briefly summarised a number of major enforcement operations conducted against local OMG from the mid-to-late 1990s, during which substantial quantities of methamphetamine were seized and clandestine laboratories manufacturing methamphetamine discovered (Horne, 1997).

A subsequent New Zealand Police report, written in 2002, explains that the police had observed a steady increase in the availability of amphetamines in New Zealand during the late 1990s (New Zealand Police, 2002). The increasing availability of amphetamines was reflected in a rise in seizures of amphetamines in New Zealand during the late 1990s and early 2000s (see Figure 10.1) (Ministerial Action

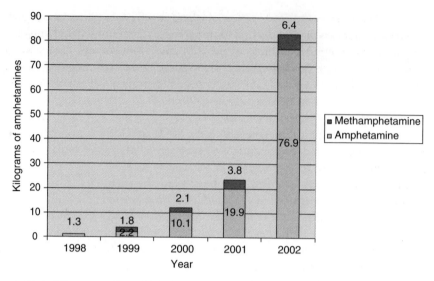

Figure 10.1 Kilograms of amphetamine/methamphetamine seized in New Zealand, 1998–2002. *Source*: Ministerial Action Group on Drugs, 2003.

Group on Drugs, 2003; New Zealand Police, 2002). It was noted in the 2002 police report that an increasing proportion of amphetamine seizures involved methamphetamine and that most of this methamphetamine was seized inside New Zealand rather than at the international border, suggesting a growing level of domestic methamphetamine manufacture (New Zealand Police, 2002). This understanding is supported by the rising number of methamphetamine laboratories detected during this time (Figure 10.2) (Ministerial Action Group on Drugs, 2003). There were also increasing numbers of arrests for both the use and supply of amphetamine-type stimulants (ATS) over this period.

Some of the police data systems used at this time did not clearly distinguish between methamphetamine and other amphetamines (Ministerial Action Group on Drugs, 2003). The ATS drug data category used by New Zealand Police at the time included all the amphetamine drugs, plus ecstasy. As the legal penalties for all amphetamines were the same at this time, there was little institutional incentive to conduct expensive scientific tests on amphetamine seizures to determine whether a seizure was methamphetamine or the traditional amphetamine sulphate (known as 'speed'). In addition, the purity of amphetamine seizures is not central to drug prosecutions, and consequently tests of the potency of amphetamines are generally only conducted for large seizures in New Zealand (see Nice, 2007).

The increase in the domestic manufacture of methamphetamine created the problem of safely dismantling methamphetamine laboratories and paying for the cleanup of buildings used for the manufacture of the drug. Methamphetamine manufacture involves the use of volatile chemicals which can cause explosions when heated incorrectly (Horne, 1997; New Zealand Police, 2002). The chemicals used in methamphetamine manufacture can also leach into the immediate environment

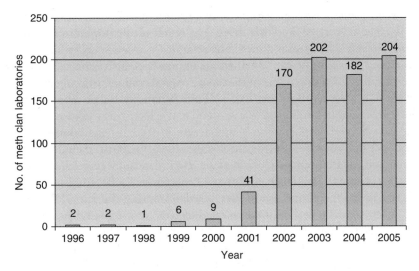

Figure 10.2 Number of clandestine methamphetamine laboratories detected in New Zealand, 1996–2005. *Source*: National Drug Intelligence Bureau, 2008.

and surrounding buildings and fixtures if not stored safely (Horne, 1997; New Zealand Police, 2002). Consequently, buildings used for the clandestine manufacture of methamphetamine, such as rental accommodation and hotel rooms, often required decontamination to make them safe for further occupation (Horne, 1997; New Zealand Police, 2002).

The 2002 New Zealand Police report discusses three factors which contributed to the rise in methamphetamine in New Zealand during the late 1990s and early 2000s (New Zealand Police, 2002). Firstly, the use of methamphetamine crossed a social divide between a largely working class criminal subculture to mainstream youth culture, as use moved from the traditional OMG subculture to people involved in the growing dance party culture. Dance party goers were using methamphetamine to sustain long periods of dancing and partying (see Klee, 1997). The high price and irregular supply of imported ecstasy (MDMA) in New Zealand may have contributed to the enthusiasm for locally made methamphetamine among the dance party fraternity (see Schmidt, 2001; Wilkins et al., 2003; Zander, 2002). Secondly, an international drug trafficking group based in Eastern Europe had begun smuggling large quantities of methamphetamine into New Zealand from Poland. Thirdly, local New Zealand OMG switched from the occasional international smuggling of methamphetamine to the large-scale domestic manufacture of methamphetamine. The 2002 New Zealand Police report claims that local OMG were instrumental in establishing the domestic manufacture of methamphetamine in New Zealand, and were thereby responsible for increasing the availability of methamphetamine which eventually came to dominate the local New Zealand amphetamine market by the early 2000s (New Zealand Police, 2002; Schmidt, 2001).

Another factor often mentioned as contributing to the popularity of methamphetamine in New Zealand is the fact that methamphetamine can be smoked rather than injected (United Nations Drug Control Programme, 2001). New Zealand had an established culture of smoking drugs as a result of the popularity of cannabis. This may have made smoking methamphetamine a more socially acceptable behaviour than injecting heroin. Methamphetamine was also reported to be much more cost-effective than cocaine in the New Zealand context, offering effects which lasted for 4–6 hours rather than half an hour (Schmidt, 2001). The international supply of methamphetamine to New Zealand is also likely to have been enhanced by the increase in methamphetamine manufacture in several neighbouring Southeast Asia and oceanic countries during the 1990s and early 2000s, including Australia, Thailand and the Philippines (Farrell et al., 2002; Matsumoto et al., 2002; Sattah et al., 2002; United Nations Drug Control Programme, 2001, 2002).

The rise in amphetamine use in New Zealand during the late 1990s was confirmed when funding was secured to conduct a second national household drug survey in 2001. Comparison of the findings from the 1998 and 2001 national household drug surveys found that past-year use of stimulants had increased from 3% in 1998 to 5% in 2001 (Wilkins et al., 2002b, 2002c). This result was particularly noteworthy as there had been no change in the population prevalence of either cannabis or LSD use (Wilkins et al., 2002b, 2002c). Analysis of the demographic characteristics of stimulant users from the 2001 national household survey found that users came from a broad range of ethnic and socio-economic backgrounds including professional and managerial occupations (Wilkins et al., 2005b). These findings supported the observation that methamphetamine use had expanded into mainstream New Zealand society. The 2001 national household drug survey also confirmed the growing availability of stimulants in New Zealand. In the 2001 survey, 47% of those who had used a stimulant in the past year reported that stimulants were 'easier' to obtain as compared to a year ago, while only 13% said they were 'harder' to obtain as compared to a year ago (Wilkins et al., 2005b).

By 2001 the New Zealand media had become aware of the rise in use of the 'new' amphetamine, referred to on the streets as P. A steady stream of articles on methamphetamine appeared in the popular press from this time onwards (see Little, 2003; Matthews, 2001; Philp, 2002; Schmidt, 2001; Zander, 2002). The initial media attention focused on the connection between amphetamines and the dance party culture in New Zealand, and on the role OMG were playing in the manufacture and trafficking of amphetamines (see Matthews, 2001; Philp, 2002; Schmidt, 2001). New Zealand Police recounted stories of OMG involvement in recent methamphetamine manufacture and trafficking and the money earned by OMG from the burgeoning methamphetamine trade (Cumming, 2002; Philp, 2002; Zander, 2002). These early media stories described the difference between methamphetamine or P and older forms of amphetamine sulphate or 'speed' which had traditionally been used in New Zealand (see Philp, 2002; Zander, 2002). Whereas methamphetamine was generally smoked in a glass pipe and sold by the 'point' (i.e. 0.1 gram) for around NZ\$100–NZ\$120 per point, the traditional amphetamine sulphate was a 'cut' powder which was snorted and sold by the gram at a cost of NZ\$120–NZ\$150 per gram (Philp, 2002; Zander, 2002).

An early research study of the impact of ATS in New Zealand completed in 2004 included the first interviews of methamphetamine users conducted in New Zealand (Wilkins et al., 2004a). A sample of frequent methamphetamine users was recruited from New Zealand's largest city (Auckland) using purposive sampling and snow-balling. The interviews confirmed that in New Zealand methamphetamine was generally smoked and consumed by the point (0.1 gram). It also documented a range of physical and psychological problems experienced by users of methamphetamine including 'teeth problems', 'trouble sleeping', 'racing heart', 'skin problems', 'anxiety', 'depression', 'mood swings', 'paranoia' and 'short temper'.

A demand side estimate of the dollar value of the amphetamine market, calculated using prevalence, quantity and price data from the 2001 national household drug survey, demonstrated the economic scale of the amphetamine trade in New Zealand (Wilkins et al., 2004a). The annual dollar value of the amphetamine market in New Zealand in 2001 was estimated to be NZ$123 million, which approached the size of the cannabis market in New Zealand, previously estimated to be worth NZ$168 million per year in 1998 using the same method (Wilkins et al., 2002a). Theses market estimates were re-calculated using data from the 2003 national household drug survey and compared to the 2001 market estimates (Wilkins and Sweetsur, 2005). While the total dollar value of the amphetamine market was approximately the same in 2003 as compared to 2001 (i.e. NZ$97 million in 2003 compared to NZ$123 million in 2001), the total quantity of amphetamine consumed fell considerably (i.e. 166 000 g in 2003 compared to 429 000 g in 2001), while the mean price of a gram of amphetamine was higher (i.e. NZ$687 in 2003 compared to NZ$245 per gram in 2001). These changes in the composition of the amphetamine market reflect the fact that increasingly the amphetamine sold in New Zealand was methamphetamine (i.e. purchased in 0.1 g 'points' for NZ$100) rather than the previous amphetamine sulphate (i.e. purchased by the gram for NZ$120–NZ$150).

The focus of media coverage of methamphetamine in New Zealand changed in 2002 as the use of methamphetamine was linked to a number of high-profile violent homicides. Methamphetamine was identified as a factor in both a triple homicide and a double homicide committed in 2002 (Gower, 2002). Both of these multiple killings were notable for their callous nature and because the perpetrators had recent histories of methamphetamine use. In January 2003, the use of methamphetamine was implicated in a bizarre samurai sword attack which left two women with their hands severed and another man murdered, and lead to a home invasion and hostage stand-off with police (Wall and Horwood, 2003). The perpetrator was reported to be under the influence of methamphetamine and was involved in methamphetamine manufacture and dealing (Wall and Horwood, 2003). Finally, in December 2003, methamphetamine use was implicated in the fatal beating of a 6-year-old child (Gardiner, 2003). The perpetrator, who was reported to have been recovering from a five-night-long binge on methamphetamine, beat his stepdaughter to death after she refused to go to school (Gardiner, 2003). These brutal crimes were widely reported as linked to methamphetamine and shocked the New Zealand public. Subsequent media coverage of methamphetamine paid greater attention to the mental health effects of methamphetamine on users and the implications of its use by criminals for violent crime (MacLeod, 2003; Zander, 2002). While the true causal role of methamphetamine in these violent crimes is difficult to determine, the resulting media coverage appeared to shift the public's perception of methamphetamine from a recreational dance party drug to a drug associated with violent crime and mental health problems (Wilkins et al., 2006). These crimes also made methamphetamine a political issue in New Zealand.

Recent trends in methamphetamine use

In 2003, a third national household drug survey was completed in New Zealand (Centre for Social and Health Outcomes Research and Evaluation (SHORE), 2004). Comparison of the level of stimulant use in the 2003 survey with the previous 2001 national household drug survey indicated there had been a levelling out in levels of stimulant use and availability (Wilkins et al., 2006). There was no statistically significantly change in the past-year prevalence of stimulant use in 2003 compared to 2001 (4 vs. 5%). The proportion of past-year stimulant users who said that the availability of stimulants had become 'harder' compared to 12 months ago was higher in 2003 compared to 2001 (25 vs. 12%). The authors of this research argued that the stabilisation of stimulant use and declining levels of availability of stimulants in New Zealand by 2003 reflected a wider public awareness of the mental health risks associated with methamphetamine use, and an increase in law enforcement and legislative focus on methamphetamine use after 2001 (Wilkins et al., 2006).

A fourth wave of national population surveying of drug use in New Zealand conducted in 2006 provided further evidence that amphetamine use had levelled out (Wilkins and Sweetsur, 2008). There was no statistically significant change in the past-year use of stimulants in 2006 compared to 2003 (3 vs. 4%). The levelling out of amphetamine use in New Zealand in the mid-2000s can be viewed as part of the natural lifespan of the methamphetamine trend. Growing awareness of the health risks of methamphetamine and increasing law enforcement focus and legal penalties imposed for methamphetamine offending are likely to have deterred occasional and experimental drug users from using methamphetamine, and have increasingly left a residual user population of heavy and dependent users (see Kleiman, 1992, pp. 287–290). As was found with cocaine in the late 1980s, the levelling out and decline in the general population use of a drug can paradoxically lead to growing social costs related to its use as dependent users can no longer support their drug use through selling drugs to occasional users (Caulkins, 2007; Kleiman, 1992, pp. 287–290). When the illegal market for a drug is contracting, dependent drug users are increasingly forced to commit more intrusive crimes such as burglary and robbery to finance their drug use (Kleiman, 1992, pp. 287–290). Consequently, while methamphetamine use in the general population may be considered to have stabilised in New Zealand, levels of use remains high by international standards and the social costs related to its use may not have changed, or may even have escalated, when compared to the peak in its is use among the general population in 2001.

In 2005, the Illicit Drug Monitoring System (IDMS) was funded by the New Zealand Government to provide annual 'snapshots' of drug trends and drug-related harm in New Zealand to inform timely responses by government and non-government agencies to drug problems (Ministerial Action Group on Drugs, 2003; Wilkins and Rose, 2003). The IDMS had a more modest budget than the national household drug surveys which allowed it to be completed on a more frequent basis than the household surveys. The IDMS interviewed three groups of frequent drug user (i.e. methamphetamine, ecstasy and injecting drug users), as well as interviews with key experts working in the drugs area, and collated secondary data sources on drug use from a range of sources. It collected both qualitative and quantitative data, which allowed emerging trends in drug use to be put in a wider context.

Findings from the first wave of the IDMS confirmed that methamphetamine was now well established in the illegal drugs market in New Zealand (Wilkins et al., 2005a). Among the frequent drug users interviewed for the 2005 IDMS, 51% described the current availability of methamphetamine in New Zealand as 'very easy', with a further 38% describing the current availability as 'easy'. When the frequent drug users were asked how the availability of methamphetamine had changed in the past 6 months, 29% said it had become 'easier', 51% said it was 'stable' and 12% said it was 'more difficult'. More recent waves of the IDMS have indicated declining availability of methamphetamine in New Zealand. A higher proportion of frequent drug users in the IDMS reported the availability of methamphetamine had become 'more difficult' in the past six months in 2008 compared to 2007 (Figure 10.3).

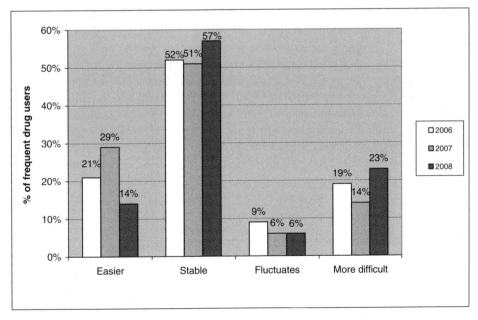

Figure 10.3 Change in the availability of methamphetamine by frequent drug users, 2006–2008. *Source*: Wilkins, Girling and Sweetsur, 2007.

Law enforcement and legislative responses to methamphetamine

The emergence of methamphetamine in New Zealand presented a number of challenges to law enforcement agencies and existing drug control legislation (Horne, 1997; United Nations Drug Control Programme, 2001; Wilkins, 2002). It was recognised that there was a need for more frequent monitoring of drug trends than had been achieved with the household drug surveys.

A range of government initiatives were enacted from 2002 onwards in response to the rise in methamphetamine use in New Zealand (Ministerial Action Group on Drugs, 2003; New Zealand Police, 2004). In 2002, a number of specialised police teams were established and trained to safely dismantle the clandestine amphetamine laboratories discovered by police. The National Drug Intelligence Bureau (NDIB) (a multi-agency government body consisting of officials from the New Zealand Ministry of Health, New Zealand Police and New Zealand Customs Service) agreed to a voluntary Memorandum of Understanding (MOU) with the New Zealand Chemical Industry Council to monitor the sale of the precursor chemicals being used to manufacture methamphetamine. At the regional level, the New Zealand Police developed voluntary agreements with their local pharmacies (see later). A national coordinator of actions against methamphetamine laboratories and a precursor analyst were appointed to enhance intelligence capacity and ensure the timely processing of evidence related to prosecutions for methamphetamine manufacture. The New Zealand Customs service paid greater attention to the importation of ephedrine, products-containing ephedrine and other chemical precursors used in methamphetamine manufacture. In early 2003, the New Zealand Parliament re-classified methamphetamine use under the *Misuse of Drugs Act 1975* from a Class B to a Class A drug offence – the highest offence class which carries a maximum penalty of life imprisonment for manufacture and trafficking. The re-classification of methamphetamine to Class A also enhanced the power of drug enforcement agencies to search suspected methamphetamine offenders and the premises used for methamphetamine manufacture and trafficking. The quantity of methamphetamine required to establish presumption of supply was set much lower, reflecting the fact that methamphetamine was sold in tenths of a gram rather than whole grams at the retail level. In early 2004, the importation of ephedrine, pseudoephedrine and methamphetamine pipes were classified as Class C offences under the *Misuse of Drugs Act 1975*, each carrying penalties of up to 8 years imprisonment.

Efforts to restrict methamphetamine precursors

The most commonly used method in New Zealand for the manufacture methamphetamine requires the precursor pseudoephedrine, which is contained in a number of 'over-the-counter' (OTC) cold remedies available in community pharmacies. Individuals have been found to go on shopping 'runs' of community pharmacies, buying large amounts of the pseudoephedrine-containing products with the intention of selling them to methamphetamine makers ('cooks') at a great profit. A pack of OTC cold remedies costing around NZ$12 could be sold on for a significant profit.

In early 2002, New Zealand Police began discussions with the pharmacy profession to raise awareness among community pharmacists of such inappropriate purchasing, and asking them to be vigilant. They also developed data collection methods for pharmacists who could then alert police by faxing identifying details of purchasers. In most cases, this required the collection of information such as name, address and photo ID. This strategy developed differently around the country and was enforced to varying extents and in different ways. A survey of New Zealand community pharmacies showed a wide variation in who was asked for ID, where and how details were recorded, and on what grounds a decision was made to send data to police (Butler et al., 2007; Sheridan et al., 2007). There were also concerns about the legality of pharmacists requesting such information in respect of New Zealand's privacy laws, although there was no question that pharmacists, under their Code of Ethics, had a responsibility to ensure OTC products were not being sold for misuse. Pharmacists also described a number of issues in undertaking this 'policing' role, including encountering aggressiveness from customers (both legitimate and otherwise), and the cost of having to take time off work to provide evidence in court and paying for locum cover, often only to have the case postponed. Furthermore, a lack of feedback from New Zealand Police had left some pharmacists feeling disempowered and undervalued. Nonetheless, the majority were still positive about their role in reducing the availability of pseudoephedrine for the illicit manufacture of methamphetamine (Butler et al., 2007; Sheridan et al., 2007).

The greater vigilance by pharmacists of pseudoephedrine sales may have made pseudoephedrine less easily available (although it could still be imported), which in turn may have contributed to the plateauing of methamphetamine laboratory detections in the later 2000s (see Figure 10.2).

Drug treatment and methamphetamine in New Zealand

In New Zealand, drug services have traditionally focussed on opioid dependence. Publicly funded drug and alcohol clinics generally operate as community alcohol and drugs services, which take in clients with problematic substance use, triaging at intake and providing targeted psychosocial interventions. In addition, for those with opioid dependence, referral for methadone treatment is possible. Some services also offer alcohol, opioid and other drug detoxification treatments.

In order to describe a treatment population in New Zealand, data from Community Alcohol and Drugs Services (CADS) Auckland have been provided. CADS Auckland is the largest service of its kind in New Zealand, with annual client numbers of around 10 000 and new open referrals to the service between 1 July 2007 and 30 June 2008 at around 9100 (some of whom referred more than once) (CADS Auckland, personal communication, 2009). At triage, clients are requested to complete a number of data collection tools, including the AUDIT Alcohol Screen (Saunders et al., 1993), the Leeds Dependence Questionnaire (Raistrick et al., 1994) which explores frequency of use, assessment of dependence using the Severity of Dependence Scale (SDS) (Gossop et al., 1995) and two questions on patterns of use: one on level of use and one on route of use, all based on average experience during the last 6 months. Questions for stimulants are around amphetamines in general, and not methamphetamine specifically, although most of the amphetamines use in New Zealand will be methamphetamine. Not all new clients complete these tools, for a number of reasons, so the following data need to be interpreted with caution.

Using data based on 26 501 new client episodes between 1 July 2004 and 30 June 2008, 15 028 completed the alcohol and drug screen, 2037 had used amphetamines (assumed to be mainly methamphetamine) and of those it was estimated that 75% ($N = 1528$) were dependent, based on an SDS score of 4 or more. Year-by-year estimates of dependence appear to have slightly decreased over the 4-year period from 80 to 73% (CADS Auckland, personal communication, 2009).

Unlike in many other countries, injecting is not the major route of administration for these clients, with smoking being far more common. Of the self-identified amphetamine users accessing CADS between 1 July 2004 and 30 June 2008, around 13% had injected, 66% smoked, 16% snorted and 5% used orally – as their main route of use in last 6 months. Year-by-year reporting indicates that the proportion of injecting and smoking remained reasonably constant over time (CADS Auckland, personal communication, 2009).

CADS Auckland offers a range of treatment options for those with problematic methamphetamine use including appropriate psychosocial interventions. A small number of inpatient beds are available for those who require inpatient detoxification. However, intensive psychosocial interventions are the main form of treatment used, although insomnia and severe agitation may be managed symptomatically with diazepam or risperidone, respectively, depending on symptoms and their severity. A detoxification of this type often involves multiple drugs, and a stay of 7–10 days is planned. No data are available for outcomes post-detoxification (CADS Auckland, personal communication, 2009). Outpatient treatment includes one-to-one as well as group-based interventions. Commonly practiced clinical modalities are motivational interviewing, cognitive behavioural therapy, dialectical behavioural therapy and 12-step facilitation. Mental and physical health interventions are offered depending on the presentation of the patients. The majority of presentations are chaotic and tend to be crisis driven. Considerable effort needs to be made to engage patients. The service aims for a family-inclusive approach.

A number of non-government organisations offer residential treatment options. They are based on therapeutic community interventions. Some will include the 12-step facilitation and a strong focus on self-help.

Injury and methamphetamine in New Zealand

Injury associated with methamphetamine can broadly be classified into three categories: injury as a result of one's own use, injury as a result of someone else's use and injury related to methamphetamine manufacture. An association between methamphetamine use and injury (but not necessarily cause and effect) has been noted in many studies, including links with interpersonal violence (Cohen et al., 2003), blunt trauma injury (Richards et al., 1999), road traffic fatalities (Drummer et al., 2004) and injuries related to clandestine manufacture (Burgess, 1997; Horton et al., 2003; Irvine and Chin, 1991).

With an increasing level of interest and concern about the impact of methamphetamine use, a study was commissioned in 2004 to explore whether methods of data collection were feasible in New Zealand, which would help establish any relationship between, or collate data on, methamphetamine use and injury. The study found that routinely collected data from hospital emergency departments were not useful when exploring this association and where data do exist, toxicological drug screens are not usually available to confirm self-report. In the qualitative part of the study, however, a member of emergency services indicated they had attended an explosion at a clandestine laboratory, where injuries to children had occurred. Others described injuries to 'cooks' – burns for example – and also injuries to those in the vicinity of the laboratory. Furthermore, key experts reported being aware of users suffering injuries such as falls after using methamphetamine, and as a result of assaults, fights and physical expressions of anger such as punching walls and windows (Sheridan et al., 2005).

Another data collection method used in this study explored the association between methamphetamine use and injury among people attending a one-day music festival. Although only a pilot study, it found that users had experienced injuries associated with their own use and the use of others, plus injuries associated with manufacture of the drug (Sheridan et al., 2008). While the study was designed to explore methodological issues, the types of injuries found were not inconsistent with international literature.

Conclusions: policy lessons from the New Zealand experience

A number of policy lessons can be taken from the recent rise of methamphetamine use in New Zealand. These observations are largely aimed at countries and places where there has been little previous experience of methamphetamine use:

(1) Law enforcement data series can be effective leading indicators of increasing methamphetamine use, including methamphetamine seizures, arrests for methamphetamine use and dealing, and detection of methamphetamine laboratories. To this end, it is important that law enforcement data systems distinguish methamphetamine from other ATS such as low-potency amphetamine sulphate (i.e. 'speed'), other designer amphetamines and ecstasy. However, there is a need to interpret trends in drug enforcement statistics with caution, as they are affected by the priority and resources drug enforcement agencies dedicate to detecting a particular drug type.

(2) Specialised drug research capacity is required to ensure that a rise in methamphetamine (or other synthetic drug types) can be distinguished from other traditional low-potency amphetamines. Established population level drug surveys may not include precise enough drug categories to distinguish methamphetamine from general amphetamines, and may not be conducted frequently enough to provide timely information about emerging drug trends. An ongoing drug monitoring research system (such as the IDMS in New Zealand), which interviews frequent drug users and includes information from key experts and secondary data sources on drug use, is highly desirable as a means of tracking changes in drug use, including the emergence of new variants of existing drugs. These research programmes tend to be smaller than household drug surveys, which means they can be conducted more frequently and be more flexible and responsive to changes in the drug use environment. Drug monitoring programmes should include detailed quantitative data on aspects of drug use, such as means of administration, and unstructured qualitative information, which can add depth to the understanding of emerging drug trends.

(3) A strong law enforcement and legislative response to methamphetamine appears to have made some impact on the trajectory of methamphetamine use in New Zealand. This includes appropriate classification of methamphetamine in drug control legislation to reflect the fact that methamphetamine is a greater health risk than traditional amphetamines, and amendments to quantity-related clauses to reflect the fact that methamphetamine is used and sold in much smaller quantities than traditional amphetamines. An effective law enforcement response should also include the monitoring and control of chemical precursors used to manufacture methamphetamine. This will require legislative amendments to include penalties for illegally importing key precursor chemicals, and institutional capacity to monitor the importation and sale of key precursors. In New Zealand, it is not entirely clear how effective the voluntary MOU with the chemical industry and voluntary regional agreements with pharmacies were at restricting access to pseudoephedrine-based products, and whether a more formal legislative system of control might be required (see Butler et al., 2007; Nice, 2007; Sheridan et al., 2007). The law enforcement response to methamphetamine will be most effective during the early stages of the spread of methamphetamine use when supply is in its infancy and the user base is small. A rapid response by law enforcement to a rise in methamphetamine use requires timely information of drug trends and the budgetary and legislative support of the government of the day.

(4) The New Zealand experience suggests that media stories, which included descriptions of the serious mental heath effects of chronic methamphetamine use and made the link between methamphetamine use and violent crime and drug addiction, may have been effective at undermining the reputation of methamphetamine as a 'safe' recreational drug, and thereby assisted in the containment of its spread. In other countries which have experienced problems with methamphetamine use, shocking crimes committed by methamphetamine users have been reported to galvanise public aversion to the drug and spurred

further action by the authorities (Kleiman and Satel, 1997, Kleiman, 1992, Matsumoto et al., 2002). A drug's reputation is considered central to fuelling a drug epidemic by encouraging the curious to start use, and reinforcing the desire current users to continue and escalate their use (Caulkins, 2007, Klee, 1997, Kleiman, 1992).

(5) The establishment of large-scale domestic methamphetamine manufacture appears to have been central to the ease of availability of methamphetamine in New Zealand and other countries. A focus on preventing local methamphetamine manufacture would appear to be a key strategy in containing methamphetamine use.

Acknowledgements

The authors would like to thank the Community Alcohol and Drugs Services (CADS), New Zealand Police and the National Drug Intelligence Bureau (NDIB) for providing data used in this Chapter. The New Zealand National Household Drug Survey was funded by the Ministry of Health and Health Research Council (HRC) of New Zealand. Secondary analysis of the household drug survey findings was funded by the New Zealand National Drug Policy Discretionary Fund. The IDMS is supported by a number of New Zealand government agencies including Police, Ministry of Health and Customs Service.

References

Adamson, S. and Sellman, D. (1998) The pattern of intravenous drug use and associated criminal activity in patients on a methadone waiting list. *Drug and Alcohol Review* 17: 159–166.

Australian Bureau of Criminal Intelligence (2002) *Australian Illicit Drug Report 2000–2001*. Australian Bureau of Criminal Intelligence.

Black, S. and Casswell, S. (1993) *Drugs in New Zealand: A Survey 1990*. The University of Auckland, Auckland: Alcohol & Public Health Research Unit.

Burgess, J. L. (1997) *Methamphetamine Labs: Community Risks and Public Health Responses*. Washington Public Health. Available at http://healthlinks.washington.edu/nwcphp/wph97/methlab.html. Accessed 3 March 2004.

Butler, R., Sheridan, J. and Kairuz, T. (2007) New Zealand community pharmacists, experiences in collecting information from purchasers of pseudoephedrine-containing products: findings from a qualitative study. *Pharmaceutical Journal* 278: 491–494.

Caulkins, J. (2007) The need for dynamic drug policy. *Addiction* 102: 4–7.

Cohen, J. B., Dickow, A., Horner, K., Zweben, J. E., Balabis, J., Vandersloot, D. and Reiber, C. (2003) Abuse and violence history of men and women in treatment for methamphetamine dependence. *American Journal on Addictions* 12(5): 377–385.

Cumming, G. (2002) Gangs mean big business. *New Zealand Herald*, 16 February 2002.

Drummer, O. H., Gerostamoulos, J., Batziris, H., Chu, M., Caplehorn, J., Robertson, M. D. and Swann, P. (2004) The involvement of drugs in drivers of motor vehicles killed in Australian road traffic crashes. *Accident Analysis & Prevention* 36(2): 239–248.

Expert Advisory Committee on Drugs (2002) *The Expert Advisory Committee on Drugs (EACD) Advice to the Minister on: Methamphetamine.* Wellington: Expert Advisory Committee on Drugs.

Farrell, M., Marsden, J., Ali, R. and Ling, W. (2002) Methamphetamine: drug use and psychoses becomes a major public health issue in the Asia Pacific region. *Addiction* 97: 771–772.

Field, A. and Casswell, S. (1999a) *Drug Use in New Zealand: Comparison Surveys 1990 and 1998.* The University of Auckland, Auckland: Alcohol and Public Health Research Unit.

Field, A. and Casswell, S. (1999b) *Drugs in New Zealand: A National Survey 1998.* The University of Auckland, Auckland: Alcohol and Public Health Research Unit.

Gardiner, J. (2003) How Williams killed Coral after night on P. *New Zealand Herald*, 11 December 2003.

Gossop, M., Darke, S., Griffiths, P., Hando, J., Powis, B., Hall, W. and Strang, J. (1995) The Severity of Dependence Scale (SDS): psychometric properties of the SDS in English and Australian samples of heroin, cocaine and amphetamine users. *Addiction* 90(5): 607–614.

Gower, P. (2002) 'P' is for psychotic – users linked with rising violence. *New Zealand Herald*, 14–15 December 2002.

Horne, B. (1997) *Policing the Illicit Use of Amphetamine Related Drugs in New Zealand.* New Zealand Police, Wellington: Wellington Regional Drug Squad.

Horton, D. K., Berkowitz, Z. and Kaye, W. E. (2003) Secondary contamination of ED personnel from hazardous materials events, 1995–2001. *American Journal of Emergency Medicine* 21(3): 199–204.

Irvine, G. and Chin, L. (1991) The environmental impact and adverse health effects of clandestine manufacture of methamphetamine. In: Miller, M. A. and Kozel, N. J. (eds), *Methamphetamine Abuse: Epidemiologic Issues and Implications.* Research Monograph 115. Rockville, MD: National Institute on Drug Research, pp. 33–46. Available at http://www.nida.nih.gov/pdf/monographs/115.pdf. Accessed 6 April 2009.

Klee, H. (ed.) (1997) *Amphetamine Misuse: International Perspectives on Current Trends.* Amsterdam: Harwood Academic Publishers.

Kleiman, M. (1992) *Against Excess: Drug Policy for Results.* New York: Basic Books.

Kleiman, M. and Satel, S. (1997) Methamphetamine returns. *Drug Policy Analysis Bulletin* 1, January 1997.

Little, P. (2003) Speed limits. *New Zealand Listener* 188(5–11 April): 17–21.

MacLeod, S. (2003) P is for paranoia. *New Zealand Herald*, 12 October 2003.

Matsumoto, T., Kamijo, A., Miyakawa, T., Endo, K., Yabana, T., Kishimoto, H., Okudaira, K., Iseki, E., Sakai, T. and Kosaka, K. (2002) Methamphetamine in Japan: the consequences of methamphetamine abuse as a function of route of administration. *Addiction* 97: 809–817.

Matthews, P. (2001) The lost war on drugs. *Listener*, 19 May.

Ministerial Action Group on Drugs (2003) *Methamphetamine Action Plan.* Wellington: New Zealand Government.

National Drug Intelligence Bureau (2008) *Illicit Drug Assessment.* Wellington: National Drug Intelligence Bureau.

Newbold, G. (2000) *Crime in New Zealand.* Palmerston North: Dunmore Press.

New Zealand Customs Service (2002) *Review of Customs Drug Enforcement Strategies 2002.* Project Horizon Outcome Report. Wellington: New Zealand Customs Service.

New Zealand Police (2002) *Preliminary Assessment of Substance Proposed for Classification or reclassification Under Sections 4–4B of the Misuse of Drugs Act 1975 ('the Act') – Methamphetamine (Confidential).* Wellington: New Zealand Police.

New Zealand Police (2004) *Safety Tips: What is Methamphetamine? What Police are Doing.* Available at http://www.police.govt.nz/safety/meth.php#WhatPolicearedoing. Accessed 7 April 2005.

Nice, M. (2007) *New Zealand Methamphetamine Purity Trends: Technical Report.* A Technical Report for the New Zealand Police, The National Drug Intelligence Bureau, the Centre for Social and Health Outcomes Research and Evaluation (SHORE) at Massey University, the Institute of Environmental Science and Research (New Zealand), and in support of the requirements for the Ian Axford New Zealand Fellowship in Public Policy. Ian Axford New Zealand Fellowships in Public Policy.

Philp, M. (2002) Gangland rising. *Metro*, June 2002.

Raistrick, D., Bradshaw, J., Tober, G., Weiner, J., Allison, J. and Healey, C. (1994) Development of the Leeds Dependence Questionnaire (LDQ): a questionnaire to measure alcohol and opiate dependence in the context of a treatment evaluation package. *Addiction* 89(5): 563–572.

Richards, J. R., Bretz, S. W., Johnson, E. B., Turnipseed, S. D., Brofeldt, B. T. and Derlet, R. W. (1999) Methamphetamine abuse and emergency department utilization. *Western Journal of Medicine* 170(4): 198–202.

Sattah, M., Supawitkul, S., Dondero, T., Kilmarx, P., Young, N., Mastro, T., Chaikummao, S., Manopaiboon, C. and van Griensven, F. (2002) Prevalence of and risk factors for methamphetamine use in northern Thai youth: results of an audio-computer-assisted self-interviewing survey with urine testing. *Addiction* 97: 801–808.

Saunders, J. B., Aasland, O. G., Babor, T. F., de la Fuente, J. R. and Grant, M. (1993) Development of the Alcohol Use Disorders Identification Test (AUDIT): WHO collaborative project on early detection of persons with harmful alcohol consumption: II. *Addiction* 88: 791–804.

Schmidt, V. (2001) The energy and ecstasy. *Metro*, January 2001.

Sheridan, J., Kairuz, T. and Butler, R. (2007) Reporting purchasers of pseudoephedrine products to police: New Zealand community pharmacists' experiences. *Journal of Pharmacy Practice and Research* 37: 19–21.

Sheridan, J., McMillan, K., Wheeler, A., Lovell, C., Lee, A. and Ameratunga, S. (2008) Methamphetamine and injury – a survey of individuals attending a one-day music festival in New Zealand: piloting a new methodology. *Journal of Substance Use* 12(1): 49–56.

Sheridan, J., McMillan, K., Wheeler, A., Lovell, C., Lee, M. and Ameratunga, S. (2005) *Exploring Methamphetamine and Injury: Feasibility Studies of Data Collection Methods. A Report for the Accident Compensation Corporation (ACC).* Centre Report Series No. 108. The University of Auckland, Auckland: Injury Prevention Research Centre.

Centre for Social and Health Outcomes Research and Evaluation (SHORE) (2004) *2003 Health Behaviours Survey: Drug Use Methodology Report.* Auckland: SHORE, and Te Ropu Whariki, Massey University.

United Nations Drug Control Programme (2001) *Global Illicit Drug Trends 2001.* Oxford, NY: United Nations Office on Drug Control and Crime Prevention.

United Nations Drug Control Programme (2002) *Global Illicit Drug Trends 2002.* Oxford, NY: United Nations Office on Drug Control and Crime Prevention.

United Nations Office on Drugs and Crime (UNODC) (2003) *Ecstasy and Amphetamines – Global Survey 2003.* New York: UNODC.

Wall, T. and Horwood, A. (2003) Drug 'Pure' linked to sword attacks and gunshot death. *New Zealand Herald*, 25 January 2003.

Wilkins, C. (2002) Designer amphetamines in New Zealand: challenges and policy initiatives. *Social Policy Journal of New Zealand* 19: 14–27.

Wilkins, C., Bhatta, K. and Casswell, S. (2002a) A demand side estimate of the financial turnover of the cannabis black market in New Zealand. *Drug and Alcohol Review* 21: 145–151.

Wilkins, C., Bhatta, K. and Casswell, S. (2002c). The emergence of amphetamine use in New Zealand: findings from the 1998 and 2001 national drug surveys. *The New Zealand Medical Journal* 115(1166): 256–263.

Wilkins, C., Bhatta, K., Pledger, M. and Casswell, S. (2003) Ecstasy use in New Zealand: findings from the 1998 and 2001 National Drug Surveys. *The New Zealand Medical Journal* 116: 383–393.

Wilkins, C. and Casswell, S. (2003) Organised crime in cannabis cultivation in New Zealand: an economic analysis. *Contemporary Drug Problems* 30: 757–777.

Wilkins, C., Casswell, S., Bhatta, K. and Pledger, M. (2002b) *Drug Use in New Zealand: National Surveys Comparison 1998 and 2001*. Auckland: Alcohol & Public Health Research Unit.

Wilkins, C., Girling, M. and Sweetsur, P. (2007) *Recent Trends in Illegal Drug Use in New Zealand, 2006 – Findings from the Combined Modules of the 2006 Illicit Drug Monitoring System (IDMS): Final Report*. Auckland: SHORE and Te Ropu Whariki, Massey University.

Wilkins, C., Girling, M., Sweetsur, P. and Butler, R. (2005a) *Methamphetamine and Other Illicit Drug Trends in New Zealand, 2005: Findings from the Methamphetamine Module of the 2005 Illicit Drug Monitoring System (IDMS)*. Auckland: SHORE and Te Ropu Whariki, Massey University.

Wilkins, C., Reilly, J., Rose, E. and Casswell, S. (2005b) Characteristics of amphetamine-type stimulants (ATS) use in New Zealand: informing policy responses. *Social Policy Journal of New Zealand* 25: 142–153.

Wilkins, C., Reilly, J., Rose, E., Roy, D., Pledger, M. and Lee, A. (2004a) *The Socio-Economic Impact of Amphetamine Type Stimulants in New Zealand: Final Report*. Auckland: Centre for Social and Health Outcomes Research and Evaluation, Massey University. Available at http://www.shore.ac.nz/projects/ATS%20research.htm; http://www.police.govt.nz/resources/2004/meth-impact/. Accessed 3 April 2009.

Wilkins, C. and Rose, E. (2003) *A Scoping Report on the Illicit Drug Monitoring System (IDMS)*. Auckland: SHORE, Massey University.

Wilkins, C. and Sweetsur, P. (2005) *The Dollar Value and Seizure Rates of the Illicit Markets for Amphetamine and Ecstasy in New Zealand in 2003*. Auckland: SHORE and Te Ropu Whariki.

Wilkins C. and Sweetsur P. (2008) Trends in population drug use in New Zealand: findings from national household surveying of drug use in 1998, 2001, 2003 and 2006. *New Zealand Medical Journal* 121, 61–71.

Wilkins, C., Sweetsur, P. and Casswell, S. (2006) Recent population trends in amphetamine use in New Zealand: Comparisons of findings from national household drug surveying in 1998, 2001 and 2003. *The New Zealand Medical Journal* 119(1244). Available at http://www.nzma.org.nz/journal/119-1244/2285/.

Yska, R. (1990) *New Zealand Green: The Story of Marijuana in New Zealand*. Auckland: David Bateman.

Zander, B. (2002) Speed freaks. *Listener* 6–12 April.

Chapter 11

JAPAN'S LONG ASSOCIATION WITH AMPHETAMINES: WHAT CAN WE LEARN FROM THEIR EXPERIENCES?

Akihiko Sato

In 2005, the Japanese government revised the prison policies for the first time in nearly 100 years. It adopted a policy to promote education about drug addiction in prisons. (This seemed very late, but hopefully not too late, for the addicts who still remain in prison.) Some typical interventions used with methamphetamine and amphetamine use in Japan are reviewed in this chapter. The reasons why such late revisions have finally occurred after a long history of methamphetamine and amphetamine use and control are discussed.

Interventions in Japan today

Legal and health

Today, in Japan interventions for methamphetamine use (including amphetamine) can be classified in one of the two ways, legal and health. While legal interventions also include a health aspect, there are still many aspects which remain exclusively legal in nature, but conversely there remain instances where health interventions make difference outside of the legal system. The two areas have just begun to merge in Japan.

The Japanese government revised the Prison Law in 2005. This was in response to many criticisms about the conditions and the managements of prisons, which had been made following revelations that prison officers had assaulted some inmates. In the process of the revision of Prison Law, a number of correctional and educational components were revised.

The revised 'Law Concerning Penal Institutions and the Treatment of Sentenced Inmates' was enacted and the application started as of 24 May 2006. It contains the chapter (Chapter 82) that orders all penal institutions to educate inmates who suffer from drug addiction. This provision was brought about for the first time since enactment of the old Prison Law in 1908.

Since 2006 there has been debate concerning those who are arrested for the violation of Stimulants Control Law, triggered by an overflowing prison population. The Council of Legislation at the Ministry of Law has discussed whether it would be appropriate to adopt the policy that those who are arrested for the violation of the law could attend rehabilitation programmes in self-help groups in exchange for custody. The decision to date has been not to approve these sorts of changes partly because there has been a shortage of institutions for them, but mainly because some members of council still have doubts about the effectiveness of rehabilitation in self-help groups (Minutes of the Council of Legislation, 2006).

It appears that the sentencing of those who violated the Stimulants Control Law has been, on average, more severe than in Western countries. This might reflect some people's notion that severe punishment has been the main way, even the only way, to deal with methamphetamine abuse and addiction. In the past several years, some alternative systems such as Drug Courts have been examined as alternatives for Japan.

To date, the Ministry of Health, Labour and Welfare (MHLW) has not yet adopted any standardisd policy or guidelines concerning the rehabilitation of persons with methamphetamine addiction. The Ministry of Health and Welfare (MHW, now MHLW) has promoted 'consultations for drug-related problems' since 1999, and has ordered every local authority (prefecture) to accept drug-related consultations in its mental health centre. This, however, has been just for consultations and not for rehabilitation. Discussion about the standardisation of the rehabilitation of drug addiction continues.

Drug Addiction Rehabilitation Centre and Narcotics Anonymous

Outside the penal system, interventions for methamphetamine have been left primarily to hospitals and doctors. Interventions vary in nature, but one of the most popular and influential treatment programmes for methamphetamine addiction today is by attending self-help activities, represented by two popular groups: Drug Addiction Rehabilitation Centre (DARC) and Narcotics Anonymous (NA). Both have been tightly connected with each other since their inception.

DARC is pronounced and written as 'da-ru-ku' in Japanese. It was founded by a former methamphetamine addict, Tsuneo Kondo, in 1985 in Tokyo, and is a self-help activity centre operated mainly in an intermediate institution (halfway house). The road to establish DARC was a hard one; it had been believed for a long time, even by recovered alcoholics and those supporting recovery of alcoholism, that drug addicts could not be recovered like alcoholics. Kondo underwent a 12-step recovery programme at Meryknoll Alcohol Center in Sapporo City and noticed the effectiveness of the programme even for methamphetamine addicts. He established DARC home for drug addicts with support from Father Roy Assenheimer of Meryknoll Mission. Kondo found that first 3 steps of the 12 were especially crucial for DARC and adopted them as the main principles without any rules, except attending group meetings (Kondo, 1997, 2000).

The recovered addicts of DARC home began to establish DARC and DARC-style rehabilitation programmes in other areas, and there are now up to 36 institutions all over Japan. One of the main programmes in DARCs is a group meeting, two or three times a day, with 12 steps. All lodgers of DARCs have an obligation to attend group meetings, which run in the institution every morning and afternoon, and NA meetings every evening, which are run outside of the institutions. Attending NA meetings is said to be important for recovery for addicts especially after leaving the institutions (Kondo, 1999). Interestingly, staff and members have a flexible attitude to 'relapse', which is often interpreted as just one step towards recovery (Kondo, 2004).

Almost all DARCs are operated by ex-DARC lodgers or ex-addicts who act as the models for recovery, but every DARC is slightly different in some way because the circumstances and the conditions of the institutions differ from each other. For example, many DARCs adopt sports programmes as one of the most important activities (as physical exercise therapy), which means that DARCs choose different events that are available in their (natural) environments. There are also some DARCs just for day care with no accommodation. Some DARCs are funded by the local authority through funds for certified institutions for people with mental health problems, but others are not.

Although DARCs look like therapeutic communities and some doctors regard them as such (Nagano, 1996), they have no professional staff for support. Every DARC has its own network for medical and other support in its area, helping users deal with flashbacks or other medical or psychological problems. Medical institutions that support DARCs are also supported by DARCs in the sense that they can introduce DARCs and/or NA meetings to patients. All of these features and the differences among DARCs show that DARC is not a united organisation but that every DARC is a node of social networks for rehabilitation of drug addiction.

Entering and staying in DARC costs, on average, approximately 150 000 yen (approximately US$1500) per month. Some of the lodgers pay for it with the livelihood protection which they receive from the local authority and others are paid for by their families. Research shows that 54% of residents receive livelihood protection (Morita, 2004). Some of the DARC staff and ex-lodgers who work as volunteers in and out of DARC often visit penal institutions to deliver the 'message' based on the educational programmes in the institutions.

One study showed that the proportion of lodgers of DARCs who originally came from the same prefectures as their DARC was 8%. This low rate is interpreted as one of the reasons for the effectiveness of DARCs since it shows that many lodgers can get out of the relationships that are connected to drugs (Ichige, 2002). Another study found that the average age of the residents of DARC is 31.6 years and most lodgers are between late 20s and late 30s (Kondo, 2004; Kondo et al., 2004). One statistic from a DARC (Ibaragi DARC) shows that the rate of the graduates (those who have stayed until the end of the 9-month period) was approximately 38% from 1992 to 2000 (Ichige, 2002), but DARC does not officially show rates of recovery (Ichige, 1998).

Another self-help activity centre NA has no intermediate institution associated with it, but instead uses various sites for meetings: churches, public halls and hospitals. NA Japan began in 1981 and is now registered with 131 groups with 324 weekly meetings all over Japan (March 2009). As noted above, the lodgers of DARCs have an obligation to attend NA meetings every evening, which means that NA has been supported by DARC. That is sometimes said to reflect the weakness of activities of NA in Japan (Kondo, 1999; Masui et al. 2006); it also means that DARCs function improperly without NA meetings (Assenheimer, 1991).

DARC and NA are not just for methamphetamine users, but many members have used methamphetamines and/or volatile solvent, which have been popular with young people in Japan since the 1970s. One study shows that the proportion of methamphetamine addicts in DARC is over 50%, and some of them used volatile solvents before using methamphetamine (Morita, 2004).

The way to recovery

One of the typical ways to access self-help programmes has been by way of hospitals and doctors. A prospective patient is often brought to see a doctor by his or her family, and if there is something wrong with the patient the family often agrees with legally protective ('enforced') hospitalisation. If there are hallucinations and/or delusions, intraveneous haloperidol is often prescribed. However, there is a tendency to avoid prescribing minor tranquiliser and anti-anxiolytic drugs as benzodiazepines because they may result in a secondary addiction. The patient is encouraged to attend the meetings of self-help groups, which is often the main treatment programme, and to attend DARC if this is thought suitable. Once the patients are believed to be abstinent from drugs, they can leave hospital but must continue to attend meetings regularly (Iwashita and Yonemoto, 1996; Yuzuriha, 2003).

One hospital has requested that the narcotic agents of MHLW, who have the right to arrest, be called in to pressure patients to stay sober and continue in treatment programmes. This is not a popular position, but some doctors claim that it is effective (Hirai, 2001a, b). There are also some doctors who call the police based on an agreement with the patients' families, especially when the patients have been connected to violent gangs ('Bou-ryoku-dan' in Japanese) (Yuzuriha, 2003). Many doctors (75%; Konuma, 1999) do not call for police when they see a patient who has used methamphetamine (there is no legal duty to do so). These doctors believe that medical intervention is better than a penal intervention, and because they believe that the relationship of mutual trust between the doctor and the patient is one of the most important factors in keeping patients in programmes (Konuma, 1999).

It is clear from this overview of present interventions in Japan that there is no special or unique treatment for methamphetamine users in Japan even after a long association. Why has a unique intervention not been developed in Japan and why have revisions to educational components in the Prison Law come so late?

Discovery and use of methamphetamine in Japan

Discovery of methamphetamine and the Second World War

Methamphetamine was discovered in 1888 (published in 1893) by a Japanese pharmacologist, Dr Nagayoshi Nagai, in the course of researching extracts of Maou (Ephedrae Herba). Methamphetamine was not used in Japan until the 1940s, when some researchers who had read pharmaceutical articles published in the West thought it would be useful for some patients (Horimi et al., 1940; Miura, 1941). There were 24 kinds of patent medicines containing methamphetamine or amphetamine on sale at that time, for example, Hospitan (methamphetamine), Takarapin (methamphetamine), Philopon (methamphetamine), Zedrin (amphetamine), Agotine (amphetamine) and Neoagotine (methamphetamine) (Ikuta, 1951). This list shows that methamphetamine was (probably still is) more popular than amphetamine in Japan.

One of the most famous and popular medicines was Philopon, which was put on sale in 1941. 'Philopon' is said to be a word coined by combining the Greek words 'philo (love)' and 'ponos (labor)', which had been synonymous with stimulants for a long time.

One of the biggest usages of methamphetamine at that time was thought to be in military, the Imperial Japanese Armed Forces. For example, the soldiers on sentry duty were supplied with the tablets called Cat-eye tablet ('Neko-me-jou' in Japanese). One of the most famous uses was for the special forces such as Kamikaze; the drug was mixed with green tea and stamped with Emperor's crest, named Storming tablet ('Totsugeki-jou' or 'Tokkou-jou').

During the social upheaval following the Second World War, medicines in stock with the Armed Forces were distributed to the general population. One old man who was a telegraph operator in the Air Force reported that he brought these back to university to use them for studying all night. Similar comments have been given by several old men, all of them were very surprised to hear that the medicine they had been given was the stimulants that was said to make users psychotic. There was no abuse of methamphetamine reported immediately after the Second World War.

Emergence of the condemnation of methamphetamine users

While there was no abuse of methamphetamine at that time, condemnation of methamphetamine *users*, especially writers and performers, began. For example, a poet who wrote in a magazine about a problem of Philopon connected to the post-war (Après-guerre) literature movement (Hirano, 1949) claiming that he met a demonic man during the war who had sold Philopon, even though he was informed that it made young people who took it continue to fight against their will till death (Kamikaze). The poet considered Philopon as a symbol of the darkness of the war and condemned the movement and people using Philopon for their demonic and backward looking ways. Users such as stand-up comedians were looked down on as immoral (Suzuki, 1949; Takeyama, 1949). Methamphetamine was condemned at this time not because of its effects but because of its symbolic meaning and because those who used it were looked down upon as deviants.

Change of medical knowledge on methamphetamine

Similar trends in attitudes to methamphetamine can be found in medical journals of the 1940s as well. There were some researchers who examined methamphetamine and amphetamine in terms of the effect on the body and the mind; their articles always referred to beneficial effects such as avoiding sleepiness, treating narcolepsy and so forth as well as to side effects like sleeplessness, mood swings and habituation.

After the famous and popular comedian named Miss Wakana died from a heart attack in 1946, attitudes began to change. One of the earliest changes was at the conference of the Japanese Society of Internal Medicine. Two young doctors presented a case which was presumed to be acute poisoning by Philopon (Nakazaki and Mori, 1947). This case would have been unremarkable because it was just one example of the side effects of the drug which were already known to researchers. Several researchers who had published the papers on methamphetamine commented on the case, observing that this was a fatal feature of methamphetamine, as witnessed by the death of the comedian and other 'immoral users' (Horimi, 1947; Iwata, 1947). Other researchers at that time still continued to discuss both positive and negative effects of methamphetamine in a balanced way (Higo, 1949; Tanaka, 1948).

In following years, changing attitudes to methamphetamine were found in the field of psychopathology. Papers referred to the 'immoral' users such as performers who were considered to have some psychopathological problems which would combine with methamphetamine to produce fatal results. The extent of change in attitudes can be seen in the review and the summary of methamphetamine research appeared in the *Journal of the Japan Medical Association* in 1950 (Kasamatsu and Kurino, 1950). It discussed many aspects of methamphetamine and concluded that it produced habituation on the basis that 'no one doubted the habitual nature of methamphetamine today' with no verification of this claim of particular note, the review also stated that methamphetamine habituation occurred only as a result of the psychopathology of some 'immoral' users, so that so-called normal people could use it without any problems.

Following the review, all of the research which tried to demonstrate the habituation associated with methamphetamine failed to do that except in cases where there was some psychopathology (Kawamura, 1953; Tai et al., 1955a, b). One of the most influential and famous pieces of research in the 1950s was published as a psychopathology book (Tatetsu et al., 1956). Consequently, methamphetamine became something which inevitably caused psychosis by way of the addiction, because researchers in psychopathology had always proposed a continuum from use to psychosis via addiction (Kasamatsu and Kurino, 1950; Saito, 1952; Tatetsu et al., 1956). While psychopathologists themselves often pointed out in their research that the relationship was only one of probability, at the same time they always explored the concept of continuity because they were attracted by the notion that researching methamphetamine psychosis would reveal the secrets of psychosis. The continuum of use and psychosis was then seen as the destiny of all users, despite the fact that this was not the case for so-called normal people such as workers who regularly used it without signs of psychosis.

Legalisation of methamphetamine control and after

Stimulants Control Law

The process of legislating the status of methamphetamine reflected what people at that time considered the drug to be. The first reference to methamphetamine use in the National Diet was in 1949. The minutes of the Diet show that the first step in calling methamphetamine use into question was related to the circumstances around street children using methamphetamine, most of whom had lost their parents in the Second World War (National Diet, 1949). The representatives of the Diet and the staff of the government shared the opinion that those who were to be blamed were not the street children using methamphetamine but the smugglers and the adults who gave methamphetamine to them. The children stole goods in exchange for methamphetamine so that they were thought to be victims (National Diet, 1949; *Asahi Shimbun*, 1949a, b). Food shortages also meant that street children used methamphetamine to boost energy levels depleted by food shortages.

Methamphetamine control was thus established on the basis that young people using methamphetamine were victims of the drug smugglers. Two psychopathologists were called to the Diet to testify about the problems and features of methamphetamine use including psychosis (National Diet, 1951a), but the purpose of methamphetamine control was not to punish the users but to maintain strict control over smugglers (National Diet, 1951b). The Stimulants Control Law was established in June 1951. The law contained the clause that prohibited the possession of the drug, but the clause was inserted in order to arrest the smugglers who often insisted that their drugs were just for their own use and not for sale (National Diet, 1951c, 1951d).

The change of narrative on methamphetamine use

The process whereby the Stimulant Control Law 1951 was established was quite different from what it would be in Japan today. Indeed, to understand what people think about methamphetamine today we need to look at another process which led to changes in narratives about the drug after the 1951 law was established. The new narratives of methamphetamine use have shaped policy and people's notions since 1954.

As noted above, methamphetamine use by so-called normal adults was not regarded as critically as it is today. For example, in the discussion about the legislation of control over stimulants, it was stated that the New Police Forces had a plan to use stimulants themselves (National Diet, 1951a). While this was criticised by the psychopathologists involved with the hearing, it shows that using stimulants did not necessarily bring about strong reactions and that the police forces themselves talked about the good effects. Another example was an essay, published in a medical journal, which showed that all the journalists attending a press conference used methamphetamine regularly (Japanese Medical Association, 1950). A famous novelist,

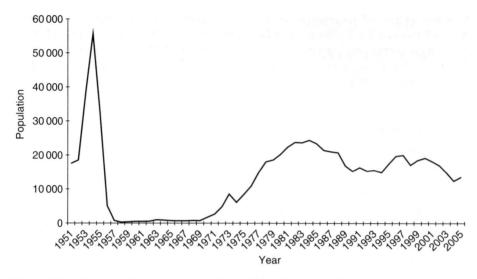

Figure 11.1 Number of arrests for violation of stimulant control law.

Ango Sakaguchi, wrote that, based on his experience, sleeping tablets were much more harmful than methamphetamine (Sakaguchi, 1950).

In 1954, an 11-year-old schoolgirl named Kyoko was killed in her primary school; at first this incident was treated as the result of the teacher's carelessness. After it was revealed that the offender had used methamphetamine, a movement against the drug was launched with psychopathologists denouncing methamphetamine for its harmful effect of making users psychotic (Hayashi, 1954). The incident led to the campaign by the government launched in 1954 for the eradication of methamphetamine use, which resulted in 55 664 arrests in 1954, the largest number in the history of the number of arrests for violation of Stimulants Control Law (see Figure 11.1). From 1954 onwards, narratives on methamphetamines converged, becoming consistently negative.

This campaign also resulted in a change of the narratives of the users of methamphetamine. After 1954, all the narratives that appeared in documents of the government, newspapers and magazines followed this new pattern's common features:

(1) Users had begun to use methamphetamine not because of habit or to commit antisocial acts.
(2) They could not stop using the drug.
(3) Many problems were associated with use, such as hallucinations and violence.
(4) They were finally arrested and became aware that they had been intoxicated.
(5) They would often express their gratitude to police for their arrest (Sato, 2006).

Importantly, this pattern of narratives showed that what was to be blamed was not users themselves but methamphetamine. In other words, the fatal feature of methamphetamine was a way to show that the users were a kind of victim, avoiding responsibility for their past problems and showing that they were now normal after all (Sato, 2006). This pattern has been repeated ever since and provided the standpoint from which Japanese drug policy over methamphetamine use had been justified since 1954, especially in 1970s, the so-called second wave of stimulants (Sato, 2006).

This historical perspective shows the emergence of the view that all people who use methamphetamine inevitably become insane and cannot recover – which most Japanese people believe today. It also accounts for the basis of the doubts about the effectiveness of recovery that was shown by members of the Council of the Legislation.

Nationalist talk

There has been another and more important aspect of the discourse around methamphetamine use in Japan: the view that methamphetamine abuse has been caused by hostile forces from outside the country. This accounts for the strength of the campaign launched in 1954 after a schoolgirl was killed. When the campaign was launched, the chief of the crime prevention division of the Metropolitan Police commented that they would tighten control over the smugglers even when power-ful Korean figures influences tried to influence their investigations (*Asahi Shimbun*, 1954; Metropolitan Police, 1955). Smuggling methamphetamine had been associ-ated with the *Red powers* of (North) Korea and China, who were thought to be invading Japan at that time. The introduction of the report on smuggling began with the emphasis on the purity of Japanese people (Metropolitan Police, 1955), and in the middle of the report the following statement was made:

> In addition, 70 percent of these smugglers, unlawful producers, and bootleggers consist of Korean people and they gnaw at the bodies and spirits of probably 1,500,000 of our fellow countrymen. In extreme, we seem to be living with a large crowd of acquired insane and brutal offenders and spending everyday with a lot of producers of such offenders...Our fellow countrymen who are the victims of Korean people seeking after their own interests, especially young people who will take our future generations, will become sick and decline in health, and finally addicts will destroy of our social order...Korean people who are well informed of the dangers of stimulants rarely use it by themselves nor allow their children to use it (Metropolitan Police, 1955).

The source of '70%' referred above was the result of the focused inspections of Korean villages by Metropolitan Police in 1953 (National Diet, 1953), which also accounts for an upward curve of the number of arrests in 1953 (Figure 11.1).

These sort of nationalist outpourings have been strong and popular in Japan since 1953. The revision of Stimulant Control Law in 1954 was discussed with the revision of Immigration Law, including enforced repatriations of Korean people (National Diet, 1954). These could be thought as one of the results of the anti-communist movements known as Red Purge, which begun in 1950 with suggestions of General Douglas MacArthur of General Headquarters/Supreme Commander for the Allied Powers that had occupied and controlled Japan after the Second World War.

Over time, the 'hostile forces' involved with methamphetamine use in such discourses have included Japanese violent gangs, people from Iran who came to get jobs and North Koreans of today. Discussions about methamphetamine have often involved something threatening to the Japanese people, which is why methamphetamine use and addiction have been punished more severely than necessary and treatment has not developed until recently. In addition, the policy of MHW and MHLW has reflected these discourses. Narcotic agents of MHW and MHLW have been working not for promotion of treatment or rehabilitation of addiction but for exposure of possession and use. The policy of MHLW has sometimes been criticised for policing order rather than promoting health (National Diet, 2002).

Conclusion

Probably it has been believed that Japan had a recognisable methamphetamine problem immediately after the Second World War because of the disorder of post-war circumstances, which produced an epidemic of methamphetamine psychosis. Indeed, some psychopathologists, criminologists and government officials have written about the history of methamphetamine in Japan as above without any careful examinations of the historical documents. However, when you carefully analyse the details of the historical processes associated with methamphetamine, you can find another appearance of history and other processes of interventions and policy in the past (Sato, 2006).

There is no doubt about the importance of advertising and emphasising the dangers and risks of methamphetamine use, especially for young people. However, distorted information about drugs and the justification of the policy through the 'terrors' of use often produce more harmful consequences than benefits. Japanese experiences with methamphetamine use could be thought as one of such examples.

Fortunately, these trends have now been slowly changing, typically represented by the revision of the Prison Law. However, the changes have not been based on any humanitarian notions or careful re-examination of the policy in the past. It might be said that such introduction is accidental and fortunate.

DARC and other self-help groups have been unique in the history of Japan's long association with methamphetamine use in the sense that they have been changing the belief that recovery from methamphetamine addiction is not possible. They have led the change in the way that methamphetamine addicts are dealt with by both the penal system and the health policy in Japan.

References

Asahi Shimbun (1949a) *Asahi Shinbun*, Tokyo, Morning Edition, 19 October 1949.
Asahi Shimbun (1949b) *Asahi Shinbun*, Tokyo, Morning Edition, 22 November 1949.

Asahi Shimbun (1954) *Asahi Shinbun*, Tokyo, Evening Edition, 15 October 1954.

Assenheimer, R. (1991) Four conditions for institution for rehabilitation. In: DARC Editorial Committee (ed.), *Why We Stay in DARC: Records of a Private-Run Drug Addiction Rehabilitation Centre*, Tokyo: DARC, pp. 16–24.

Hayashi, S. (1954) Comments in *Asahi Shimbun*. Morning Tokyo Edition, 7 May 1954.

Higo, M. (1949) Influences of phenylmetylamine and histamine to the respiration of brain tissue. *Folia Pharmacologica Japonica* 45: 94–95.

Hirai, S. (2001a) Cooperation of control and support in the measures to cope with drug abuse. *Hou to Seishin Iryou* 14: 19–38.

Hirai, S. (2001b) Psychotherapy for young people using illegal drugs. *Japanese Journal of Psychotherapy* 27(6): 53–63.

Hirano, I. (1949) Philopon disaster. *World View*, December 1949, pp. 68–71.

Horimi, T. (1947) Additional comment. *The Journal of the Japanese Society of Internal Medicine* 36: 69.

Horimi, T., Hashimoto, S., Inoue, K., Soya, K. and Egawa, S. (1940) On the action of 'Hospitan' to mental conditions. *Mitteilungen der Medizinischen Gesellschaft zu Osaka* 39: 827–837.

Ichige, K. (1998) *At the End of Drift*. Tokyo: Tsutsui Shobo.

Ichige, K. (2002) *We Are on the Way to Recovery*. Ibaragi: Nakashobo.

Ikuta, B. (1951) On stimulants. *The Science and Crime Detection* 4(2): 28–53.

Iwashita, S. and Yonemoto, T. (1996) Pharmacological therapy. In: Fukui, S. and Konuma, K. (eds), *Handbook of Drug Addiction*, Tokyo: Kongo Shuppan, pp. 77–98.

Iwata, S. (1947) Warning for continual uses of philopon. *The Journal of the Japanese Society of Internal Medicine* 36: 98–99.

Japan Medical Association (1950) Editorial: Where does Philopon go. *The Journal of Japan Medical Association* 24(2): 141.

Kasamatsu, A. and Kurino, R. (1950) Phenylmetylamine (philopon) toxicosis. *The Journal of Japan Medical Association* 24(2): 92–101.

Kawamura, M. (1953) A supplement to information about actions of phenylmetylamine. *Folia Pharmacologica Japonica* 49: 382–389.

Kondo, T. (1997) *Drug Addiction*. Tokyo: Taikaisha.

Kondo, T. (1999) Practices and problems of self-help activities of drug addictions. *The Journal of Public Health Practice* 63(2): 93–97.

Kondo, T. (2000) *Beyond Drug Addiction*. Tokyo: Kaitakusha.

Kondo, T. (2004) Roles of a private-run drug addiction rehabilitation center 'DARC' to support recovery from drug addiction. *Seishinka Rinshou Sabisu* 4: 31–34.

Kondo, C., Kouda, M., Shibata, O. and Wada, K. (2004) A study of effectiveness of recovery from drug dependence by participates with 'DARC'. *Japanese Journal of Alcohol and Drug Dependance* 39(2): 118–135.

Konuma, K. (1999) Research on functions and roles of national and public mental hospitals for drug addicts. In: Wada, K. (ed.), *Epidemiological Research on Drug Addictions and Research on Adequate Medical Treatments for Patients with Intoxicated Psychosis*. Report for MHLW Grants of Scientific Research, pp. 99–108.

Masui, M., Kawano, Y. and Masami, M. (2006) A new self-help support system for the recovery process at drug addiction rehabilitation centers. *Bulletin of Nagoya City University School of Nursing* 6: 13–24.

Metropolitan Police Headquarters to Measure for Stimulants (1955) *The Harm of Stimulants (Phipolon) and the Measures to Cope with It*. Tokyo: Metropolitan Police.

Minutes of the Council of Legislation (2006) *Meetings on the Policy to Make Proper the Populations of Penal Institutions*, 3. Ministry of Law, 15 December 2006.

Miura, K. (1941) On the stimulants derived from Ephedrae Herba. *Jikken Ihou* 28: 7–12.

Morita, N. (2004) Research on the actual conditions of self-help groups. In: Wada, K. (ed.), *Research on the Actual Conditions of Drug Abuse and Addiction, Their Social Influences and Measures to Cope with Them*. Report for MHLW Grants of Scientific Research, pp. 121–135.

Nagano, K. (1996) Milieu therapy: treatments in therapeutic community. In: Fukui, S. and Konuma, K. (eds), *Handbook of Drug Addiction*. Tokyo: Kongo Shuppan, pp. 172–187.

Nakazaki, T. and Mori, H. (1947) One case of an acute poisoning of Philopon. *The Journal of the Japanese Society of Internal Medicine* 36: 98.

National Diet (1949) *Minutes of the Committee of Welfare of the 5th House of Councillors*, No. 7, 24 October 1949.

National Diet (1951a) *Minutes of the Committee of Welfare of the 10th House of Councillors*, No. 6, 15 February 1951.

National Diet (1951b) *Minutes of the Committee of Welfare of the 10th House of Councillors*, No. 8, 22 February 1951.

National Diet (1951c) May 23, *Minutes of the Committee of Welfare of the 10th House of Councillors*, No. 29, 23 May 1951.

National Diet (1951d) *Minutes of the Committee of Welfare of the 10th House of Councillors*, No. 31, 25 May 1951.

National Diet (1953) *Minutes of the Committee of Welfare of the 17th House of Councillors*, No. 1, 30 October 1953.

National Diet (1954) *Minutes of the Committee of Welfare of the 19th House of Councillors*, No. 45, 25 May 1954.

National Diet (2002) *Minutes of the Special Committee for Youth Problems of the 154th House of Representatives*, No. 5, 13 June 2002.

Saito, M. (1952) Phenylmetylamine and its social significance. *Kyoto Igaku Zassi* 3: 30–34.

Sakaguchi, A. (1950) Drug, suicide and religion. *Bungei Shunjuu*, January 1950.

Sato, A. (2006) *Drug and Discourse: Methamphetamine in Japan*. Tokyo: Toshindo.

Suzuki, S. (1949) Performers and Philopon. *The Journal of Japan Medical Association* 23(7): 474.

Tai, H., Ezoe, T. and Kato, N. (1955a) Biochemistorical research on stimulant intoxication (1). *Psychiatria et Neurologia Japonica* 57(3): 115–124.

Tai, H., Ezoe, T. and Kato, N. (1955b). Biochemistorical research on Stimulant Intoxication (2). *Psychiatria et neurologia Japonica* 57(3): 124–130.

Takeyama, T. (1949) Philopon and Righteousness. *Kaizo*, December 1949, pp. 88–90.

Tanaka, K. (1948) Research on individual differences of reactions to drugs. *Folia Pharmacologica Japonica* 44: 85.

Tatetsu, S., Akio, G. and Tsuyoshi, H. (1956) *Stimulant Intoxication*. Tokyo: Igaku Shoin.

Yuzuriha, T. (2003) Research on modelling of treatment institutions for drug addictions. In: Murakami, S. (ed.), 2002, *Research on Modelling of Preventations, Medical Treatments and Aftercare of Drug Addicts*. Report for MHLW Grants of Scientific Research, pp. 87–94.

Chapter 12

THE EMERGENCE OF METHAMPHETAMINE IN THAILAND: INTERVENTIONS AND TREATMENT

Anjalee Cohen and Catherine McGregor

Introduction

This chapter examines the growing supply and demand for methamphetamine pills in Thailand since the mid-1990s, and the attempts made by the Thai government, as well as users themselves, to control methamphetamine use. We explore the diversification of the illicit drug trade in the Golden Triangle, in which opiate producers branched out and began producing methamphetamine to cater for a flourishing local and sub-regional market. Initially this market comprised workers such as truck drivers and labourers but soon extended to a burgeoning number of student users. We consider the appeal methamphetamine has among Thai youth in the context of a globalised commodity culture and a Thai desire for all things modern. The positive images associated with methamphetamine among young Thai population have emerged in stark contrast to the negative images of methamphetamine portrayed by the Thai media. Young people and their use of methamphetamine have been depicted as uncontrollable and as a significant threat to Thailand's social order. This moral panic is reflected in Thailand's anti-drug campaigns and interventions, particularly the 2003 Thai 'war on drugs'. We argue that the drug war was an overreaction to Thailand's methamphetamine problem and that the harm it brought to individuals and communities outweighed any positive short-term reductions achieved in methamphetamine consumption.

The diversification of the illicit drug trade in the Golden Triangle

The Golden Triangle (a region encompassing northeast Burma, northern Thailand and northern Laos) was the world's largest producer of opium for about four decades after World War II. By the end of the 1950s, the Golden Triangle produced roughly 700 tons of opium. Production peaked in 1989 at 3050 tons and increased from 50 to 72% of the world's illicit supply (McCoy, 2003). There are a number of political and economic reasons for this. Firstly, during the 1950s there was a significant decline in opium cultivation in traditional growing areas in China and the Middle East due to prohibition and strict law enforcement. Secondly, the Chinese Nationalist Army (Kuomintang or KMT), which fled into Burma from Yunnan in 1949 in the aftermath of the Chinese Revolution, expanded opium cultivation and trafficking in order to help finance their war against Mao's China. This was supported by the Criminal Intelligence Agency as the KMT helped to patrol the border with communist China. Increased opium production was also stimulated by the growth of a large local market for heroin among US troops in Vietnam in the 1960s and early 1970s, as well as continued armed revolt by ethnic minorities (such as the Shan) in northeast Burma who were fighting for independence against the Burmese government. Like the KMT, these minority armies financed themselves through opiate trafficking (McCoy, 2003; Yawnghwe, 2005).

From about the mid-1970s to the mid-1990s, the dominant drug lord in the Golden Triangle region was Khun Sa. In January 1996, Khun Sa and his Mong Tai Army surrendered to the Burmese Army which led to a heroin drought and a steep rise in the price of heroin. This provided a stimulus to methamphetamine production, as heroin users in Thailand resorted to methamphetamine as a substitute drug. However, even prior to his surrender Khun Sa had turned to the production of methamphetamine which was in part a response to Burmese military attacks on his caravan routes and the saturation of international heroin markets (McCoy, 2004). Thus, it is important to emphasise that the rapid expansion of methamphetamine production was not to the exclusion of opiates, rather it was the pursuit of new market opportunities and market diversification. Heroin production continued for the global market and methamphetamine production was increased to meet the demand of the local and sub-regional market.[1]

After Khun Sa's surrender, the United Wa State Army and other armed groups in Burma exploited and expanded the methamphetamine market in Thailand. Apart from the growing demand for methamphetamine in the region (especially Thailand), the production of methamphetamine appealed to producers because of the limited precursor chemicals needed and the ease of access to the main precursor chemical ephedrine from China. As it is more easily synthesised in comparison to amphetamine, methamphetamine is more readily available in the illicit market (Sulzer et al., 2005). Other factors that made the production of methamphetamine appealing were the simplicity of production techniques which require minimal chemical knowledge and equipment, the fact that production is not affected by weather conditions and availability of suitable land (as in the case of opium), the low costs of manufacture and high profitability (Chouvy and Meissonier, 2004).

The proliferation of methamphetamine use in Thailand was a consequence of not only mass production in Burma but the way the drug is marketed, which is largely through a decentralised four-tiered pyramid system (Lewis, 2003) and, more recently, through mobile phone dealer transactions (German et al., 2006). New customers have often been solicited through the offer of free samples. Also, dealers may offer sizeable discounts for the purchase of larger quantities, thus tempting consumers to buy more tablets than they need for themselves. Consumers then readily become small-scale dealers by selling the excess to new customers. Whilst many small dealers turned to trading as a means of supporting their habit, others were forced into trading due to poverty, unemployment and indebtedness, which was exacerbated by Thailand's worst-ever economic crisis in 1997 (Emmons, 1999). In fact, the high levels of unemployment triggered by the Asian economic crisis contributed to the spread of methamphetamine use in rural areas as many methamphetamine-using labourers were pressured to return home from Bangkok and provincial cities to their villages, where they introduced the drug to local agricultural workers (Surached, 2004).

The rising demand for methamphetamine in Thailand

From 1960–1970, methamphetamine in the form of Methedrine could be legally purchased in Thai pharmacies during which time it was colloquially referred to as a 'diligent drug' (*ya khayan*), particularly by truck drivers, as it enabled them to work for longer hours. However, methamphetamine pills were more frequently labelled the 'horse drug' (*ya ma*) due to the logo of the original (legal) importer and due to the strength it gave to the user (Farrell et al., 2002; Pasuk and Baker, 2004). By 1999, an estimated 257 000 workers, including truck drivers, factory hands and labourers, were regular amphetamine users (McCoy, 2004). Abuse of the drug later resulted in government controls and the beginning of an underground methamphetamine trade. Subsequent media publicity and warnings regarding the dangers of methamphetamine use, coupled with widespread availability, aroused curiosity among Thai youth and as methamphetamine use shifted from being mostly an occupational drug to a leisure drug so too did its name, image and status. It was not until the 1990s when use of the drug began to reach 'epidemic' proportions among students that methamphetamine pills were strategically renamed the 'crazy drug' (*ya ba*) by the government. Interestingly, methamphetamine was less of a perceived threat when workers used it predominantly as an occupational drug. The 'diligent drug' or 'horse drug' was transformed from a relatively acceptable work stimulant that assisted workers to enhance labour performance to a 'crazy' drug linked with a rebellious and hedonistic youth culture.

From the mid-1990s, student consumption of methamphetamine began to take off and to surpass that of other occupations. Schools, vocational colleges and universities became a prime target for traffickers and dealers. In 1991, students comprised 2.6% of those admitted to drug dependence treatment centres for amphetamine-type stimulant (ATS) problems. This proportion had increased to 45.3% in 1998. From 1995 to 1999, the greatest proportion of admissions for ATS problems were in the 15–19-year-old age group, followed by the 20–24-year-old age group (Poshiyachinda et al., 2000, p. 392). A 1999 survey of 1725 students attending vocational schools in Chiang Rai, northern Thailand, found that 41.3% of male students and 19% of female students had used methamphetamine, according to self-reported history or urine tests or both (Sattah et al., 2002).

Methamphetamine, consumerism and modernity

The growing demand for methamphetamine pills, particularly among Thai youth, coincided with a growing consumer culture and a desire for global youth cultural commodities. From the mid-1980s to the mid-1990s, Thailand had one of the fastest growing economies in the world (Pasuk and Baker, 1998). Various Thai media and businesses fostered by economic development have been crucial to the formation of a Thai youth culture. Thailand's increasing exposure to global mass media and global culture is palpable as the Thai youth embrace Western and Japanese popular music, film and fashion. Global brand names have become symbols of modernity, and consuming these modern products is perceived by many Thai people to lead to a life of success and happiness (Kasian, 1996; Ubonrat, 2000). Methamphetamine as a modern global commodity is no exception; as Lyttleton points out, ATS across Southeast Asia symbolise a social ethos geared to a 'consumer culture oriented to the pursuit of pleasure through purchase' (Lyttleton, 2004, p. 916). The growing popularity of methamphetamine in Southeast Asia, including Thailand, is in part a reflection of the changing social values that have accompanied capitalist development. As a stimulant, methamphetamine use is consistent with Thailand's new fast-paced, achievement- and consumer-driven society – in this context, methamphetamine is the ideal capitalist drug.

For many young Thai, methamphetamine has become the drug of choice because of its low price, availability, accessibility and, in particular, the multiple purposes for which it may be used. As a social drug, methamphetamine is used to enhance the pleasurable experience of a range of leisure and recreational activities such as card playing, computer games, dancing, listening to music or just spending time with friends. The Thai youth also utilise methamphetamine for functional purposes including work or house chores, whilst many students consume methamphetamine to improve their academic performance. It is common for students to take up methamphetamine during the very demanding and competitive university entrance examinations, as it enables them to stay awake and study for extensive periods. The drug is also consumed by adolescents to improve performance in sports such as soccer or to give them an edge in competitive activities such as motorbike racing. Some users turn to methamphetamine to enhance sexual performance, whilst others consume it to lose weight. The important point is that among Thai youth methamphetamine is highly valued for its multi-faceted purposes.

As methamphetamine is a synthetic drug and produced in the form of a pill, consumers associate it with modern medicine (Chouvy and Meissonier, 2004). Thai consumers place great faith in pills due to a culturally constructed belief in their efficacy and power (van der Geest and Reynolds Whyte, 1989). This is evident in Thai people's widespread purchase of pharmaceuticals. For example, during the 1980s Thailand had the highest per capita drug (i.e. pharmaceutical) consumption of all ASEAN (The Association of Southeast Asian Nations) countries (Cohen, 1989, p. 164).

The fact that amphetamines are products of modern technology and, in addition to illicit production, are manufactured by legitimate pharmaceutical companies backed by medical authorities contributes to the perception among many users that they are safe (Grinspoon and Hedblom, 1975, p. 288). The problem with this attitude is that young Thai people tend to underestimate the potential dangers of uncontrolled and excessive methamphetamine use. Arguably, methamphetamine's image as a modern synthetic product or as a 'postmodern commodity'[2] appeals to many young Thai people in their desire to be *thansamai* (up to date). Many young Thai users perceive methamphetamine as 'cool' and fashionable. In Chiang Mai, opium and heroin are mostly used by people above 30 years of age (Chouvy and Meissonier, 2004, p. 62) and are therefore associated with an older and 'uncool' generation. Thus, it is the modern image associated with ATS, rather than simply the pharmacological properties of the drug, that impels many Thai youth to take up methamphetamine.

Methamphetamine and youth harm reduction

Whilst there is a tendency for users to underestimate methamphetamine-related harms because of the positive images described above, the Thai government and media have clearly exaggerated the attendant dangers and social upheaval created by methamphetamine consumption. In their study of methamphetamine use in Thailand, Chouvy and Meissonier noted that '[m]ethamphetamine is certainly not harmless, but when used moderately it is unlikely to cause social disruption. Workers, drivers and employees who do use it regulate their consumption' (Chouvy and Meissonier, 2004, p. 72). Those who consume methamphetamine solely for occupational work are not the only users capable of controlling their use. Chouvy and Meissonier ignore the ways in which young people who use methamphetamine recreationally may also regulate consumption.

There is a significant proportion of young people who do not experience serious problems from methamphetamine use, apart from sleeplessness and suppressed appetite, culminating in general fatigue (Cohen, 2006). This is in part due to controlled use and the social context in which the drug is predominately used. Smoking[3] or inhalation of vapour is the preferred way of using methamphetamine in Thailand (Humeniuk and Ali, 2004). The fact that methamphetamine is commonly smoked among Thai youth makes methamphetamine use particularly conducive to sharing. Among Thai adolescents, methamphetamine pills are typically shared by a group of four to five people in someone's dorm room and passed around one by one for each individual to smoke. Cohen's ethnographic study (2006) of methamphetamine use among young northern Thai supports Zinberg's (1984) argument that the peer group is the most crucial source of instruction and practices for drug control (Zinberg, 1984). As one young Thai male noted, '[t]hose who go crazy or paranoid are usually those who take it alone. You don't usually get this way when you use in a group' (Cohen, 2006, p. 165). Cohen found that many of the problematic users she interviewed consumed methamphetamine alone so that they did not have to share and could consume as much as they desired. Consequently, users generally consume more methamphetamine when they use the drug in isolation. Thus, it is the social use rather than solitary use of methamphetamine that, in part, helps to moderate consumption and minimise harm.

Zinberg (1984) suggests that the sanctions and rituals of drug-using groups help prevent the abuse of illicit drugs. For Zinberg, the combination of values and rules of conduct (social sanctions) and patterns of behaviour (social rituals) act as informal social controls among drug users.[4] Cohen (2006) found that young Thai methamphetamine users employed various measures (or social rituals) to reduce or to avoid some of the negative short-term side effects of methamphetamine. For example, to avoid fatigue from lack of sleep or severe weight loss due to suppressed appetite, some of Cohen's informants reported taking methamphetamine in the early morning rather than evening so that they could sleep at night. Others reported drinking alcohol with methamphetamine[5] or smoking marijuana after using methamphetamine since these central nervous system depressants counteract the stimulant effects of methamphetamine that, in turn, enables users to 'come down' and sleep. To avoid excessive weight loss, some informants would take methamphetamine after a main meal or drink milk throughout the day. There was also a common rule among informants not to purchase methamphetamine from dealers, as they did not know in case the drug had been adulterated, although it is difficult to verify how common this practice is.

It should be noted, however, that not all social sanctions and rituals help reduce harm or are intended to (Grund, 1993; Zinberg, 1984). In some instances, specific routes of methamphetamine administration increase the adverse effects of the drug. For example, both smoking and injection of methamphetamine can lead to dependence, but injection carries a greater risk of contracting blood-borne viruses such as HIV. Both smoking and injection of methamphetamine produce rapid and intense reinforcing effects that are more likely to produce dependence on the drug. In contrast, when taken by mouth, the effects of methamphetamine do not peak for $1^{1}/_{2}$ to 2 hours (Cook et al., 1993).

Furthermore, some users took methamphetamine as soon as they began to 'come down' in order to avoid the unpleasant feelings associated with this experience, thus leading to repeated use. This use pattern indicates the onset of withdrawal symptoms when methamphetamine use is reduced or stopped and is one of the criteria for the diagnosis of dependence (DSM-IV-TR, 2000). Whilst some patterns of behaviour may increase the harms associated with methamphetamine use, the majority of users did appear conscious of controlling their use through various rituals and sanctions to minimise harm to their health and without causing significant social disruption.

Despite many young Thai people's ability to regulate methamphetamine consumption, their use of the drug is nonetheless perceived by the general public as uncontrollable and excessive, causing a national hysteria which culminated in the 'war on drugs'. This moral panic seems unwarranted given that the numbers of dependent methamphetamine users is lower than is generally claimed in the media, with some reporting figures of well over 2 million 'addicts'. Drawing on figures from the Ministry of Health, research indicates that out of the 2.5 million estimated methamphetamine users, 2 million consume an average of 1–2 tablets per month and half a million are dependent (Lewis, 2003; Pasuk, 2003). Moreover, the use of methamphetamine is arguably less life-threatening compared to other illicit drugs, such as heroin, or legal drugs such as alcohol and tobacco, which are associated with much higher mortality rates (AIHW, 2007; Bartu et al., 2004). Additionally, withdrawal from amphetamines is relatively mild (McGregor et al., 2005). This is not to deny that the use of methamphetamine may cause serious health risks such as psychosis (Srisurapanont et al., 2003), but that the extent of the deleterious effects of the drug and the social disruption it causes has been overstated in public discourses.

Interventions and treatment

In 2001, the Thai government declared ATS abuse to be the number one national security threat. Border patrols were increased and negotiations began with neighbouring countries (Laos, Cambodia and Burma) in an attempt to curb the manufacture of methamphetamine. At the same time, a propaganda campaign exaggerating the psychotic effects of methamphetamine was launched, depicting images of drug-crazed murderers running rampant. Despite its efforts, the government's lack of success in reducing the use of methamphetamine was noted by the King in his birthday speech in December 2002. The King's concerns were no doubt triggered by the release of statistics from the Office of Narcotics Control Board (ONCB) and the Ministry of Health, which estimated that approximately 2 million people had some experience with methamphetamine, of whom a significant majority were reportedly secondary school students (Pasuk and Baker, 2004).

On 1 February 2003, the Prime Minister of Thailand, Thaksin Shinawatra, declared a punitive and ruthless 3-month 'war on drugs' (*songkhram prappram ya sephtit*). The priority of the government's anti-drug campaign was to target the use and abuse of methamphetamine among students. In relation to methamphetamine dealers and traffickers, police officials nationwide were set targets for the number of arrests and seizures they were to meet within the 3 months and were even offered bonuses for the number of arrests made. Provincial governors and police chiefs who failed to meet targets were threatened with dismissal. Given Thaksin's demands, it was not surprising that many extra-judicial killings took place, with 2637 people reportedly killed during the 3-month period (Pasuk and Baker, 2004, p. 163). Thaksin responded to accusations against police regarding the large number of extra-judicial killings by claiming that most of the deaths involved dealers shooting other dealers in order to silence them and protect themselves. Thaksin's 2003 drug war was met with concern and criticism from local and international organisations (including Amnesty International and the United Nations) regarding the violation of human rights (Amnesty International, 2004).

During and following the 'war on drugs', the potential for stigmatisation and recrimination was particularly marked in small rural communities with relatively stable resident populations. These communities came under substantial pressure as local leaders were expected to provide the authorities with lists of resident drug users and dealers (Vongchak et al., 2005). Identified dealers and drug users were either imprisoned or coerced into treatment.

Prior to 2001, drug treatment in Thailand was provided largely through public inpatient units, outpatient clinics and community drop-in centres. Some monasteries also provided withdrawal treatment consisting of a combination of religious vows and meditation. Whilst many clinics had untrained staff, other clinics, particularly those in the large centres, had trained staff offering medically supported withdrawal, psychosocial therapy and rehabilitation (including therapeutic communities) for a range of illicit and licit drug problems.

As part of the response to the increasing prevalence of methamphetamine use in Thailand, in 1998, the Government of Thailand began the implementation of the Matrix Model treatment in substance abuse treatment facilities across the country. Developed in the USA, this manualised 16-week intensive outpatient intervention is an abstinence-based model that uses a cognitive behavioural therapy approach incorporating stimulant education, family education, 12-step programmes and positive reinforcement for behaviour change and treatment compliance. To implement the use of the Matrix Model in Thailand, Thai clinicians and counsellors underwent training at the Matrix Institute clinics in Southern California, whilst clinicians from the Matrix Institute travelled to 12 primary sites in Thailand to provide additional training. It was planned that these primary sites would then train an additional 800 clinicians over approximately 3 years (Obert et al., 2003).

Preliminary results of an outcome study of the Matrix Model in a Thai population were promising with 80% of those who remained in treatment providing methamphetamine-free urine samples at their final assessment (Obert et al., 2003). However, concerns have been raised that abstinence-based behavioural interventions largely developed in the USA may not translate well to an Asian culture (Ahmad, 2003). To establish a benefit for this treatment approach in a Thai population, outcome evaluation studies comparing the Matrix Model to a standard treatment are needed.

Such evaluation studies have been conducted in the USA where the Matrix Model was compared with treatment as usual in a multi-site, randomised clinical trial involving 978 treatment-seeking methamphetamine-dependent individuals. Treatment retention, clinic attendance, incidence and duration of methamphetamine abstinence (confirmed by urinalysis) was significantly greater in those individuals assigned to receive treatment using the Matrix Model. However, whilst gains in terms of improvements in substance use and psychosocial functioning remained, group differences did not persist at 6-months follow-up (Rawson et al., 2004).

In 2002, mandatory drug use treatment in camps operated by the Royal Thai Armed Forces was initiated as part of the 'war on drugs'. As a result, a large number of new treatment centres were established within community hospitals, and health centres, as well as short-term military style drug rehabilitation 'boot camps', where physical activity, discipline and abstinence from drugs were enforced. Treatment in the camps was provided by military personnel from all three services who were given a 'Fast Model' 4-week training course in drug treatment and rehabilitation (BINLEA, 2004). Treatment lasted for 4–21 days in the camps where, in addition to traditional boot camp physical activities, training in 'life skills' was provided to enable them to maintain a drug-free lifestyle in the community following discharge. Mandatory treatment for identified drug users resulted in an increase in methamphetamine treatment admissions from 21 665 to 480 711 between 2002 and 2003

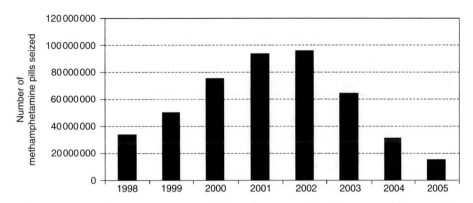

Figure 12.1 Number of methamphetamine pills seized in Thailand, 1998–2005. *Source*: ONCB Thailand (2006).

(ONCB Thailand, 2002). These camps have largely been discontinued (German et al., 2006). It is difficult to assess the impact of treatment in both drug treatment centres and camps due to a general lack of follow-up in Thailand's rehabilitation programmes (Lewis, 2003, p. 55). However, the lack of expertise among treatment personnel and the frequency of repeat admissions suggest that methamphetamine treatment in Thailand is still in an early stage of development.

Despite the callous approach with which the 'war on drugs' was fought, it had a significant effect on the supply of methamphetamine. The annual number of indictments for this drug declined from 187 676 cases in 2002 to 38 130 cases in 2004 (Poshyachinda et al., 2005, p. 462). The amount of methamphetamine pills seized in the same period also dropped from 8622 kg to 2759.3 kg. Figure 12.1 above indicates a significant increase in seizures from 1998 and a substantial decline following the drug war in 2003.

Whilst the 'war on drugs' may have led to a decline in the supply of methamphetamine and, consequently, increased prices, consumption remains widespread (German et al., 2006),[6] many substituted methamphetamine with other drugs such as alcohol or benzodiazepines (Vongchak et al., 2005) and there was an increase in seizures and arrests relating to crystal methamphetamine (Aramrattana, 2004). In 2003, 48.8 kg of crystal methamphetamine were confiscated by authorities, rising to 93.1 kg in 2006, whilst arrests for crystal methamphetamine-related charges rose from 70 cases in 2003 to 906 cases in 2006 (ONCB, 2007). It is difficult to determine the current level of consumption of crystal methamphetamine, but these statistics suggest use is likely to have increased since the 2003 'war on drugs'.

Conclusion

Among consumers of the drug, methamphetamine has a positive image as a modern, 'cool' and multi-purpose drug. Therefore, anti-drug campaigns that demonise the drug and exaggerate its deleterious effects are unlikely to resonate with users, particularly among controlled users who do not experience serious adverse effects. Methamphetamine use can lead to dependence, but there are many occasional users who are capable of regulating methamphetamine use through group rituals and sanctions and who do not pose a significant threat to society. The Thai government's punitive 'war on drugs' was an extreme response to methamphetamine use in Thailand. This arose in part out of a moral panic surrounding the proliferating use of methamphetamine among Thai youth. Whilst methamphetamine use has been associated with a range of harms to the individual and the community, the 'war on drugs' caused the deaths of over 2000 people and resulted in widespread fear of and discrimination against all drug users. Although there was a decline in the supply of methamphetamine following the 2003 drug war, there are substantial concerns around the wider impact of supply reduction strategies such as the Thai 'war on drugs' particularly in relation to the effects of these strategies on the families and communities involved. Adopting a more comprehensive public health approach that incorporates a greater balance of harm reduction, demand reduction and supply reduction strategies would minimise the impact on individuals and the wider community.

Notes

1. For example, an investigation of 93 drug laboratories (run by the United Wa State Army and 18 other armed groups) in the Shan State in March 2003 found that 59 laboratories produced both heroin and methamphetamine and 34 produced methamphetamine only SHAN (2003).
2. Lyttleton argues ATS may be seen as a postmodern commodity due to the fact millions of the pills are mixed with imported substances by small mobile factories and subsequently marketed through transnational flows (Lyttleton, 2004, p. 931).
3. Methamphetamine vapour is readily released by heating pills on foil or in a pipe and inhaling the vapour.
4. For more examples of controlled drug use see Moore (1993) and Grund et al. (1994).
5. Many suggested one of the advantages of methamphetamine was that it enabled users to drink more alcohol which may actually increase harm over the long term. Many also reported smoking more cigarettes following methamphetamine use, which also poses greater health risks (Cohen, 2006).
6. Although some studies have identified a decrease in the prevalence of methamphetamine use and initiation (Daosodsai et al., 2007).

References

Ahmad, K. (2003) Asia grapples with spreading amphetamine abuse. *Lancet* 361: 1878–1879.

AIHW (2007) *Statistics on Drug Use in Australia 2006*. Drug Statistics Series No. 18. Cat. No. PHE 80. Canberra: Australian Institute of Health and Welfare.

Amnesty International (2004) *Thailand Memorandum on Human Rights Concerns*. AI Index: ASA 39/013/2004. 27 October 2004.

Aramrattana, A. (2004) Ice. In: *2nd National Conference on Substance Abuse*, Khon Kaen, Thailand.

Bartu, A., Freeman, N. C., Gawthorne, G. S., Codde, J. P. and Holman, C. D. (2004) Mortality in a cohort of opiate and amphetamine users in Perth, Western Australia. *Addiction* 99: 53–60.

BINLEA (2004) *Thailand: International Narcotics Control Strategy Report – 2003 Bureau for International Narcotics and Law Enforcement Affairs*. Washington, DC: US Department of State.

Chouvy, P.-A. and Meissonier, J. (2004) *Yaa Baa: Production, Traffic and Consumption of Methamphetamine in Mainland Southeast. Asia Singapore*: Singapore University Press.

Cohen, A. P. (2006) *Youth Culture and Identity: Consumerism, Drugs and Gangs in Urban Chiang Mai, Northern Thailand*. Unpublished PhD Thesis, Macquarie University, Sydney.

Cohen, P. T. (1989) The politics of primary health care in Thailand, with special reference to non-government organisations. In: Cohen, P. T. and Purcal, J. T. (eds), *The Political Economy of Primary Health Care in Southeast Asia*. Canberra: Australian National University.

Cook, C. E., Jeffcoat, A. R., Hill, J. M., Pugh, D. E., Patetta, P. K., Sadler, B. M., White, W. R. and Perez-Reyes, M. (1993) Pharmacokinetics of methamphetamine self-administered to human subjects by smoking S-(+)-methamphetamine hydrochloride. *Drug Metabolism and Disposition: The Biological Fate of Chemicals* 21: 717–723.

Daosodsai, P., Bellis, M. A., Hughes, K., Hughes, S., Daosodsai, S. and Syed, Q. (2007) Thai war on drugs: measuring changes in methamphetamine and other substance use by school students through matched cross sectional surveys. *Addictive Behaviors* 32: 1733–1739.

DSM-IV-TR (2000) *Diagnostic and Statistical Manual of Mental Disorders*, 4th edn, Text Revision. Washington, DC: American Psychiatric Association.

Emmons, K. (1999) Suffer the children. *Far Eastern Economic Review*, 15 April 1999.

Farrell, M., Marsden, J., Ali, R. and Ling, W. (2002) Methamphetamine: drug use and psychoses becomes a major public health issue in the Asia Pacific region. *Addiction* 97: 771–772.

German, D., Sherman, S. G., Sirirojn, B., Thomson, N., Aramrattana, A. and Celentano, D. D. (2006) Motivations for methamphetamine cessation among young people in northern Thailand. *Addiction* 101: 1143–1152.

Grinspoon, L. and Hedblom, P. (1975) *The Speed Culture: Amphetamine Use and Abuse in America*. Cambridge, MA: Harvard University Press.

Grund, J. P. G. (1993) *Drug Use as a Social Ritual: Functionality, Symbolism and Determinants of Self-Regulation*. Rotterdam: Erasmus University.

Grund, J. P. G., Kaplan, C. D. and De Vries, M. (1994) Rituals of regulation: controlled and uncontrolled drug use in natural settings. In: Heather, N. (ed.), *Psychoactive Drugs and Harm Reduction: From Faith to Science*. London: Whurr.

Humeniuk, R. and Ali, R. (2004) Amphetamines in Asia: the value of information networks. *Drug and Alcohol Review* 23: 235–237.

Kasian, T. (1996) Cultural forces and counter-forces in contemporary Thailand. In: Thumboo, E. (ed.), *Cultures in ASEAN and the 21st Century*. Singapore: UniPress, pp. 239–265.

Lewis, D. R. (2003) *The Long Trip down the Mountain: Social and Economic Impact of Illicit Drugs in Thailand*. Bangkok: UN Office on Drugs and Crime, Regional Centre for East Asia and the Pacific.

Lyttleton, C. (2004) Relative pleasures: drugs, development and modern dependencies in the golden triangle. *Development and Change* 35: 909–935.

McCoy, A. (2003) *The Politics of Heroin: CIA Complicity in the Global Drug Trade, Afghanistan, Southeast Asia, Central America, Colombia*, Revised edition. Chicago: Lawrence Hill.

McCoy, A. (2004) The stimulus of prohibition: a critical history of the global narcotics trade. In: Steinberg, M. K., Hobbs, J. J. and Mathewson, K. (eds), *Dangerous Harvest: Drug Plants and the Transformation of Indigenous Landscapes*. New York: University Press.

McGregor, C., Srisurapanont, M., Jittiwutikarn, J., Laobhripatr, S., Wongtan, T. and White, J. M. (2005) The nature, time course and severity of methamphetamine withdrawal. *Addiction* 100: 1320–1329.

Moore, D. (1993) Social controls, harm minimisation and interactive outreach: the public health implications of an ethnography of drug use. *Australian Journal of Public Health* 17: 58–67.

Obert, J., Rawson, R., McCann, M., Laob, S. and Ling, W. (2003) Matrix model for methamphetamine treatment: the Thai experience. In: *65th Annual Scientific Meeting of the College on Problems of Drug Dependence*, Bal Harbour.

ONCB (2007) Statistics on numbers of drug cases throughout the country during 2003–May 17 2007. Available at http://www1.oncb.go.th/document/Annual_cases.pdf. Accessed 22 September 2007.

ONCB Thailand (2002) Thailand Narcotics Control Annual Report 2002. Report No. 1-03-2545. Bangkok: Office of the Narcotics Control Board, Ministry of Justice of Thailand.

ONCB Thailand. (2006). Thailand Narcotics Control Annual Report 2005. Bangkok: Office of the Narcotics Control Board, Ministry of Justice, Thailand.

Pasuk, P. (2003) Drug policy in Thailand. In: *Senlis Council International Symposium on Global Drug Policy*, Lisbon, Portugal, 23–25 October 2003.

Pasuk, P. and Baker, C. (1998) *Thailand's Boom and Bust*. Chiang Mai: Silkworm Press.

Pasuk, P. and Baker, C. (2004) *Thaksin: The Business of Politics in Thailand*. Chiang Mai: Silkworm Books.

Poshiyachinda, V., Perngparn, U. and Danthamrongkul, V. (2000) The amphetamine-type stimulants epidemic in Thailand: a case study of the treatment, student, and wage labourer populations. In: *Epidemiologic Trends in Drug Abuse, Volume II: Proceedings of the Community Epidemiology Work Group National Institute on Drug Abuse*, Bangkok.

Poshyachinda, V., Na Ayudhya, A. S., Aramrattana, A., Kanato, M., Assanangkornchai, S. and Jitpiromsri, S. (2005) Illicit substance supply and abuse in 2000–2004: an approach to assess the outcome of the war on drug operation. *Drug and Alcohol Review* 24: 461–466.

Rawson, R. A., Marinelli-Casey, P., Anglin, M. D., Dickow, A., Frazier, Y., Gallagher, C., Galloway, G. P., Herrell, J., Huber, A., McCann, M. J., Obert, J., Pennell, S., Reiber, C. and Vandersloot, D., Zweben, J. (2004) A multi-site comparison of psychosocial approaches for the treatment of methamphetamine dependence. *Addiction* 99: 708–717.

SHAN (2003) *Show Business: Rangoon 'War on Drugs' in Shan State*. Shan Herald Agency for News, December 2003, Rangoon.

Sattah, M. V., Supawitkul, S., Dondero, T. J., Kilmarx, P. H., Young, N. L., Mastro, T. D., Chaikummao, S., Manopaiboon, C. and Griensven, F. (2002) Prevalence of and risk factors for methamphetamine use in northern Thai youth: results of an audio-computer-assisted self-interviewing survey with urine testing. *Addiction* 97: 801–808.

Srisurapanont, M., Ali, R., Marsden, J., Sunga, A., Wada, K. and Monteiro, M. (2003) Psychotic symptoms in methamphetamine psychotic in-patients. *International Journal of Neuropsychopharmacology* 6: 347–352.

Sulzer, D., Sonders, M. S., Poulsen, N. W. and Galli, A. (2005) Mechanisms of neurotransmitter release by amphetamines: a review. *Progress in Neurobiology* 75: 406–433.

Surached, L. (2004) *A Comparative Study of Technical College Students and Rubber Plantation Labourers' Attitudes towards Methamphetamine Use in Chumpon Province, Thailand*. Unpublished MA Thesis, Macquarie University, Sydney.

Ubonrat, S. (2000) The ambiguity of the 'emerging' public sphere and the Thai media industry. In: Wang, G., Servaes, J. and Goonasekera, A. (eds), *The New Communications Landscape: Demystifying Media Globalization*. London: Routledge.

Van Der Geest, S. and Reynolds Whyte, S. (1989) The charm of medicines: metaphors and metonyms. *Medical Anthropology Quarterly* 3: 345–367.

Vongchak, T., Kawichai, S., Sherman, S., Celentano, D. D., Sirisanthana, T., Latkin, C., Wiboonnatakul, K., Srirak, N., Jittiwutikarn, J. and Aramrattana, A. (2005) The influence of Thailand's 2003 'war on drugs' policy on self-reported drug use among injection drug users in Chiang Mai, Thailand. *International Journal of Drug Policy* 16: 115–121.

Yawnghwe, C. (2005) Shan state politics: the opium-heroin factor. In: Jelsma, M., Kramer, T. and Vervest, P. (eds), *Trouble in the Triangle: Opium and Conflict in Burma. Chiang Mai: Silkworm Books*. Chiang Mai: Silkworm Books.

Zinberg, N. E. (1984) *Drug, Set and Setting: The Basis for Controlled Intoxicant Use*. New Haven, CT: Yale University Press.

Chapter 13

STIMULANT USE IN CENTRAL AND EASTERN EUROPE: HOW RECENT SOCIAL HISTORY SHAPED CURRENT DRUG CONSUMPTION PATTERNS

Jean-Paul Grund, Tomas Zabransky, Kevin S. Irwin and Robert Heimer

Overview

Current patterns of production and consumption of amphetamine-type stimulants (ATS) in Central and Eastern Europe (CEE) are best understood in historical context. ATS drug use, control and treatment in the region can be largely comprehended as artefacts of the social and political economies and ideologies of the former Soviet Union and its satellite countries. In this chapter, we draw upon our own studies and the available data regarding ATS use from several countries in the CEE region. We review the continuity and distinctions in the social structure of ATS; this use continues to be dominated by localised home-made production and small-group consumption patterns that were a product of the austere and controlled conditions of Communism. We then describe the health consequences for current users of ATS. These consequences are shaped by a legacy of punitive prohibition and drug treatment aimed at controlling individuals' threat to the collective interests of the state as suggested by the totalitarian regime. As the CEE geopolitical landscape grows ever more complex, multiple forms of reliable data are crucial to ensure state responses to ATS use that reflect fidelity to sound public health policy and programming, as well as evidence-based treatment.

Introduction: illicit drug use and recent social history in CEE

The recent social history of Central and Eastern Europe (CEE) has significantly influenced the use of psychotropic substances in this region and continues to do so today. Before the rise of communism, patterns of drug use in CEE were much like those in Western Europe. In the early twentieth century, drugs like opiates and cocaine were unregulated and their use in patent medicines was widespread (de Kort, 1995). In parts of Europe where poppy seeds remain a staple of the dessert menu, opiates were part of folk medicine and represented monetary value in many rural communities. Stricter regulation of psychoactive drugs gradually resulted in drug trafficking and use moving further underground, but illicit drugs remained part of trendy nightlife in most European capitals and major ports. Drugs – whether cannabis, cocaine, morphine or heroin – were often found where *high life* met *low life* and left their traces in music, literature and art. The establishment of the Soviet Union and its post–World War II expansion of hegemony westward resulted in CEE going in distinctly different directions, not only politically and economically but also culturally, from Western Europe.

With respect to the theme of this volume, we first of all argue that during the 1970s and 1980s a Soviet drug culture developed that was radically different from Western countries. In part, this development was fed by the different concepts of youth that emerged after World War II on different sides of the Iron Curtain. While in the market economies of the West new youth cultures developed in a time of increasing prosperity and decreasing parental control, the Eastern youth were subjected to state control through the *Pioneers, Komsomol, Socialist Youth Union* and other Communist Party youth movements.

When countercultures, such as the beat generation and the hippies, popularised drug use among youth in the Western hemisphere, few Eastern youngsters caught on and most made do with alcohol. Those that did catch on (and developed a drug appetite) had a problem: the drugs known from Western media and popularised by Soviet anti-drug propaganda that linked Western drugs to the needle were not readily available. While in the West an illicit global industry started catering to the drug tastes of the hippies and successive customers, the closed borders in the East resulted in a situation in which young people who were intent on using drugs had to turn to alternatives that were locally available or could be produced locally.

At first, just as drug experimenters in Europe and the USA used the Merck Manual to identify psychoactive compounds in the 1960s and 1970s, drug users in CEE during the late 1970s and 1980s gained knowledge of the psychoactive properties of various medications such as morphine (*Steklo*[1]), tramadol (Tramal), phenmetrazine (Fenmetrazin, *Dex*), codeine and phenobarbital containing composite analgesics (e.g. Alnagon or ketamine (Ketalar)). All of these diverted drugs have found their way into syringes and veins.

During the 1980s, various simple chemical recipes for producing potent injectable drugs, using natural ingredients or diverted medications and household chemicals, spread through underground drug user networks throughout the Communist world. In Poland, the production of an injectable opioid cocktail from poppy straw, called *kompot* (*cheornaya* in Russian because of its black colour), was traced back to chemistry students in Gdansk (Alcabes et al., 1998). In Czechoslovakia, in addition to an opioid mixture made of pharmaceuticals containing codeine (called *braun* because of its brown colour*)*, the recipe for *pervitin* or *piko* (methamphetamine) was attributed to a *Capo* of one of Prague's *squads* (see below) with the pseudonym *Freud* who had taken a few semesters of chemistry at technical university (Zábranský, 2007). The widespread presence of drug user/producer collectives across CEE suggests that in many places creative drug users turned to their chemistry class books to emulate the drugs of the West.

Later in this same time period, similar activity occurred elsewhere in the region regarding the production of amphetamine-type stimulants (ATS) derived from ephedrine or pseudoephedrine. Following the publications of a number of informative books about *vint* culture in Russia, such as *Nizshij pilotazh* (*Low Flying*) by Shiryanov in 2001, an important vehicle for the dissemination of information on the preparation of these compounds in the Russian-speaking world became the internet, especially the now defunct website www.vintclub.ru. Thus, drug users throughout this region gave their parents' tradition of *самогон* (*samagon*, Russian for moonshining or bootlegging alcohol) a whole new level of meaning. One of the most troubling aspects of this development is that most recipes resulted in drugs that were meant to be injected instead of being consumed by less dangerous and less addictive routes.

The Soviet Union developed specific drug laws and systems of substance abuse control and treatment (Butler, 2003). Inspired by the Communist ideology, Soviet drug legislation, its enforcement and the *narcology* system emphasised state control over the individual. Cloaking state control with the white coat was an almost universally accepted practice in communist psychiatry. As we explain below, the Soviet idea of treatment for substance abuse (and other *social diseases*) was characterised by a sequential execution of increasingly punitive and compulsory measures. Its involuntary nature reveals that legislators and health authorities had little confidence in voluntary actions of citizens.

Narcology and Soviet drug legislation served as models for most CEE countries after World War II (Grund, 2003). Thus, most countries inherited severely repressive legislation pertaining to drug users and other minorities considered deviant. Unlike the positive movements in various CEE countries concerning the civil rights of, for example, homosexuals or more pragmatic approaches to prostitution, the situation regarding drug control remains repressive and prohibitionist. In sum, the transition away from the Soviet system did little to reverse restrictive and counterproductive laws and policies related to drugs.

While few reliable data are available, the 1970s and 1980s in most Central European countries saw drug use remaining largely part of a subcultural undertow. But in Central Asia, use of opium, and subsequently heroin, turned out to be a growing side effect of the Afghan War (1979–1989), while in Russia veterans who had picked up an opiate habit during their service introduced drugs and drug knowledge to the friendship networks to which they returned. During the turbulent 1990s, the use of home-made opiates and amphetamines increased drastically throughout the region. Whereas Czech Police and medical authorities estimated the number of *all* illegal drug users[2] to be around 30 000 in the Czechoslovak Socialist Republic (population 15 million) of the 1980s (Nožina, 1997), in 1998 the estimated number of *problem* drug users (90% injectors) in the Czech Republic (population 10 million) was 33 000 (Mravčík and Zábranský, 2001). Only halfway through the 1990s did this come to the attention of the police, researchers and health authorities. When agencies such as the World Health Organisation (WHO) and United Nations Programme on HIV/AIDS (UNAIDS) realised the scope of the problem, yet another level was added to the meaning of *samagon*, as throughout the former Soviet Union (FSU) largely ignored epidemics of drug injection had set the stage for the epidemics of HIV and hepatitis C infection that now afflict the region.

Without a doubt, the introduction of the market economy and open borders has significantly expanded the drug economies in CEE countries, but this seems to have particularly affected the opiate economy. Heroin trafficking and use has replaced traditional home-made injectable opiates from poppies or pharmaceuticals (in, e.g., western Russia, Ukraine, Poland, Czech Republic, Slovakia and the Baltics) or opium gum (in, e.g., central Asia and Asiatic Russia), although outside central Asia this is often limited to the larger and more prosperous cities; in poorer cities and in rural areas users still primarily inject home-made opiates.

In most CEE countries, a similar trend towards criminal professionalisation around the production and distribution of ATS is far less apparent. *Therefore, the tradition of kitchen production continues to dominate stimulant use throughout the CEE region.* Consistent across the region is the use of ephedrine or pseudoephedrine as the starting material; what differs is whether the starting material is reduced to methamphetamine or oxidised to methcathinone. Also important in the context of recent and future European Union (EU) expansion is that use of ATS is more widespread in the western parts of the former East Block, that is in nations now inside or bordering the EU. Over time, this may influence patterns of drug use in the entire EU.

In this chapter, we focus on the two aspects that distinguish amphetamine and other drug use in CEE from that in Western Europe: the tradition of kitchen-produced amphetamines and opiates use and the Soviet narcology approach. We describe the production processes of methamphetamine and methcathinone, the networks that market them, and their consumers. We then describe the treatment available to stimulant users.

Data sources

Data on methamphetamine use in CEE are limited. This chapter is based on a review of published and grey literature, and the authors' research and policy work (both published and unpublished) in the region, which often included observational field notes and transcripts of interviews with drug users. The Eurasian Harm Reduction Network (EHRN) facilitated a call for methamphetamine-related information from the region that resulted in a number of unpublished manuscripts. We have also checked a number of points with prevention and treatment professionals from the region. Specifically in preparation for this chapter, interviews were conducted in Prague with a former methamphetamine user and with an outreach worker who has worked at 'cooking flats' for the last 15 years.

Self-produced methamphetamine and methcathinone: a primer on kitchen chemistry

Both methamphetamine and methcathinone are ephedrine-derived stimulants that appear to exert their psychopharmacological effect by a common mechanism that promotes the release of dopamine in the brain. Methamphetamine is known in the CEE region under names like *pervitin*,[3] *vint* or *bielie* (white); methcathinone

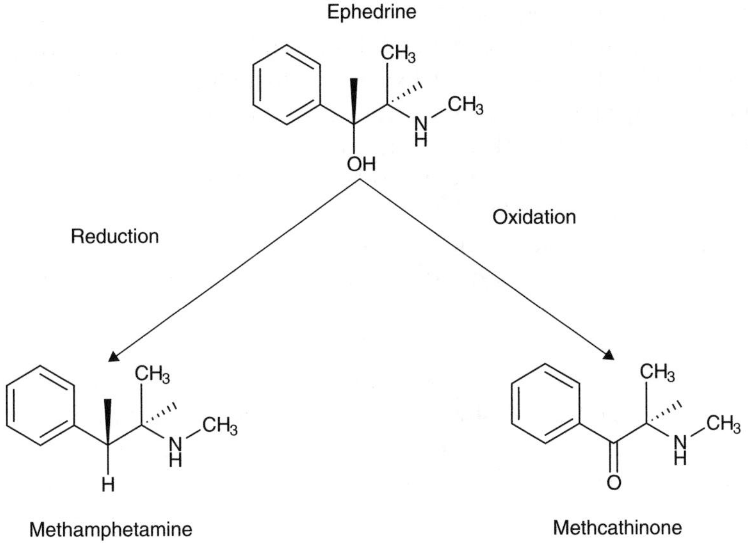

Ephedrine

Reduction

Oxidation

Methamphetamine

Methcathinone

Figure 13.1 Ephedrine-based stimulants.

is commonly referred to as *jeff* or *boltushka*.[4] The results of consuming these drugs, at least initially, include senses of well-being, physicality (including sexual stimulation), increased energy and increased attention. While the chemical structures of methamphetamine and methcathinone are similar, there are differences in the duration of the effects of each drug, the extent to which each heightens the above-mentioned psychological effects and the process required for their chemical synthesis. Methamphetamine is produced by reduction while methcathinone is produced by oxidation, which is a simpler, less dangerous but less favoured chemical reaction. The starting material, either ephedrine or pseudoephedrine, can be recovered from diverted decongestant and cold medications or from Chinese herbal preparations of ephedrine.[5] Here, we describe the processes that drug users use to produce these powerful stimulants (Figure 13.1).

Extracting ephedrine

Ephedrine and pseudoephedrine are used in a variety of common prescription medications and over-the-counter preparations in the CEE region, including cough syrups (Solutan), tablets, herbal energisers, crèmes and ointments. As one methamphetamine cook from the Russian city Kazan pointed out, extracting ephedrine from such preparations that are mixtures of many ingredients with a wide range of solubilities and viscosities requires specific knowledge, skills and ingredients:

After evaporating the alcohol, the content of a (50 ml) bottle of Solutan is mixed with an alkali (e.g. NaOH) and gasoline and shaken vigorously. After shaking, the liquid separates into 2 layers; the top yellow one contains the ephedrine, and the bottom, dark red one contains the waste. The yellow separation is filtered and funneled into another bottle, where HCl is added followed by further intense shaking. As a result, crystalline flakes appear at the base of the bottle, ranging in color from white (best) to light red (poorer quality). The gasoline is poured off and evaporated. The flakes are subsequently added to about 5 ml of water. More shaking results in a white liquid ephedrine solution, which then is dried on a standard ceramic plate or lab glass over moderate heat, leaving a soft crust of white ephedrine crystals. One bottle of Solutan will produce about 0.8 gr. of these ephedrine crystals, ready for making *vint*. (KSI field note excerpt, Kazan, Russia, 2004.)

There are many local recipes for extracting (pseudo)ephedrine across CEE. For example, in the Czech Republic, toluene or tetrachlorethylene is usually used instead of gasoline. Czech pervitin cooks consider gasoline inferior, 'unimaginable guck' according to one Czech pervitin cook (TZ, interview with ex-user, Zlin, Czech Republic, 2008).

Preparation of methamphetamine

Sergei arranged his materials on the kitchen table. He tapped out about 1 g of ephedrine crystals onto a magazine, then added red phosphorous powder from a small plastic bottle, about 3/4 the volume of crystals. He mixed these together and poured the mixture into a small brown bottle. After adding a few granules of iodine, he put on the bottle cover without the tube and holding his thumb over the opening swirled the contents vigorously, saying that the goal is to homogenise and start the reaction. Soon thereafter the mixture started bubbling. Small silver balls formed, which then formed one larger ball. After about 5–6 minutes he was satisfied with a dark and slightly reddish substance. He lit a candle, took off the stopper, added a few drops of sulphuric acid, put the pipette into the rubber stopper and re-capped the bottle. Holding the bottle by the stopper, he moved and turned the bottle over the flame, explaining that the goal is to cook without too much intense heat and to obtain a specific aroma, reminiscent of apples or violets. He smelled the mixture repeatedly, explaining that being able to recognise the appropriate smell is the key to making good *vint*. After about 15–20 minutes he removed the cover and blew the smoke away a few times. He then added 5 cm^3 of water into the reactor bottle, placed his thumb over the top and shook it hard. By now the colour was lighter, almost greenish. Slava then slightly bent the tip of the needle on the 20-cm^3 syringe and rolled up a ball of cotton over the tip. He said this is the *mitla*, or, the broom. Sergei drew up the solution from the reactor bottle, swiping the sides of the bottle clean, and then squeezing the cotton with his fingers to extract the last little bit. He discharged the solution into the water glass and added about a gram of soda, which started a slight reaction. Slava then made another broom and drew the final solution back up into the 20-cm^3 syringe. He said that they will wait for Sergei's wife to return from work before injecting the *vint*. (KSI field note excerpt, Kazan, Russia, 2004.)

In total the preparation of methamphetamine in this field note took about 45 minutes. Normally, this may be somewhat shorter as Sergey and Slava made extensive efforts to explain the cooking process. While the preparation of *vint* requires a level of sophistication in chemistry and cooks prefer the protected environment of an apartment's kitchen, *vint* can also be cooked outside as the first author observed on the bank of the Pskova river in Pskov, Russia in 1999.

The preparation of methamphetamine witnessed in the Czech Republic during field research by the second author was of the same chemical nature with slight variations in chemicals used, but the kitchen laboratory equipment was slightly more sophisticated. Czech *pervitin* cooks see a thermometer as imperative for the proper preparation of the drug, which relies, according to Czech traditional drug lore, for a large part on the 'magical temperature of 127°C'. 'Over 132°C everything would be fucked up' (field notes of the researcher). Another difference is that Czech *pervitin* cooks normally crystallise the solution Sergey and Slava ended up with and subsequently use fresh (sometimes distilled or even physiological saline) water to dissolve the crystals and inject. Injecting the cooked solution immediately is frowned upon by Czech *pervitin* users. As one injector explained, 'That is something too bad to do even in the worst cold turkey – you can wait another 15 minutes, can't you?' (field notes of the researcher). Crystallisation further represents a more sophisticated measure of quality control for both the cook and the user. The colour of the resulting crystals allows for assessment of quality, as another explained, '[w]hen it is yellowish, it means too much acid being added and that is no good for your veins; pink and red means remnants of phosphor and that poisons your nerves and brain; and grey pervitin means that temperatures were bad and then the effects of pervitin are bad, too: you get too jittery, and sometimes paranoia.' Last but not least, crystallised *pervitin* can be crushed and the powder snorted, which is favoured by recreational and younger Czech users.

Preparation of methcathinone

Unlike the reduction of ephedrine to methamphetamine, methcathinone is a product of oxidation of (pseudo)ephedrine. This reaction is gentler and less prone to creating a toxic working place. However, the reaction is quite exothermic and the heat generated can cause the expansion of gases that can explode closed reaction vessels. Therefore, any open glass vessel will do as seen in the following excerpt of a field note:

Denis explains that *jeff* (methcatinone) is made of ephedrine, household vinegar, permanganate and water. 'Preparing *jeff* is very easy and straightforward', he says. He puts the ephedrine powder in a drinking glass, adds water, vinegar and the permanganate. When the permanganate hits the water, the solution turns a deep purple. He stirs the mixture vigorously for some 15–20 minutes at room temperature. He looks at and sniffs the solution several times, which slowly changes color to a dark brown. When this is the case he draws the drug into a 20 ml syringe through a cotton filter, pulling up about 15 ml of clear and colorless liquid. He attaches a new (large bore) needle to the barrel and shoots the contents into a vein in his right underarm. This clearly produces a big rush as he lies down on the bed and closes his eyes, but within 10 minutes he is participating in the conversation again. (JPG field note excerpt, Pskov, Russia, 1999.)

The preparation of methcathinone takes significantly shorter time than methamphetamine, about 15–20 minutes. Despite this shorter cooking time and the more challenging chemistry of methamphetamine, (pseudo)ephedrine reduction to methamphetamine is generally favoured over methcathinone since the former produces a stronger and longer-lasting effect. Which drug is prepared largely depends on the other chemicals available and the knowledge of the chemist. Better informed respondents suggest that methcathinone is prepared when the chemicals for methamphetamine are not available or when one does not have time to prepare methamphetamine, which takes about twice as long as cooking up methcathinone. We have found that those with insufficient chemistry knowledge reported to us that they were making *vint*, but an analysis of their descriptions of the process revealed them to be making *jeff*.

The setting of home-produced stimulants: users, producers, networks and markets

Both the processes described above, with many variations, were rediscovered and adapted to the limitations of *kitchen chemistry* in the days of communism, as were the many recipes for home-made heroin from poppies, opium gum and opioid-based (e.g. codeine) pharmaceuticals. Stimulant recipes remain widely circulated up to the present day in many former Communist countries. Similarly, as drug use continues to be severely punished under post-Soviet law, manufacturing of ephedrine-based stimulants for anything more than an occasional high for a small group of friends requires a sophisticated level of underground organisation.

John (1986) described groups of drug-using friends and associates in the Prague drug scene of the early 1980s, called *squads**, in which individuals from different walks of life took on specialised roles and skills in the drug production process (supply of ingredients, chemicals, (kitchen) laboratory equipment, processing location and chemistry skills) were divided between squad members. Before the political changes, methamphetamine was almost exclusively produced and available in these tight-knit friendship groups. According to Zábranský (2007), the 'social inclusiveness' of the *squads**, in which youth and young adults from families of workers, intellectuals and Communist *nomenclatura* alike participated and collaborated, is an example of the Communist-induced *social levelling*. During the

---

* "party" [paar-teeh] in Czech.

1990s, the authors observed this phenomenon in several CEE cities, and it remains the case that many drug injectors in the larger cities are fairly well educated (Kozlov et al., 2006), although they are also unemployed or under-employed and have high levels of arrest and incarceration (Booth et al., 2008). In smaller cities and rural areas in particular, however, drug injection has over the years become increasingly associated with unemployment, poverty and social exclusion (Atrill et al., 2001; Balakireva et al., 2006; Chintalova-Dallas et al., 2006; Grund et al., 2007; Schiffer and Schatz, 2008).

As in the West, the diffusion of illicit drug patterns seems to go hand-in-hand with social descent – that is, illicit drugs are mostly introduced in rather exclusive (middle class or, as in Czechoslovakia, socially levelled) environments, but when they spread into wider society, they tend to seek out more vulnerable populations, in which they merge with more serious social and health problems. Such *disease clustering* (Knox, 1989) or *syndemics* (Singer and Clair, 2003) can often lead to increased visibility and public concern. According to March et al. (2006), personal, social and economic conditions are all linked in a process of social exclusion that compounds the problem of drug misuse. Throughout CEE minority populations are disproportionally affected by drug injection and HIV, in particular the Roma (Grund et al., 2007). In, for example, Latvia and Estonia, young Russian (and Roma) males are over-represented among problem drug users, and in Estonia HIV prevalence among drug users is concentrated in those of Russian ethnicity (Uusküla et al., 2007). This has been linked to the geopolitical changes that turned the Russians into a *new* disenfranchised minority with all the associated problems (Downes, 2003).

Minority and other problematic users mostly consume opiates in this region. As in the West, stimulants seem to attract more differentiated user populations with more varied use patterns. In the Czech Republic, *pervitin* use is reported in all social classes, while in many of the larger cities in the region (recreational) use of methamphetamine is part of the dance scene (Zábranský, 2007). Methamphetamine users are mostly younger than opiate users (Balakireva et al., 2006; Chintalova-Dallas et al., 2006). Balakireva et al. (2006) suggest that for many Ukrainian youngsters amphetamines may be the first hard drug they use, often by injection.

Our studies in Russia and other post-Soviet countries suggest that many characteristics of the social structure of methamphetamine use and production have remained largely unaltered after the regime change. Networks of methamphetamine users have become larger, but less inclusive, and more concentrated in larger social networks of often disenfranchised youth who may or may not experiment with (injectable) drugs (Balakireva et al., 2006; Des Jarlais et al., 2002; Miovský and Zábranský, 2001). In a study conducted in St Petersburg in 2002–2003, 37% of the drug users had injected a stimulant in the month prior to interview and only 4% had injected stimulants exclusively. Nevertheless, HIV incidence was associated with stimulant injection and the likelihood was highest in those who injected only stimulants (Kozlov et al., 2006).

While in Lithuania CEE laboratory-produced amphetamine sulphate seems to have become available (Kestutis Butkus, Association *TAVO DRUGYS*[6], personal communication, 2007), in most countries home production remains popular. As activities unknown during Soviet times, such as street drug markets or mobile phone-based drug markets, contribute to weaker and more diffuse drug use networks, the modus operandi of home-produced drugs requires drug users to collaborate and regularly socialise with each other. Our studies indeed indicate that most home-produced drugs are shared among the members of small, often connected networks of mostly 2–5 drug-using friends. Users pool money and collaborate in covertly organising drug production and consumption and acquiring the required precursors and chemicals. Some have access to the precursor (ephedrine) through the family medicine cabinet or (hospital) pharmacies, and others obtain processing chemicals. Another can provide his kitchen, but the cook plays a central role, as only he or she has the knowledge to 'Practice a little Witchcraft', as one Russian *vint* cook explained. Most chemicals required in the home production of ATS can in principle be purchased from pharmacies, drug stores, battery stores and gasoline stations, but in practice quite some efforts are required to obtain all chemicals, especially when purchasing on a regular basis and when there is a need to avoid drawing attention to oneself. But this is not always the case; in 2004, we witnessed open sales of all reactants necessary to make *vint* at the Lubyanka metro station in Moscow. An old woman was selling Solutan in blue bottles on one stairway, and a veteran of the Afghan War missing one leg at the knee was selling the iodine and red phosphorus on the adjacent stairway. The police regularly patrolling the station chose to ignore them, but did move to harass particular young men who approached the vendors. Exactly how the police decided whom to harass was unclear, but it was clear that not all purchasers where subject to harassment.

Since the changes in the drug laws in Russia and most other CEE countries in the second half of the 1990s, medications containing ephedrine or pseudoephedrine are officially only available by prescription. Injection drug users (IDUs) in Russia explained that nowadays Solutan and other 'precursor' medications are harder to get from pharmacies. Nevertheless, our (RH, KSI) efforts to purchase Solutan from pharmacies in St Petersburg without a prescription were successful. In far eastern Russia, Chinese ephedrine tonics still appeared to be widespread during our visit there in 2004. Stricter controls have reduced the availability of diverted pseudoephedrine-based medications and raised the price of products such as Solutan severalfold in the shadow economy, but a number of medications containing pseudoephedrine are commonly available over the counter.

Where there is a demand, it will likely be met. Over the years, methamphetamine injectors bought precursors and processing chemicals from various types of suppliers. During the second half of the 1990s, *babushki* ('grandmas' in Russian) sold their ephedrine-based prescriptions on the squares of St Petersburg. More recently users report buying ephedrine tablets and industrial crystal ephedrine, imported illegally from China, Romania and other countries. While these *babushki* disappeared from the streets in some places, ephedrine and pseudoephedrine now often reaches users through sales at unregulated 'flea markets', such as one held on Fridays and Saturdays in Yekaterinburg, from members of disenfranchised (minority) communities, or via small entrepreneurs who are used to navigating the darker shades of grey in the shadow economy. In addition, as already indicated, medications containing small doses of pseudoephedrine can be purchased over the counter, without a prescription.

The above production field notes suggest that home production of methamphetamine or methcathinone in Russia (and other FSU countries) usually ends up in a small batch (containing $\leq$ 1g of the active drug) of liquid stimulant that is injected in a group of drug-using friends – either immediately or shortly after. This fitted rather snugly with the Soviet tradition of routinely injecting antibiotics and other medications.

We have not observed users in Russia or other FSU countries who dried and crystallised their product, either for personal storage or small-scale sale to other stimulant users. In the Czech Republic – where in contrast with all other countries in the region, methamphetamine is traditionally not a secondary but the number one illicit drug – our fieldwork and focus groups with low-threshold drug workers suggest a higher degree of commoditisation. In Prague, *piko* produced by small user-producers is first crystallised and consumed after re-dissolving the crystals in water. A part may be stored 'for later' or for small-scale business. Czech 'squads', typically about 3–8 people large, often end up with 1–3 g of pervitin. Usually IDUs themselves, these small-scale producers are the source for pervitin crystals for other (known) users. Injection is also the prevailing pattern for other problem drug users (some 80% of those in contact with specialised medical and/or non-medical services).

Since 2001 the use of *pervitin* in the Czech dance scene has steadily increased (Kubů et al., 2006; Mravčík et al., 2008). Among recreational and occasional users, the drug is mostly snorted, especially within a distinct subpopulation of stimulant users, subject to different trends and influences such as the popularity of ecstasy XTC in the (international) dance scene. According to key informants from the electronic dance scene, methamphetamine has been often marketed as cocaine in the second half of 2000s (unpublished research of the second author); this fake cocaine[7] reflects the increasing popularity and higher price of yet another 'Western drug' in the Czech Republic. The increasing popularity of pervitin among recreational users in the (commercial) dance and club scene may well induce further professionalisation of production and trafficking of methamphetamine in the Czech Republic, from 'home production' to 'garage production'. In 2008, for the first time in Czech history, the Czech police reported a crackdown of two methamphetamine laboratories in garages in the Prague suburbs with a reported capacity of tens of grams of pervitin per day (see, e.g., ČTK, 2008).

Nonetheless, such market changes are difficult to assess since few actual studies have been conducted. After the shutdown of a legal pharmaceutical ephedrine factory close to Prague in 2004–2005, there was a noticeable shift towards the use of pseudoephedrine-containing medications by small-scale producers. Local police estimate that 90% of the methamphetamine on the market results from small-scale home production. However, Zábranský (2007) suggests that the proportion of home-produced methamphetamine on the Czech markets may be overestimated by the police, as they only catch small-scale producers (often after neighbourhood complaints), while the Czech customs regularly seize larger quantities (kilos) of ephedrine imported from Asia, Balkan countries and Eastern Europe that most probably have their (so far unidentified) buyers in the country.

Current epidemiology of stimulant use in selected CEE countries

Few reliable data are available on stimulant use in this region, and this review of current epidemiology is therefore limited. Here, we present data on new EU member states, Russia and a number of FSU states. Many surveys in the EU countries collapse methamphetamine and amphetamine (sulphate) into one category, making it impossible to make inferences about trends in consumption of the different ATS (European Monitoring Centre for Drugs and Drug Addiction (EMCDDA), 2008).

Czech Republic

According to a recent overview, methamphetamine use and abuse is rare compared to other illegal drugs in the EU with two marked exceptions: the Czech and Slovak Republics (Griffiths et al., 2008). The Czech Republic represents a special case, different from other CEE countries, as for the last 35 years *pervitin* has consistently been the main problem drug. Methamphetamine accounts for two-thirds of the problem drug users[8] in the Czech Republic (presently estimated at 31 000). *Pervitin* users represent the majority of those seeking drug treatment in the Czech Republic (58%, i.e. 4889 persons) and 62% (2528 persons) of first-time treatment applications in 2006, and they represent 63% (i.e. 12 100 persons) of drug injectors who used low-threshold services in 2006. *Pervitin* users in the Czech Republic seek treatment services sooner after starting to use the drug and have more treatment episodes before achieving abstinence than users of opiates and other illicit drugs. Czech pervitin injectors do not differ in seroprevalence of viral hepatitis C compared with Czech opiate injectors (both about 35%), and the prevalence of HIV is very low in both groups. Contrary to its prominence in problem drug use, pervitin is only the third cause of fatal drug overdose. In the Czech general population or school surveys, *pervitin* ranks fifth among illegal drugs consumed. Only 5% of the estimated Czech yearly consumption of pervitin (3133 kg) is in the recreational drug scene (Vopravil and Český statistický úřad, 2005), but the lifetime prevalence in clubbers is steadily increasing (Kubů et al., 2006; Mravčík et al., 2008). Overall, of the 2165 drug arrests made in 2006, 60% were associated with pervitin.

Slovak Republic

What is now the Slovak Republic never experienced major problems with methamphetamine when it was part of the Czechoslovak Federative (Socialist) Republic, during the Communist regime (until the end of 1989) or in the transition period until 31 December 1993, when Czechoslovakia was split into two separate countries. Around 2000, however, Czech know-how on methamphetamine preparation started to diffuse into Slovakia (Zábranský, 2002), soon followed by a sharp increase in both percentage and absolute number of those in abstinence-oriented medical treatment due to methamphetamines (NMCD, 2007). Methamphetamine now represents the most frequently cited *primary drug* among those seeking treatment in Slovakia and about 38% of those seeking harm reduction services are methamphetamine injectors.

The estimated number of problem users of *pervitin* is 13 000 (of the estimated 18 900 of all problem drug users) (NMCD, 2007). A study of drug-using sex workers in Bratislava also suggested a preference of pervitin over heroin: 63% of 98 sex workers used pervitin regularly, and 37% used heroin (OZ Prima, 2007). Due to major (drug) law reform in 2006, recent criminal statistics in Slovakia are not available. However, the overview of Griffiths et al. (2008) suggests that among EU countries, only Czech Republic and Slovak Republic reported dismantling of methamphetamine (kitchen) 'laboratories' in 2004 and 2005 (no newer EU-wide data available).

Other new EU Member States

Estonia reports one methamphetamine laboratory dismantled in 2005 and substantial seizures of methamphetamine (54 kg in 2004 and 13.5 kg in 2005) (Oole et al., 2006). Estonian population surveys of 1998 and 2003 and ESPAD (European School Survey Project on Alcohol and Other Drugs) surveys suggest that in the general and school populations (meth)amphetamines are most frequently used after cannabis and ecstasy. Tallinn has a vibrant club culture and, as in many other places, the consumption of illicit drugs (such as ecstasy, ATS, and cannabis) is an integral feature of this youth subculture (Allaste and Lagerspetz, 2002). In 2005, the unofficial '*guestimate*' was that there were between 10 000 and 15 000 IDUs in Estonia, primarily opiate injectors, while a significant minority injected ATS. Opiate injectors are mostly Russian speakers, while ATS injecting seems more common among ethnic Estonians. Estonian drug experts emphasised that IDUs in Estonia, in particular stimulant injectors, are very young. NGOs that organise needle exchange in Tallinn estimated that there were 6000–10 000 IDUs in the capital in 2005; of those, 60% reportedly injected heroin and 40% ATS (Grund, 2005).

According to UNODC's World Drug Report 2007, the highest prevalence of ATS use in Europe is reported in Estonia (and the UK and Denmark[9]) (UNODC, 2007), but only 1.4% of drug treatment clients in Estonia are ATS users (unpublished drug treatment data, NIHD, Estonia). First-time and repeating visitors of syringe exchange programmes in 2006 most frequently injected amphetamines (53%) in the last 4 weeks, followed by heroin (40.9%), home-produced opiates (38.9%) and fentanyl (9.1%) (Abel-Ollo et al., 2007). A behavioural respondent-driven sampling study of IDUs found that 63% had used amphetamine within the previous 4 weeks, while for 19% it was their main drug (Uusküla et al., 2005).

The Lithuanian ESPAD survey of 2003 measured 6% lifetime prevalence of amphetamine use in the school population (Hibbell et al., 2004). In 2006, 16 kg of methamphetamines was seized from Lithuanian citizens arrested abroad (in Denmark, Belarus, Sweden and Russia) for possession or smuggling of larger amounts of drugs (Lithuanian Annual Report to EMCDDA 2006). Sixty-four per cent of Latvian clients of low-threshold centres are ATS users, yet most drug treatment at the Riga Centre of Psychiatry and Addiction Disorders is provided to heroin injectors (Grund, 2007). The Latvian Organized Crime Enforcement Bureau identifies Lithuania as the source of methamphetamine (Latvian National Focal Point, 2008).

Griffiths et al. (2008) refer to 'relatively high levels of methamphetamine use among some population groups in Hungary'. According to the Hungarian Annual EMCDDA Report, the number of people in treatment due to amphetamine-type drugs almost doubled between 2000 and 2006, to about 1500 patients. In 2006, six deadly ATS overdoses were registered (Drog Fokuszpont, 2006).

A recent EMCDDA report (2008) mentioned anecdotal accounts of increasing methamphetamine use from several CEE countries including Latvia and Bulgaria.

Ukraine

A recent study from Kiev, Ukraine, suggests that 68.8% of injectors in the city have injected pseudoephedrine-based drugs in past 1 month prior to interview (Booth et al., 2008). Another Ukrainian study among 808 young (under 24) IDUs suggested that, after home-produced opiates, stimulants (both methamphetamine and methcathinone) are most frequently the first drugs injected (Balakireva et al., 2006). Another study suggests that methcathinone or *boltushka* had become increasingly popular among the very young and very poor of the city of Odessa in the late 1990s and 2000s (Chintalova-Dallas et al., 2006).

Russia

Studies of Russian IDUs suggest that ATS are an important but secondary drug among Russian IDUs. In our studies from 11 Russian cities, from 15 to 89% of IDUs had injected stimulants at least once in their lifetime and 0–43% had done so in the 30 days prior to being interviewed, whereas 90% had injected heroin in the same 30-day period (Borodkina et al., 2005). There was an association between cities with high lifetime experience of ATS injection and high levels of recent ATS injection (Spearman $p < 0.005$). The six cities in which the majority of IDUs had lifetime experience of injecting ATS also had highest levels of recent injection. In our studies conducted solely in St Petersburg, 27% of 492 IDUs we interviewed between 2005 and 2008 had injected ATS in the 30 days prior to interview (White et al., 2008). This is a decrease from 36% of IDUs who reported recent use in 2002–2003 (Shaboltas et al., 2006). Our experience in St Petersburg suggests that there is a small core of IDUs who use only ATS; during both periods, the percentage of injectors who injected only ATS was small – 5% or less of the individuals we interviewed. There is a larger number who will use both ATS and heroin, and the shift between drugs seems to depend on availability, since the period of time with the highest percentage of ATS injectors coincided with a drought in heroin brought on by the US invasion of Afghanistan.

Other FSU states

The second author's regular contacts with treatment and prevention professionals in the post-Soviet countries suggest increasing concern with methamphetamine and methcathinone use in both urban and rural areas of Ukraine (see also Booth et al., 2006, 2008) and increasing use in Moldova (Scicutelnicuc et al., 2007) . While they scored poor in terms of drug preference in a recent Georgian survey among users of harm-reduction services, ephedrine-based stimulants were the drugs most frequently used in the month before the interview (Otiashvili et al., 2008).

Interventions

Globally, the abuse of methamphetamine and other ATS has become a primary concern only in the last 10–15 years. In most countries concerns over heroin and subsequently cocaine has dominated the research, policy and treatment agendas. The effects and physical, psychological and behavioural correlates associated with stimulant use are extensively discussed by Hildrey, Thomas and Smith in Chapter 2 and Pates and Riley in Chapter 3, while various chapter authors discuss (emerging) treatment approaches towards the problem of ATS use. Worldwide, specific approaches towards ATS dependence are developing only slowly. In the CEE region not only has the shape of the drug culture been determined by the totalitarian past, but so too has the response to drug use and drug-related problems. The substance abuse treatment systems in this region have not responded well to the changing social *risk environment* (Rhodes, 2002) that was brought about by the political changes that have taken place since the early 1990s. In trying to understand this situation, we discuss the history of dependence treatment in CEE.

Historical context: narcology, the Soviet approach to drug use and deviance

Trust is good, control is better (Lenin)

Most CEE countries inherited severely repressive vice legislation pertaining to drug users, sex workers and sexual minorities. Drug legislation and control have firm roots in the models of disease and deviance control of the FSU. Health care was organised according to the same doctrine that defined the economy, the educational system, internal security and crime control, as well as just about every other aspect of public life. Prioritising collectivist ideals over individual citizens' interests and rights, the state had appropriated responsibility for many aspects of life that in truly democratic societies are left, once within the legal parameters set by an independent judiciary, to the individual, 'civil society' and the market. The response to problematic alcohol use, drug use, and psychiatric problems and, for that matter, political dissent ('social diseases') was organised on principles that left little room for the rights of the individual. Drug treatment may have been available free of charge, but in exchange individuals seeking this care were expected to give up many rights and privileges. And since drug users were viewed as deviants, little attention was paid to making drug treatment actually work. As a consequence, evidence-based treatment efforts have made only slow headway in parts of CEE.

The system of *disease control* was, at best, based on tacit consent and, at worst, mandatory measures. In cases of poor treatment outcome, relapse (drug use, casual sex) or non-compliance, health authorities quickly resorted to progressively more punitive measures in order to protect the interests of the collective and re-educate ir-responsible individuals about their responsibilities towards the collective. If deemed necessary, control was asserted with the help of the militia and ultimately through re-education in social adaptation or labour camps, run by law enforcement author-ities. The Soviet legislators and health authorities had little confidence in voluntary actions of individual citizens.

This philosophy permeated laws pertaining to drug use, prostitution, sexual minorities and infectious diseases, and was given expression through vertically or-ganised health care systems of so-called narcology[10] that remain in place in many countries in the region. The narcology approach included a *narcological commis-sion*, a system of patient triage by three senior *narcologists* and three levels of treatment: (i) (nominally) voluntary ambulatory or inpatient treatment at a *narco-logical* dispensary, (ii) compulsory inpatient treatment at a *narcological* dispensary or other psychiatric institution and (iii) incarceration in a social adaptation institu-tion, run by the Ministry of Justice or prison authorities. The latter two levels were based on court-ordered sanctions. In short, narcology, the Soviet concept of sub-stance abuse treatment, was characterised by a sequential execution of increasingly punitive and compulsory measures.

Police and narcology/psychiatry both played an important role in controlling *vice* in the CCCP[11] and its satellite regimes. 'Moral police' departments, whose primary targets were drug users, prostitutes and sexual minorities, had a sepa-rate status within the law enforcement structure. Traditionally, the police and narcology cooperated closely. Together they maintained the *Narcological Register* (*narkalagičeskiy atschot*), and the local *Chief Narcologist* kept close relationships with the chief of the (narcotics) police.

In 1996 the first author (JPG), while conducting an assessment mission in Temir-tau in northeast Kazakhstan, met with the chiefs of the AIDS centre and the nar-cology centre. He proposed to invite the chief of police:

> At next day's meeting the police chief was indeed present. The first thing he said to me was: 'How many *narcomans* do you want my men to pick up? 50? 100?' I did not respond and after a short silence he burst out in laughter and said he was only joking. Nonetheless, by arresting registered drug injectors is exactly how the authorities first found out about the HIV epidemic that was rapidly spreading in this town. (JPG, Kazakhstan mission notes, June 1996.)

Thus, disease control was part of a wider scheme of population control by the state. *Narcology* was established to control people, not really to help them. Only when they *behaved did* patients *deserve* help. Treatment of any drug problem consisted mostly of detoxification only with drug users either back on the streets after 1–3 weeks (often more vulnerable to overdose) or, in case of repeat offenders, entering compulsory treatment in closed institutions. Narcology has not been based on generally recognised evidence-based concepts of addiction and best practice in treatment, while detoxification is perhaps the least complicated (and not inevitably necessary) part. Recent interviews with Russian *narcologists* and with head narcologists in several other FSU states confirmed that they recognised the inadequacy of their approach, but a substantial number of *narcologists* also reinforced the idea that outcomes mattered less than maintaining the defence that treatment failure was the fault of the patient and not of the treatment.

From control to treatment: a long and winding road

Within the context of the closed Communist society, Lenin's adagio worked fairly well in dealing with classic infectious diseases (TB, STIs). The system never worked to control alcohol or drug abuse, and in the post-Communist era this system fell apart through chronic underfunding, decreased political support, but, above all, because of social demographic changes and increased freedom under unfortunate economic conditions. The result is a narcology system that is completely out of touch with reality, including the changing morality and practices among youth about sex and drug use.

The rise in STIs in the region during the early 1990s should have been a warning sign hinting at widespread adoption of Western liberalised behaviours, with their attendant risks. Although the post-Soviet system did manage to control the increase in STIs, it could not handle the increase in drug use. Used to treating alcoholics, the narcology system (and the completely unconnected infectious disease control system) found itself ill-equipped when in the second half of the 1990s HIV and hepatitis infections exploded in largely undetected populations of IDUs throughout much of the FSU, most notably Russia, Ukraine, Latvia and Estonia.

In contrast, similar epidemics have by and large been averted in most Central European countries. HIV has not significantly spread in the Czech and Slovak Republics, or Hungary, and its epidemic spread was controlled in Slovenia and Poland. Most Balkan countries have not reported many HIV cases either, although Serbia experienced a serious HIV epidemic among IDUs, of which the current status is not completely clear. While scientific evidence is scarce, according to Zábranský (in press) the following elements are present in discussions on the absence of HIV epidemics in Central Europe: (i) a low level of HIV seroprevalence in at-risk populations in early 1990s, (ii) the early introduction of harm reduction responses such as government- or NGO-supported needle exchange programmes (as early as 1991 in Slovenia and 1992 in Czech Republic), (iii) universal health insurance that allows at least a basic level of treatment to everyone who applies and (iv) quick reform of the centralised narcology-like system into more flexible systems of medical and social care for drug users with involvement of non-medical providers and the non-governmental sector (for that aspect see, e.g., Csémy and Elekes, 2001).

Restructuring pertinent legislation and the provision of health care, making them responsive to the large expansion of injection drug use, cannot be a stand-alone or one-time measure, but must be part of a larger, continuing, and strenuous social and economic transition process. The narcology ideology outlined above is still evident in present legislative documents and in practice, in particular those relating to disease control and citizens considered deviant – drug users, prostitutes and sexual minorities. In several post-Communist countries, involuntary measures remain the defining feature of the response to these and other vulnerable groups.

Most western European countries, confronted with evidence of epidemic spread of HIV or hepatitis among its injectors, developed policies and services that have effectively controlled this aspect of the HIV epidemic. But CEE countries and in particular those of the FSU must now develop effective measures – under great time pressure – to either curb or avert the twin epidemics of drug injecting and HIV. Soviet heritage in law and medical practice, the painful process of transition, and chronic underfunding all thwart swift implementation of necessary interventions. Furthermore, several post-Communist countries do not have a pre-1989 history of democracy. In all countries in this region, protagonists of harm reduction and evidence-based interventions must face the lingering Soviet mentality that is out of sync with the principles of modern public health.

Lithuania, the Czech Republic and several other countries in CEE have abandoned narcology-inspired substance abuse treatment after the political changes – the Czech Republic did so as early as 1992. In countries such as Latvia, Slovakia, other new EU member states and throughout the Commonwealth of Independent States/FSU (Former Soviet Union), however, different variations of the centralised narcology system survived the transition to democracy. Thus, many CEE countries still have a substance abuse treatment system rooted in totalitarianism, although – often under the influence of international organisations and funding, and to different degree in different countries – with a more human face. The narcology approach in many of these countries can hardly be labelled as addiction treatment or considered a scientifically based discipline, inspired by human rights and public health concerns. At best, it is a set of guidelines on providing detoxification, in most cases without follow-up treatment. Problem drug use, or more correctly, any form of drug use, is both criminalised and medicalised. Recreational use of illicit drugs is viewed as an early stage of disease, while doctor–patient relationships are characterised by inequality. With its history and present poor record, drug treatment for many drug users in CEE remains an *unmerry go round*, where possible to be avoided. This is evidenced by the decreasing use of narcology services in most parts of Russia (Heimer et al., 2007), which has also led to an under-reporting of the extent of the HIV epidemic, since it was through testing at narcology services that the epidemic growth of HIV among drug users first came to public attention (Feshbach and Galvin, 2005; Grund et al., 2003).

Nonetheless, several countries in the region have to various degrees introduced evidence-based prevention and treatment methods towards problem drug use and

HIV. This has remained by and large limited to opioid use. Quite a few FSU countries have introduced methadone treatment for opiate-addicted people, but only recently have some begun scaling up MMT (Fiellin et al., 2008). In the past years, substitution treatment for opiate addiction has been introduced in Estonia, Bulgaria, Ukraine, Kyrgyzstan, Georgia and Moldova, many with the support of international organisations and GFATM (Fund to Fight AIDS, Tuberculosis and Malaria) funding (Fiellin et al., 2008). Likewise, in most countries in the region (mostly NGO-based) non-medical treatment (e.g. therapeutic communities) and harm reduction (needle exchange, outreach, condom provision) interventions have been developed in response to drug injection and HIV. However, in most countries the coverage provided by these initiatives remains limited due to structural under-funding and difficulties in maintaining a regular supply of harm reduction supplies or treatment medications. In Slovakia, harm reduction services experienced a decrease in governmental funding and the needle exchange programmes network that was rather insufficient so far is close to non-existent now. Shortages of drugs to treat HIV or to provide substitution therapy for opioid addiction have recently been encountered in Moldova, Georgia, Russia and Ukraine. Without GFATM or other international funding many antiretroviral treatment activities and most harm reduction work in the region would probably vanish.

Treatment for ATS dependence

Treatment *designed for* stimulant users is non-existent in this region, except perhaps in the Czech Republic, which might have the longest history of illicit methamphetamine use (some 35 years). The difficulty in finding workable, evidence-based treatment for ATS addiction is not restricted to this region; little headway has been made anywhere in developing effective treatment approaches.

In the Czech Republic, all substance abuse treatment other than for alcoholics was developed for pervitin users, since they were dominating the Czech drug scene into the early 1990s. In Communist times, there were few users of home-made opiates in the Czech Republic, while heroin appeared only in 1992–1993. When heroin use increased, heroin users were being treated in the same institutions and mostly on the same wards as methamphetamine users. After one interrupted unofficial substitution programme in 1992 and another 2 years of 'piloting' in 1999, methadone treatment was standardised in the Czech Republic and presently over 600 heroin-dependent people are in methadone treatment, while some 2500 receive buprenorphine treatment.

At present, detoxification is the primary treatment mode for methamphetamine dependence in the Czech Republic and in other CEE countries where the abuse of ATS drugs is a problem. Detoxification services are rather widely available in the Czech Republic. Detoxified patients can be referred to either ambulatory or inpatient rehabilitation, including a wide spectrum of *treatment modalities* from therapeutic communities to ambulatory cognitive behavioural therapy. Post-detoxification drug treatment is provided by both state and NGO programmes, and in a few private institutions. Whereas in opiates detoxification inter alia opiate-type pharmaceuticals are used quite widely, stimulant abstinence syndromes are allevi-ated only with anxiolytics, hypnotics or other psychotropic drugs used in opiate detoxification as well. Few provide aftercare services such as sheltered housing or job training and placement programmes. Except for in the methadone programmes, in all drop-in centres, outreach programmes, clinics, ambulances and therapeutic communities a majority of (ex-) methamphetamine users and a minority of (ex-) opiate users continue to be treated equally, that is with the same treatment philoso-phies and approaches. Even the Czech Republic does not seem to have escaped completely from the overall trends in this region that the primary drug treatment methods are abstinence-based, have been simply adjusted from (rather unsuccess-ful) alcohol treatment and are not drug specific. That is, the part of treatments that is based in medical institutions make little distinction between alcohol, opioid and stimulant users.

If countries have implemented substance-specific treatment, it is methadone or other substitution treatment for opiate addiction. Stimulant substitution (e.g. with methylphenidate or dexamphetamine), contingency management and other treat-ment options that might work with stimulant users have only recently emerged as topics of discussion among internationally oriented treatment professionals, but they are not likely to be implemented for some time. In the Czech Republic, preparations have recently started for a clinical trial of substitution treatment with methylphenidate. Meanwhile, several Czech doctors experiment with prescribing medications such as Ritalin to their long-term, chronic patients. This practice is technically not at odds with the legal provisions concerning drug treatment, and doctors have not been charged with infractions, although it is not sanctioned by medical board guidelines (see, e.g., Hampl, 2004). A clinical trial on metham-phetamine treatment using contingency management is planned for spring 2009 in the Czech Republic and possibly in Slovakia.

Discussion

In this chapter, we have explored how the social history of CEE has influenced the use of ATS and other drugs in this region and the degree to which it continues to do so until today. We have attempted to describe a number of aspects of stimulant use, stimulant markets and provision of treatment in the CEE region, and the com-plex relation with recent social history. As researchers, we are still far away from understanding this relationship; policy makers should come to realise this when preparing drug legislation and policies. Measures aiming to repress home-based 'laboratories' that manufacture ATS may have serious unintended consequences such as a paradoxical increase in the availability of ATS due to takeover of the market by large organised criminal groups and the spread of HIV; there are quite a few examples of both from outside the region.

We described the tradition of kitchen-produced ATS in CEE and the production processes of the two most common injectable ATS (methamphetamine and meth-cathinone). During Soviet times, closed borders prevented the exchange of not only legal commodities but also illegal ones. Nevertheless, information about the Western countercultures of the 1960s and 1970s did spark an interest in drugs other than alcohol among young people throughout the region, which resulted in the emergence of small, largely underground, pockets of counterculture. Whereas their parents distilled their *samagon vodka*, Soviet youth turned to the medicine cabinets and pharmacies (of which there are many in this region) looking for local highs. For example, short-acting ketamine (Ketalar), diverted from (hospital) pharmacies, easily provided the idea of an LSD experience, in particular when injected. IDUs subsequently turned to their chemistry books. In a time that both precursors and processing chemicals were easy to obtain, Eastern drug users came up with their own version of heroin and amphetamines and soon various formulas started to circulate.

The small-scale production processes of these drugs dictated a specific type of organisation and networking around the acquisition of precursors and chemicals, and the production and consumption of the resulting drugs. Methamphetamine is usually produced in groups of about three to eight users, who all have roles in the elaborate process that results in getting high. In these groups, users not only share drugs but also many basic necessities and an important part of their time (Grund, 2001). Thus, the market conditions during the Soviet era resulted in particular drug consumption patterns that shaped the drug culture in the post-Communist countries.

Drug markets in the Western hemisphere have produced rather different forms of social organisation among drug users. In New York City, for example, Preble and Casey (1969) observed how the street heroin markets during the 1960s engendered a basic 'dyad', a partnership of two best buddies or lovers, in which both participants implicitly understand the common benefits of the partnership. Within these tight partnerships just about all commodities were shared, including drugs and needles. A combination of the explosive expansion of heroin use in the 1970s and the city's financial crises of the mid-1970s, when impoverished neighbourhoods became blighted with abandoned buildings, lead to abandoned buildings being converted into shooting galleries. In these locations, the protection of the dyad was weakened and HIV passed rapidly among the previously unconnected networks of injectors who gathered there. By the early 1980s, half of the injectors in these neighbourhoods were infected with HIV (Marmor et al., 1987).

Grund (1993) described comparatively large neighbourhood-based networks organised around the so-called house addresses in Rotterdam (and other Dutch cities), where heroin and cocaine was sold and used on the spot. These house addresses succeeded the city-centre street markets of the 1970s after law enforcement crackdowns inspired by neighbourhoods' activism against crime and nuisance. During the 1980s and 1990s, these places dominated the Dutch drug scene and they were often tolerated by the authorities when nuisance in the neighbourhoods remained manageable. While at face value the Rotterdam house addresses resembled the New York shooting galleries, the then implemented policy of normalisation of drug problems (Engelsman, 1989; van de Wijngaart, 1990) engendered quite a different HIV risk environment (Rhodes, 2002).

While, due to widespread needle exchange, needle sharing was uncommon (Grund et al., 1992), this tolerated indoor environment fostered another important HIV risk behaviour, 'frontloading' or syringe-mediated-drug-sharing within networks of drug-using friends (Grund et al., 1991, 1996). This drug-sharing behaviour was later identified in the USA (Jose et al., 1993), Russia (Des Jarlais et al., 2002; Grund, 2001) and elsewhere (Grund, 1993), and has been identified as a driving factor in the HIV epidemic in Eastern Europe (Abdala et al., 2006; Dehne et al., 1999; Des Jarlais et al., 2002; Grund, 2001).

Thus, the social context of drug use in different parts of the world and in different times seems to result in different risk environments in which the social response to and the availability of drugs and precursors (the macro-risk environment) can be seen to determine the everyday drug-taking patterns in the networks of users (micro-risk environment) (Rhodes, 2002).

The recent social history of Eastern Europe has produced its own Soviet-style patterns of stimulant and other drug use that remain poorly understood by researchers and policy makers up to the present day. While epidemiological studies have informed us about the spread of drug injecting and its connection with the HIV and hepatitis epidemics in the region, the virtual absence of ethnographic research into actual drug use patterns, motives for or the social context of drug use limits our understanding of the twin epidemic in this region. A comprehensive understanding is, however, crucial to developing effective policy responses towards illicit drug use – whether these are health or law enforcement interventions. In contrast to the stereotype presented by (post-Soviet) narcology, one of the few Russian ethnographies of drug users suggests that methamphetamine and opiate users alike are concerned about their own and friends' health, undertake efforts at controlling their drug use and are (interested in) practicing harm reduction (Sarang, 2007) – an observation confirmed by the small-scale study on Russian-speaking drug users in Czech capital Prague (Zábranský and Janíková, 2008). HIV prevention programmes could extend their reach by using the networks of drug user/producers in the proliferation of harm reduction information and supplies. In Rotterdam, the Netherlands, the so-called collective needle exchange, in which active injectors distributed sterile injection equipment to their peers, accounted for more than half of the city's needle exchange volume in 1989 (Grund et al., 1992). In Kazan, Russia, *pritons* (the Russian equivalent of shooting galleries) provided the local harm reduction project an important venue to contact and reduce the risky injection practices of the *priton* clientele (Irwin et al., 2006).

We have also described how efforts to control methamphetamine's precursor ephedrine and the required processing chemicals have resulted in shifts towards its diastereomer pseudoephedrine and more frequent application of the simpler oxidation to methcathinone. Whether such measures contribute to decreases in the use of (home-produced) stimulants remains a question, but reports (Chintalova-Dallas et al., 2006) suggest that young users in Odessa, Ukraine, have turned to potentially even more harmful patterns of stimulant preparation. Lacking (pseudo)ephedrine, they have shifted to using OTC medications containing phenylpropanolamine (PPA) in the preparation (oxidation) of *boltushka* (*mix*), which contains cathinone[12]

(Chintalova-Dallas et al., 2006). PPA has been associated with increased risk for haemorrhagic stroke (Horwitz et al., 2000).

Furthermore, participation in home production itself poses an increased risk of long prison terms. UNODC reported that most of the seized methamphetamine laboratories in Europe are small kitchen laboratories (UNODC, 2007). In most CEE countries, a charge of drug production does not differentiate between production for personal (friends) consumption and large-scale production. It remains widespread in the region to strictly interpret the articles on drug production of the UN drug conventions and apply them to drug users engaging in self-preparation of drugs. This does not do justice to the social–ecological context of illicit drug consumption. It is unlikely that the international legislators who drafted the UN drug conventions had considered the rather particular situation in the CEE region, where the majority of IDUs cook injectable stimulants and opiates for their own use, without the intent to sell or make a profit. Furthermore, this strict interpretation does not serve public health goals, such as prevention of HIV, overdose and other morbidity associated with problem drug use. Incarceration puts drug users and their families at risk of HIV, HCV, TB and other health risks or trauma.

Finally, we sketched the history of drug treatment, which, in our opinion, cannot be dissociated from the social doctrine that dominated every aspect of life in this region during the larger part of the last century. Drug use and other deviancies (whether alcoholism, psychiatric problems or political dissent) were considered a threat to the collective. The primary goal of the Communist response to these 'social diseases' was to undo or isolate such threats. Treatment outcome or individual human rights were secondary to *blaming the victim*. As in all other areas of life, an inertia that is a residue of Communist attitudes lingers in those narcology institutions that continue to be dominated by old school clinicians. Young progressive doctors often feel frustrated with what in their eyes are antiquated and harsh approaches towards treatment of dependency.

One can argue that legislation in Western capitalist democracies developed equally harsh drug laws, but in Eastern Europe this development was determined by a Soviet ideology that was applied to all forms of deviance and collaboratively implemented by closely connected agents of state control – narcology and law enforcement. In the West, most drug treatment has, in the main, been developed separate from law enforcement. From the 1970s until quite recently, many Western drug treatment providers saw their work as different from drug enforcement, and in many countries police and drug services still see each other as serving opposite goals. Only more recently, cooperation between legal and treatment approaches towards addiction become more common (e.g. drug courts in the USA; repressive multi-agency individual treatment plans for *chronic, nuisance addicts* in the Netherlands).

Furthermore, many European countries have developed a variety of non-repressive measures towards drug users. According to a 2002 publication of the European Monitoring Center for Drugs and Drug Addiction on the topic of drug users and the law, many EU countries have reconsidered their position on the simple possession of drugs for private consumption and drug laws in the EU increasingly seek to strike a balance between punishment and treatment (EMCDDA, 2002). These trends may soon spread within the westernised countries of the former Soviet bloc.

Nevertheless, treatment developed for methamphetamine addiction is virtually absent in the CEE region, with perhaps the Czech Republic being the only exception. But this is not much different from the situation that exists in most Western European countries or the USA. Research to find effective treatment specific to stimulant addiction has only recently surfaced in the English language scientific literature. Studies of cognitive behavioural therapy combined with contingency management suggest that this combined treatment may be effective in 40% of methamphetamine patients (Lee and Rawson, 2008), which is substantially more than the 'guesstimated' 5% achieved with mere detoxification and 2 weeks of 're-habilitation' (*personal communication of the second author with narcologists in the FSU countries*).

Although few, there are fortunately signs that more evidence-based approaches towards problematic methamphetamine use are being considered in some countries in the region and the Czech Republic may be on the frontier of change. Trials on contingency management and methylphenidate substitution for problem methamphetamine users are planned or in preparation, while individual doctors experiment with prescribing methylphenidate (Ritalin) to long-term, chronic methamphetamine users (see, e.g., Hampl, 2004). The First Global Conference on Methamphetamine held in Prague, Czech Republic in September 2008, will hopefully stimulate similar developments in the region.

During the 1990s, the use of illegal drugs increased drastically throughout CEE. The arrival of the market economy and open borders has affected patterns of drug use – for example, in many places powder heroin has replaced homemade opiates. Quite surprisingly, this has had much less effect on the shadow economy around the production and consumption of ATS, which remain mostly produced and consumed in small groups of consumers. While methamphetamine has also popped up in the nightlife of various Eastern European cities – where ecstasy has certainly lowered the threshold for stimulants – the tradition of kitchen-produced amphetamines continues to dominate stimulant use throughout the region.

In Western Europe, generally there is at present no evidence of widespread use of methamphetamine. While use of home-made ATS is substantial in Eastern Europe, in particular in countries now bordering the EU, the concern for the EU is the extent to which the problems in the CEE states will move westward. Concern about methamphetamine is slowly entering the consciousness of the EU and in member states. It is impossible to predict the future diffusion of methamphetamine use without concerted research. Griffiths et al. (2008) suggest that methamphetamine diffusion in Western Europe is impeded by a market dominated by other stimulant drugs such as cocaine and ecstasy. Dutch prevention officers feel that the relatively well-educated recreational drug consumers in their country will eschew methamphetamine. The availability and popularity of other drugs, the perception of methamphetamine among drug users, and travel and migration to and from the enlarged union could all influence future spread of methamphetamine (Griffiths et al., 2008). The situation in the Czech Republic that exported its 'know-how' to Slovakia already, and the situation in many FSU states, the USA and Asia, shows the potential appeal of methamphetamine. Obtaining pertinent data and mounting appropriate responses will depend to a considerable degree on input from new member states and countries that border on the EU.

Acknowledgements

We would like to acknowledge the support and contributions to this chapter of Viktor Mravcik (Czech National Focal Point for Drugs and Drug Addictions), Josef Wünsch (Drop-In Drug Services and Municipality of 3rd Prague District), Ernestas Jasaitis (Lithuanian National Focal Point), Olga Borodkina (Department of Sociology, St Petersburg State University), Simona Merkinaite and Anya Sarang of the Eurasian Harm Reduction Network (EHRN). We are grateful to the active drug users and ex-users in the Czech Republic, Russia, Ukraine and other countries of the region who kindly shared their experiences.

Notes

1. 'Glass' in Russian.
2. All illegal drug use, from marihuana and (diverted) psychofarmaca, alone and combined with alcohol, to *braun* and *pervitin*.
3. The German name for the drugs used from 1930s; in Czech and Slovak Republics commonly abbreviated to *piko*.
4. Russian word for 'chatterbox'.
5. Pseudoephedrine is a diastereomer of ephedrine (natural stimulant found in *Ephedra sinica, E. equisetina, E. gerardiana* and other *Ephedras*). It is also produced industrially using yeast of the *Saccharomyces coreanus* strain. It is an active ingredient of many de-congestants of different formulas (Sudafed, Modafen, Adcil Allegra, Claritine, Panadol, Sinifed, Zyrtec and many others). For the reduction of both pseudoephedrine and ephedrine into methamphetamine the so-called Birch reaction is used. In the USA, Asia and elsewhere, until the late 1990s P2P (phenyl-2-propanone) was used as a precursor instead of pseudo-ephedrine in a slightly different reaction, resulting in a comparatively mellow product (a racemate of D- and L-optical isomers, whereas the Birch reaction results in a pure D-isomer, which is much more potent).
6. TAVO DRUGYS is a Lithuanian drug user advocacy and self-support organisation.
7. Such fake cocaine is called *pikain* – which is a combination of the terms *piko* and *kokain* – in the recreational drug scene.
8. According to the EMCDDA definition (EMCDDA, 1999).
9. It is not always clear whether the term 'Amphetamines' used in the WRD 2007 refers to all amphetamines. In the presented prevalence estimates it obviously does not consider the use of methamphetamine in the Czech Republic.
10. That is of medical discipline that has been seen as sub-discipline of psychiatry in (for-mer) Soviet Union and has been dealing with **narcomans** (users of NARCOTICS/illegal drugs).

11. Abbreviation in *azbuka (cyrilic)* for Союз Советских Социалистических Республик (Union of Soviet Socialist Republics).
12. PPA oxidizes to cathinone and reduces to amphetamine (benzedrine).

References

Abdala, N., Grund, J.-P. C., Tolstov, Y. and Heimer, R. (2006) Can home-made injectable opiates contribute to the HIV epidemic among injection drug users in the countries of the former Soviet Union? *Addiction* 101: 731–737.

Abel-Ollo, K., Talu, A., Vals, K. and Vorobjov, S., Paimre, M., Ahven, A., Neuman, A., Denissov, G. (2007) Report on the drug situation in Estonia 2007. 2007 National Report (2006 data) to the EMCDDA by the Reitox National Focal Point. Available at http://eusk.tai.ee/failid/ESTONIA_2007_NATIONAL_REPORTING_Final.pdf. Accessed 8 April 2009.

Alcabes, P., Grund, J.-P. C., Beniowski, M., Bozek, B., Kaciuba, A. and Zielinski, A. (1998) Possible epidemic spread of HIV by syringe-based drug sharing in Poland: paradigm for the new AIDS frontier. In: 12th World AIDS Conference, Geneva, June 1998, Abstract 13186.

Allaste, A. A. and Lagerspetz, M. (2002) Recreational drug use in Estonia: the context of club culture. *Contemporary Drug Problems* 29: 183–200.

Atrill, R., Kinniburgh, J. and Power, L. (2001) *Social Exclusion and HIV*. London: Terrence Higgins Trust.

Balakireva, O. M., Grund, J. P. C., Barendregt, C., Rubanets, Y. V., Ryabova, M. V., Volyk, A. M., Levchuk, N. M., Mieshierina, O. V., Bondar, T. V. and Dikova-Favorska, D. M. (2006) *Risk and Protective Factors in the Initiation of Injecting Drug Use: Analytical Report on a Respondent Driven Sampling Study & Strategy Paper Preventing the Initiation of Injecting Drug Use among Vulnerable Adolescents and Young People. Final Report.* Kiev: UNICEF/UISR.

Booth, R. E., Lehman, W. E., Kwiatkowski, C. F., Brewster, J. T., Sinitsyna, L. and Dvoryak, S. (2008) Stimulant injectors in Ukraine: the next wave of the epidemic? *AIDS and Behavior* 12(4): 652–661.

Borodkina, O. I., Baranova, M. V., Girchenko, P. V., Irwin, K. S., Heimer, R. and Kozlov, A. P. (2005) The correlation between the type of drug use and HIV prevalence of IDU in different Russian cities. *Russian Journal of HIV/AIDS & Related Problems* 9(3): 57–47.

Budnick, N. (2007) One meth problem leads to another. As state labs begin to disappear, Mexican drug cartels gladly fill the void. *The West Linn Tidings*, 29 November 2007.

Butler, W. (2003) *HIV/AIDS and Drug Misuse in Russia: Harm Reduction Programmes and the Russian Legal System*. London: International Family Health.

Chintalova-Dallas, R., Lutzenko, D., Lazzarini, Z. and Case, P. (2006) Boltushka: use of homemade amphetamine in Odessa, Ukraine. *Presented at the 17th International Conference on the Reduction of Drug Related Harm*, Vancouver, 30 April 2006–4 May 2006. Available at http://www.temple.edu/lawschool/phrhcs/rpar/about/RPAR%20and %20RAR%20Reports%20and%20Presentations/RPAR%20and%20RAR%20Slides %20and%20Posters/17th%20Conference%20on%20the%20Reduction%20of %20Drug%20Related%20Harm,%20Vancouver/Boltushka%20in%20Odessa.PPT. Accessed 8 April 2009.

Csémy, L. and Elekes, Z. (2001) What are the interrelationships between drug problems and drug policy? Lessons from the analysis of the institutional context. In: Kenis, P., Maas, F. and Sobiech, R. (eds), *Institutional Responses to Drug Demand in Central Europe an Analysis of Institutional Developments in the Czech Republic, Hungary, Poland and Slovenia*. Brookfield, VT: Ashgate, pp. 277–290.

ČTK (Czech Press Agency) (2008). *Policisté objevili laboratoř vyrábějící pervitin pro Británii* [Cops found lab producing pervitin for UK]. Available at http://www.lidovky.cz/policiste-objevili-laborator-vyrabejici-pervitin-pro-britanii-ps2-/ln_domov.asp?c=A080404_144226_ln_domov_mel. Accessed 8 April 2009.

de Kort, M. (1995) *Tussen patiënt en delinquent, geschiedenis van het Nederlandse drugs-beleid*. Hilversum: Verloren Uitgeverij.

Dehne, K. L., Grund, J.-P. C., Khodakevich, L. and Kobyshcha, Y. (1999) The HIV/AIDS epidemic among drug injectors in Eastern Europe: patterns, trends and determinants. *Journal of Drug Issues* 29(4): 729–776.

Des Jarlais, D. C., Grund, J.-P. C., Zadoretzky, C., Milliken, C., Friedmann, P., Titus, S., Perlis, T., Bodrova, V. and Zemlianova, E. (2002) HIV risk behaviour among participants of syringe exchange programmes in central/eastern Europe and Russia. *International Journal of Drug Policy* 13: 165–174.

Downes, P. (2003) *Living with Heroin – Identity, Social Exclusion and HIV among the Russian-Speaking Minorities in Estonia and Latvia*. Tallinn: Legal Information Centre for Human Rights.

Drog Fokuszpont (2006) 2006 Annual Report to the EMCDDA – Hungary.

EMCDDA (1999) *Study to Obtain Comparable National Estimates of Problem Drug Use Prevalence for all EU Member States*. Lisbon: EMCDDA.

EMCDDA (2008) *Drug Profile: Methamphetamine*. http://www.emcdda.europa.eu/html.cfm/index25480EN.html#prevalence. Accessed 8 April 2009.

Engelsman, E. L. (1989) Dutch policy on the management of drug-related problems. *British Journal of Addiction* 84(2): 211–218.

EMCDDA (2002) *Prosecution of Drug Users in Europe: Varying Pathways to Similar Objective*. EMCDDA Insights Series No. 5. Luxembourg: Office for Official Publications of the European Communities.

Fiellin, D. A., Green, T. C. and Heimer, R. (2008) *Combating the Twin Epidemics of HIV/AIDS and Drug Addiction Opportunities for Progress and Gaps in Scale*. Washington, DC: Center for Strategic and International Studies.

Feshbach, M. and Galvin, C. M. (2005). *HIV/AIDS in Russia – An Analysis of Statistics*. Washington, DC: Woodrow Wilson International Center.

Griffiths, P., Mravcik, V., Lopez, D. and Klempova, D. (2008) Quite a lot of smoke but very limited fire – the use of methamphetamine in Europe. *Drug and Alcohol Review* 27(3): 236–242.

Grund, J.-P. C. (1993) Drug use as a social ritual: functionality, symbolism and determinants of self-regulation. Rotterdam: Addiction Research Institute (IVO). Avialable at http://www.drugtext.org/library/books/grund01/grundcon.html; http://www.drugpolicy.org/library/grundcon.cfm. Last date of access of both websites: 20-05-2009.

Grund, J.-P. C. (2001) A candle lit from both sides: the epidemic of HIV infection in Central and Eastern Europe. In: McElrath, K. (ed.), *HIV and AIDS: A Global View*. Westport, CT: Greenwood Press.

Grund, J.-P. C. (2003) Towards an enabling legal and policy environment. HIV prevention among vulnerable populations in the Republic of Moldova: an assessment of the legislative environment and recommendations for legal reform. Consultation Report to the PCIMU Moldova/World Bank, 30 September 2003.

Grund, J.-P. C. (2005) Staying on track: suggestions towards the new Estonian HIV/AIDS prevention strategy 2006–2015. Report of a Mission to Estonia, 28 March 2005– 1 April 2005. Consultation Report to the Estonian Ministry of Social Affairs & UNAIDS Geneva, June 2005.

Grund, J.-P. C. (2007) Focusing the response: strategies for addressing the twin epidemics of drug injecting and HIV in Latvia: situation analysis and summary of proposed interventions. Annex to Latvia (final) draft Strategy HIV/AIDS Program, 2008–2012, prepared for UNODC Baltic Office, Vilnius and the World Bank, Utrecht, CVO, 17 December 2007.

Grund, J.-P. C., Blanken, P., Adriaans, N. F. P., Kaplan, C. D., Barendregt, C. and Meeuwsen, M. (1992) Reaching the unreached: targeting hidden IDU populations with clean needles via known users. *Journal of Psychoactive Drugs* 24(1): 41–47.

Grund, J.-P. C., Botschkova, L., Kruglov, Y., Martsynovskaya, V., Scherbinskaya, A. and Anduschak, L. (2003) *A Case Study of the Ukrainian HIV Case Registration System*. Kiev: Ukrainian AIDS Center, Ministry of Health.

Grund, J.-P. C., Friedman, S. R., Stern, L. S., Jose, B., Neaigus, A., Curtis, R. and Des Jarlais, D. C. (1996) Drug sharing among injecting drug users: patterns, social context, and implications for transmission of blood-borne pathogens. *Social Science and Medicine* 42(5): 691–703.

Grund, J.-P. C., Kaplan, C. D., Adriaans, N. F. P. and Blanken, P. (1991). Drug sharing and HIV transmission risks: the practice of 'frontloading' in the Dutch injecting drug user population. *Journal of Psychoactive Drugs* 23: 1–10.

Grund, J.-P. C., Öfner, P. J. and Verbraeck, H. T. (2007) Marel o Del, kas kamel, le Romes duvar [God hits whom he chooses; the Rom gets hit twice]. In: *An Exploration of Drug Use and HIV Risks among the Roma of Central and Eastern Europe*. Budapest: L'Harmattan.

Hampl, K. (2004) Substituční léčba závislosti na pervitinu [Substitution treatment of pervitin addiction]. *Česká a slovenská psychiatrie* 100(5): 274–278.

Heimer, R., Booth, R. E., Irwin, K. S. and Merson, M. H. (2007) HIV and drug use in Eurasia. In: Twigg, J. L. (ed.), *HIV/AIDS in Russia and Eurasia*. Basingstoke, Hampshire, UK: Palgrave Macmillan.

Hibbell, B., Andersson, B., Ahlström, S., Bjarnason, T., Ahlström, S., Balakireva, O., Kokkevi, A. and Morgan, M. (2004) The 2003 ESPAD report. In: *Alcohol and Other Drug Use among Students in 30 European Countries*, 1st edn. Stockholm: CAN & Pompidou Group, p. 387.

Horwitz, R. I., Hines, H. H., Brass, L. M., Kernan, W. N. and Viscoli, C. M. (2000) Phenylpropanolamine and risk of hemorrhagic stroke. Final Report of the Hemorrhagic Stroke Project. Yale University School of Medicine, 10 May 2000. Available at http://www.fda.gov/ohrms/dockets/ac/00/backgrd/3647b1_tab19.doc. Accessed 8 April 2009.

Irwin, K., Karchevsky, E., Heimer, R. and Badrieva, L. (2006) Using secondary syringe exchange for HIV prevention in Kazan, Russia. *Substance Use Misuse* 41: 979–999.

John, R. (1986) *Memento*, 1st edn. Praha: Československý spisovatel.

Jose, B., Friedman, S. R., Neaigus, A., Curtis, R., Grund, J.-P. C., Goldstein, M. F., Des Jarlais, D. C. (1993) Syringe-mediated drug sharing (backloading): a new risk factor for HIV among injecting drug users. *AIDS* 7: 1653–1660.

Knox, E. G. (1989) Detection of clusters. In: Elliott, P. (ed.), *Methodology of Enquiries into Disease Clustering*. London: Small Area Health Statistics Unit, pp. 17–20.

Kozlov, A. P., Shaboltas, A. V., Toussova, O. V., Verevochkin, S. V., Masse, B. R., Perdue, T., Beauchamp, G., Sheldon, W., Miller, W. C., Heimer, R., Ryder, R. W. and Hoffman, I. F. (2006) HIV incidence and factors associated with HIV acquisition among injection drug users in St Petersburg, Russia. *AIDS* 20(6): 901–906.

Kubů, P., Škařupová, K. and Csémy, L. (2006) *Tanec a drogy 2000 a 2003 – Výsledky dotazníkové studie s příznivci elektronické taneční hudby v České republice [Dance and Drugs 2000 and 2003 – Results of the Questionnaire Survey in Fans of Electronic Dance Music in the Czech Republic]*, 1st edn. Praha: Úřad vlády ČR (Office of the Czech Government).

Latvian National Focal Point (2008) *2006 National Report (2005 Data) to the EMCDDA by the Reitox National Focal Point, Latvia: New Development, Trends and In-Depth Information on Selected Issues.* Riga: The State Addiction Agency.

Lee, N. K. and Rawson, R. A. (2008) A systematic review of cognitive and behavioural therapies for methamphetamine dependence. *Drug & Alcohol Review* 27(3): 309–317.

March, J. C., Oviedo-Joekes, E. and Romero, M. (2006) Drugs and social exclusion in ten European cities. *European Addiction Research* 12: 33–41.

Marmor, M., Des Jarlais, D. C., Cohen, H., Friedman, S. R., Beatrice, S. T. and Dubin, N. (1987) Risk factors for infection with human immunodeficiency virus among intravenous drug abusers in New York City. *AIDS* 1(1): 39–44.

Miovský, M. and Zábranský, T. (2001) Přehled výsledků substudie provedené s uživateli nelegálních psychoaktivních látek a pracovníky zdravotnických zařízení a významnými poskytovateli služeb uživatelům nelegálních drog [Summary of results of a substudy carried out with users of illicit psychoactive drugs and workers at medical facilities and significant providers of services for illicit drug users]. *Adiktologie Suplementum (Vybrané substudie analýzy dopadů novelizace drogové legislativy v ČR [Selected Substudies of the Impact Analysis Project of New Drugs Legislation in the Czech Republic]* 1(1): 41–75.

Mravčík, V., Škařupová, K. and Orlíková, B. (2008) Rekreační užívání drog: Užívání drog v prostředí noční zábavy a existující intervence v ČR [Recreational drug use: drugs in the nightlife and avalable interventions in Czech Republic] [review]. *Zaostřeno na drogy [Focused on Drugs]* 3(6): 1–16.

Mravčík, V. and Zábranský, T. (2001) Prevalenční odhad problémových uživatelů drog v ČR – syntéza dostupných dat (The prevalence estimate of problem drug use in Czech Republic – synthesis of available data). *Adiktologie Suplementum (Vybrané substudie analýzy dopadů novelizace drogové legislativy v ČR [Selected Substudies of the Impact Analysis Project of New Drugs Legislation in the Czech Republic]* 1(1): 22–43.

NMCD (2007) *Výročná správa o stave drogovej problematiky na Slovensku v roku 2006, Národné monitorovacie centrum pre drogy.* Bratislava: Úrad vlády SR.

Nožina, M. (1997) Drogová historie (Drug History). In: Nožina, M. (ed.), *Svět drog v Čechách [The World of Drugs in Czechia]*, 1st edn. Praha, and Orlík nad Vltavou: KLP – Koniasch Latin Press & Livingstone, pp. 49–126.

Oole, K., Talu, A., Vals, K., Paimre, M., Ahven, A., Neuman, A., Denissov, G. and Able, K. (2006) *Report on the Drug Situation in Estonia 2006.* Tallin: NIHD, Estonian Drug Monitoring Centre.

Otiashvili, D., Zábranský, T., Kirtadze, I., Pirashvilli, G., Chavchanidze, M. and Miovsky, M. (2008) Nonmedical use of burenorphine (Subutex) in the Republic of Georgia – a pilot study. In: *Book of Abstracts*, 2008 NIDA International Forum: Globally Improving and Applying Evidence-Based Interventions for Addictions, pp. 69–70.

Preble, E. and Casey, J. J. (1969) Taking care of business – the heroin user's life on the street. *International Journal of the Addictions* 1: 1–24.

OZ Prima [NGO Prima] (2007) Charakteristika klientov nízkoprahových programov (prieskum Bordernet). Správa pre NMCD [Characteristics of clients of low-threshold pro-grammes run by NGO Prima in Bratislava (Bordernet Study). Report for Slovak National Drug Observatory].

Rhodes, T. (2002) The risk environment: a framework for understanding and reducing drug-related harm. *International Journal of Drug Policy* 13: 85–94.

Sarang, A. (2007) *Models of Drug Use and Mechanisms of Regulation and Control*. Unpub-lished Masters thesis, London School of Health and Tropical Medicine.

Schiffer, K. and Schatz, E. (2008) *Marginalisation, Social Inclusion and Health. Ex-periences Based on the Work of Correlation – European Network Social Inclu-sion and Health*. Amsterdam: Regenboog AMOC, Correlation Network. Available at http://79.170.40.55/correlation-net.org/products/marginalisation.pdf. Accessed 8 April 2009.

Scutelniciuc, O., Coscodan, C., Postoronca, D., Slobozian, V., Susanu, A., Iarovoi, P., Rim-ish, C. and Gutu, L. (2008) *Annual Report 2007: Drug Situation in the Republic of Moldova*, Chisinau: UNDP/BUMAD.

Shaboltas, A. V., Toussova, O. V., Hoffman, I. F., Heimer, R., Verevochkin, S. V., Ryder, R. W., Khoshnood, K., Perdue, T., Masse, B. R. and Kozlov, A. P. (2006) HIV prevalence, sociodemographic, and behavioral correlates and recruitment methods among injection drug users in St Petersburg, Russia. *Journal of AIDS* 41: 657–663.

Shiryanov, B. (2001) *Nizshij pilotazh [Low Flying]*. Moscow: Ad Marginem.

Singer, M. and Clair, S. (2003) Syndemics and public health: reconceptualizing disease in bio-social context. *Medical Anthropology Quarterly* 17(4): 423–441.

UNODC (2007). World Drug Report 2007. Available at http://www.unodc.org/unodc/en/data-and-analysis/WDR-2007.html. Accessed 8 April 2009.

Uusküla, A., Abel, K., Rajaleid, K. and Rüütel, K., Talu, A., Fischer, K. and Boborova, N. (2005) *HIV and Risk Behavior Among IDUs in Two Cities (Tallinn, Kohtla-Järve) in Estonia*. National Institute for Health Development, University of Tartu, Imperial College London. Available at http://www.tai.ee/failid/IDU_risk_behaviour_and_HIV_prevalence_study_2005.pdf. Accessed 8 April 2009.

Uusküla, A., McNutt, L. -A., Dehovitz, J., Fischer, K. and Heimer, R. (2007) High prevalence of blood-borne virus infections and high risk behaviour among injecting drug users in Tallinn, Estonia. *International Journal of STD and AIDS* 18: 41–46.

van de Wijngaart, G. (1990) The Dutch approach: normalization of drug problems. *The Journal of Drug Issues* 20(4): 667–678.

Vopravil, J., Mravčík, V., Petroš, O., Zábranský, T., Berszi, G., Malinová, H., Švec, J. and Holíková, N. (2005) *Project Data Collection: Illegal Activities*. Multi-beneficiary Statistical Co-operation Programme 2002 Research Reports. Luxembourg: Eurostat.

White, E., Niccolai, L., Paintsil, E., Barbour, R., Heimer, R., Toussova, O., Verevochkin, S. and Kozlov, A.. (2008) *Methamphetamine use and networks of drug injectors in St Petersburg, Russian Federation*. Prague, Czech Republic: First Global Conference on Methamphetamine.

Zábranský, T. (2002) Problem drug use and treatment responses. In: *2002 Report on the Drugs Situation in Candidate Central and Eastern European Countries*. Lisbon: EMCDDA, pp. 15–28.

Zábranský, T. (2007) Methamphetamine in the Czech Republic. *Journal of Drug Issues* 37(1): 649–674.

Zábranský, T. (in press). *Drogová epidemiologie* [Drug Epidemiology], 2nd revised edition, Czech Republic: University Palacky Press.

Zábranský, T. and Janíková, B. (2008) *Séroprevalence krevně přenosných virových infekcí mezi ruskojazyčnými injekčními uživateli na drogové scéně v hl. m. Praze (RUS-IDU-PHA)' [Seroprevalence of Blood-Borne Diseases in the Russian Speakers Injecting Drugs in Prague]*. Prague: Centre of Addictology, p. 32.

Chapter 14

SWEDEN'S LONG EXPERIENCE OF AMPHETAMINE PROBLEMS

Kerstin Käll

Introduction

Sweden was one of the countries with an early experience of amphetamine misuse, which emerged soon after the introduction of amphetamine on the pharmaceutical market in 1938. In 1943 the National Medical Board of Health issued a warning of increasing abuse, and restrictions were put on the sale of amphetamine. At this time the problem was mainly a widespread misuse of legally prescribed pills in the general population. This epidemic peaked in 1959 when as many as 6.4% of the population, age 15–64 years, had experience of amphetamine use; by 2000 this figure was down to 0.4% (United Nations Office on Drug and Crime, 2006).

In the mid-1940s, another kind of drug use epidemic became apparent. This epidemic started in a group of artists, musicians and poets and soon spread to criminally active youth. By 1954 the illegal sale of amphetamine had become quite extensive, and the first sentence for illegal dealing with central stimulants was delivered. In 1958 amphetamine was classed as a narcotic drug in Sweden, soon to be followed by other amphetamine-type stimulants (ATS). The epidemic continued to grow, and in the 1960s the epidemic gained further impetus from the international movement of 'Flower Power'. By this time an intensive media debate on drug policy had started, and it resulted in an experiment with legal prescription of narcotic drugs to drug users that lasted from 1965 to 1967. It was not a success, and during this period the drug use epidemic continued to grow. Instead of decreasing and finally quitting their drug use as intended the patients tended to increase the doses and often distributed some of their dose to friends, thereby further fuelling the epidemic. The death from overdose of a young girl, who received her drugs from one of the 'legal' users, led to the experiment being scandalised in the media and contributed to its demise (Käll, 1997).

Sweden's drug policy

The 1970s were characterised by an intense debate on drug policy in Sweden, and by the end of the decade the main elements of the present drug policy were put in place. The overriding strategic goal was to be 'a drug free society', meaning a zero tolerance of all non-medical use of narcotic drugs. The means to achieve the goal should rest on three 'pillars'. The first pillar was prevention of drug use, both initiation (primary prevention) and early detection with distinct consequences of experimental or recreational use (secondary prevention). The second 'pillar' was law enforcement of all dealings with narcotic drugs, including production, smuggling, wholesale, street peddling and possession (later on also consumption). The third 'pillar' was treatment of already addicted users. There was also a debate on whether all treatment should be voluntary, which in 1982 resulted in a law stipulating compulsory treatment for drug users who refused voluntary treatment in spite of an abundance of physical, mental and/or social consequences of their drug use. In 1988 the consumption of illegal drugs was criminalised, and in 1993 this law was sharpened so that it was possible for the police to take a urine sample from a person with signs of drug intoxication (United Nations Office on Drugs and Crime, 2006).

In terms of primary prevention of drug use, Sweden has been remarkably successful as was reported in the recent report from the United Nations (United Nations Office on Drugs and Crime, 2006). The ESPAD Report 2007 shows that among 15–16-year olds the percentage with experience of drugs other than cannabis was 4% compared to, for example, 11% in France and 9% in the UK. As for cannabis, the most common drug of initiation, the difference was even more striking: 7% in Sweden compared to 33% in Switzerland and 29% in the UK (Hibell et al., 2009). This is all the more surprising in the light of the globalised youth culture and the enormous economic power of the international drug trade and implies that prevention is possible with a successful national strategy on drug prevention.

The aim of the above-mentioned sharpening of the law on drug consumption was to make secondary prevention among young drug experimenters possible. The idea was to deliver consequences severe enough to make young drug users choose to quit drugs before they developed drug dependency. Recently, a study was conducted on the effect of early police intervention among young people in the fifth largest commune in Sweden. All persons between the age of 15 and 25 arrested for minor drug offences during 2001 were followed in police registers and social and medical files until 2005. As can be seen in Figure 14.1, the most commonly used drug in this cohort was amphetamine, closely followed by cannabis. Multiple drug use was very prevalent, but it still points to the strong position of amphetamine among young drug users in Sweden. The outcome of the study was that among the youngest (age 15–20), half had quit drugs and crime by the end of 2005, the girls more so than the boys; in the older part of the cohort, 35% had quit. The strongest predictor for not doing well was severe school problems early in life. Since the study did not include a control group, it does not prove that recovery was due to the police intervention. As was pointed out in the study, the close cooperation between police, social workers and dependency clinic in delivering adequate consequences, such as urine test control, was probably as important as the police intervention itself, but in many cases would not have been put in place unless the drug misuse had been disclosed by the police (Bergsten and Käll, 2007).

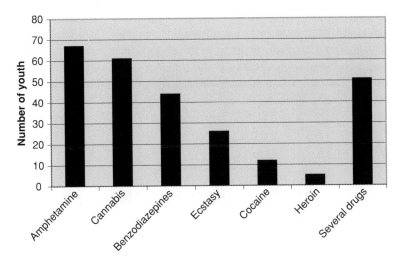

Figure 14.1 Illicit drugs used in the cohort of persons between the age of 15 and 25, arrested for minor drug offences during 2001 in a Swedish commune (several drugs: two illicit drugs or more, or one illicit drug and alcohol).

HIV among injecting drug users in Sweden

The 1980s brought the HIV epidemic into the populations of injecting drug users (IDUs) in Sweden, and a new debate emerged on drug policy where the concept of 'harm reduction' was introduced. The restrictive drugs policy outlined above was challenged in the light of this life-threatening disease spreading among IDUs. The long experience of the harms caused by illegal drug use even before HIV made both the public and the decision makers reluctant to give up the strategy of zero tolerance of drug misuse. This was particularly so since it had been rather successful in bringing down the rates of experimentation with drugs among young people, from 15% of 15–16-year-old students reporting ever testing drugs in 1971 to 8% in 2007 (Hibell et al., 2009).

The HIV epidemic among the IDUs of Sweden started among the heroin injectors in Stockholm in 1983, and when commercial tests became available in 1985 about 50% of the heroin injectors were found to be infected. Among the amphetamine injectors, who dominate the scene of IDUs in Stockholm, very few were infected at this time. In 1987 an epidemiological study of HIV among incarcerated IDUs started in Stockholm (the Remand Prison Study), and in 1988 the HIV prevalence among heroin users in the study was 45.5% compared to 5.9% among the amphetamine users (Käll and Olin, 1990). The strategy to meet the HIV epidemic among IDUs in Sweden was to put high emphasis on routine HIV testing, education of IDUs as well as prison and treatment staff, extra funding for drug treatment and increased access to methadone maintenance treatment for heroin users, but with a maintained high threshold. Two experimental sites with needle exchange

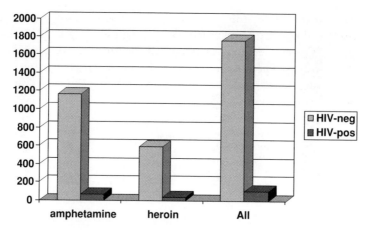

Figure 14.2 IDUs participating in the Remand Prison study in Stockholm 2002–2008 (*N* = 1501). Amphetamine, 69/212 (5.7%); heroin, 49/636 (7.6%); all, 118/1865 (6.3%).

were introduced in the South of Sweden, but not in Stockholm, where most of the HIV cases had occurred. During the following years, there was a sharp decrease in the HIV incidence among heroin users, and most of the newly infected IDUs in Stockholm were amphetamine users. In the latest data from the Remand Prison Study, there is no significant difference in HIV seroprevalence between heroin and amphetamine injectors (between 6 and 8%) as shown in Figure 14.2 (unpublished data from the Remand Prison Study). In 2006 the Swedish Parliament, relying on the recommendations from WHO, decided that needle exchange programmes could be started anywhere in Sweden on a regular basis provided that certain conditions were fulfilled, such as cooperation between health care and social service in providing drug detoxification and treatment in connection with the needle exchange. Until April 2009, no new needle exchange programmes have yet been started (V. Urwitz, personal communication, 2009). Among social workers, there is a fear that needle exchange services would signal to young people an ambiguous attitude from society concerning drug use that goes contrary to the zero-tolerance strategy. At present, there is strong political resistance on the local level against needle exchange programme in Stockholm, the opponents pointing to what they claim to be weak scientific evidence on any positive effect on HIV incidence of needle exchange programmes (Käll et al., 2007).

Treatment of amphetamine misuse

Until recently there has been no evidence-based treatment specifically aimed at amphetamine misuse. In a sense, most treatment of drug misuse in Sweden has however been aimed at amphetamine misuse, since amphetamine has been the dominating drug among heavy users, although cannabis is the most widely used illegal drug. The first treatment institutions for drug users were designed as therapeutic communities, and there are still some of these in operation. The next ideology was the Hassela pedagogic treatment for young drug users (Käll, 1997). In the last 15 years, the dominating ideology in treatment institutions has been the 12-step Minnesota programme. There are also some churches delivering drug treatment. Most of the treatment institutions are private initiatives with little incentive to do scientific evaluation, and consequently there is a lack of hard evidence on the effectiveness of institutional care of drug users. The trend in the last decades has been to try outpatient care to a larger extent, since this has proved more cost-effective with alcohol-dependent patients (Room et al., 2003). The clinical experience, however, is that outpatient care is usually not as effective with hard drug users as with alcohol-dependent patients, with the exception of maintenance treatment of opiate-dependent patients. The trend today is to recommend at least 6 months of institutional care for severe amphetamine addiction, usually the 12-step programme followed up with Narcotics Anonymous (NA) contact for several years. For the less dependent patients who receive outpatient treatment, cognitive behavioural therapy and motivational interviewing are the most prevalent new evidenced-based methods recommended in clinics for dependency disorders (Socialstyrelsen, 2007). By international standards, Sweden allocates a lot of money for drug treatment (Room et al., 2003), but this has varied with the budgetary situation and today it is not as easy to receive institutional treatment as it was in the 1980s. In most cases, the cost for institutional drug treatment is covered by the social service, but much treatment is also delivered within the criminal justice system, either in special treatment prisons, or wings of prisons, or outside prison where part of or the whole sentence can be served in a treatment institution.

The following interview is a rather typical life story of an amphetamine-addicted woman in Sweden. She is now a recovered addict and very proud of her achievements and has agreed to appear with her real name.

Helene, age 43

Helene grew up in the South of Sweden with both her parents and two elder brothers. Neither of her parents misused drugs or alcohol, and her childhood was happy until age 10 when her parents divorced. The divorce was traumatic for Helene, and she felt that her father was mean to her mother and herself during the divorce process. She could never forgive him for that and had very little contact with him after the divorce. He is now dead. Helene was very fond of her mother with whom she lived after the divorce. They moved to a city very close to Denmark that could be reached by a ferry in about 20 minutes.

At 14, Helene started to go to parties. She was not very fond of alcohol, but at a party in Denmark, she was introduced to amphetamine and told that it would allow her to dance all night. She took it orally and really enjoyed it. From now on she and her friends went to Denmark at weekends and partied with amphetamine. At first her mother knew nothing about the drugs, but when she found out Helene chose to run away from home to another city where she lived with friends and took amphetamine. No other drugs interested her. Soon she started to inject, which was common among her new friends. She enjoyed the rush and after that she always injected the drug. She was away from home for 6 months in spite of the fact that her mother did her utmost to find her through social workers, police and the media. Finally, Helene called her and said she wanted to come home.

When she came home she was immediately put in a child psychiatric clinic, and later she was transferred to a treatment unit under the law of compulsory care of minors. She ran away several times and took up drugs, and at one time she hit a staff member with a bottle in the head when they tried to stop her from escaping. She was then sentenced to a closed institution with high security, where she stayed until she was 19. When she was released she immediately took up amphetamine again. To support her habit, she developed skills in forging cheques and stealing credit cards, which rendered her a number of prison sentences. She has been in prison about 20 times and has served between 9 and 10 years inside. Sometimes, she has used amphetamine inside prison as well.

At the age of 28, she met a man who did not use drugs and they started a relationship. Helene quit amphetamine without any treatment and remained drug free for 5 years. She got a job in a second-hand shop. She thought she had left drugs behind her when she fell in love with a customer in the shop who was an ex-user of amphetamine. She broke up from her relationship and moved in with her new man. But when he relapsed, so did she and soon she was back on the track with daily injections, frauds and prison sentences.

In the beginning of her amphetamine career, Helene used to take about 1 g of amphetamine per day and that would keep her awake around the clock. As she grew older, she could take more and she could sleep in spite of the drug. When high on amphetamine she particularly enjoyed housecleaning and driving, although she never had a driver's licence. Her apartment was always clean and tidy and she has always been careful about her hygiene and appearance. She was never hanging out much with other users and she never did any prostitution.

Finally at 38, she was fed up with her drug use and criminal lifestyle and applied for treatment. She started out 2 months in a 12-step treatment unit, but she did not fit in and was instead given the opportunity to go to a family treatment unit, where she got along very well. She continued going to NA, which she has had much help from and still attends. She has not relapsed but has served one more prison sentence for old crimes.

After the last prison sentence, Helene decided to move to another part of Sweden. She had met a man who lived there, but she also wished to come to a city where she did not know other drug users. Today, she no longer has a relationship with this man, but they are good friends. She has slowly built up a new life with a nice apartment, two cats and a part time job in a café. She has a good relationship with one of her brothers and his family, and she also keeps contact with the family where she had treatment. She goes to NA and has friends there too.

Four years ago, Helene was involved in a car crash and got a head injury after which she suffers from a minor speech impediment and reduced ability to concentrate. She also has some reduced force in her right hand. She has a chronic hepatitis C infection, for which she is due for treatment in the near future. She has a reduced lung capacity and easily catches respiratory infections after a long smoking career, and she is trying to quit smoking. She has difficulties in falling asleep and needs to take sleeping pills now and then. She has minor depressive episodes and she is still very unhappy that her mother did not live to see her drug free. She has gained 15 kg of weight after quitting amphetamine, which she does not like, but she prefers the extra weight to her life with amphetamine.

Helene has now been drug free for 5 years and is very determined never to go back to drugs. She values her new life and she does not want to disappoint her relatives once more. She has new good friends and she has taken up travelling, which she has always liked. She has been to Egypt seven times in 2 years. She loves the sun, swimming and snorkelling. She has finally applied for a driver's licence.

Helene's life story illustrates the intricate patterns of factors influencing both quitting and relapsing in drug misuse. The first treatment attempts had no effect at all and when she quit the first time she did it without treatment, due to a drug-free partner. Her relapse was also related to a partner. She now appears stable and she took help from treatment and NA, but she wishes to emphasise her own choice of her new drug-free lifestyle.

New trends in treatment

There are some new initiatives concerning treatment of amphetamine misuse in Sweden. The most recent attempt at pharmacological intervention is with naltrexone, a non-selective opioid antagonist. In one study, it was shown that pre-treatment with 50 mg naltrexone daily in healthy volunteers attenuated the subjective activation and arousal induced by amphetamine. (Jayaram-Lindström et al., 2004). In a following open clinical trial, 20 amphetamine-dependent patients were treated with naltrexone and relapse prevention therapy during 12 weeks. Naltrexone was well tolerated and only three dropped out due to adverse events (headache, nausea and abdominal pain). Five persons relapsed and were lost to follow up. Two patients achieved complete abstinence from amphetamine, and in nine patients there was a significant reduction in level of consumption and frequency of use. A pronounced decrease in craving was noted during the course of treatment. The hypothesis is that naltrexone reduces the subjective effect of amphetamine by attenuating the amphetamine-induced release of dopamine (Jayaram-Lindström et al., 2005). Finally, it was shown in a randomised, placebo-controlled trial that naltrexone reduced amphetamine use in amphetamine-dependent individuals. Eighty amphetamine-dependent patients were randomised to 12 weeks of double-blind naltrexone (50 mg) or placebo treatment. Overall, 55 patients completed the trial and the naltrexone group had a significantly higher number of amphetamine-negative urine samples compared to the placebo group and they also reported significantly less craving and consumption of amphetamine (Jayaram-Lindström et al., 2008).

Medical use of amphetamine or ATS to children with attention-deficit and hyperactivity disorder (ADHD) and related disorders has long been accepted, and lately it has also become evident that many of these children need to continue their medication into adulthood (Nutt et al., 2007).

It has also been noted that persons with untreated ADHD, particularly if they also develop conduct disorder in school, are at high risk of substance abuse later in life (Ersson, 2006). There are studies indicating that as many as 25% of inmates in Swedish prisons suffer from ADHD (Ericsson et al., 2001). In some Swedish dependency clinics, there are now projects going on trying to diagnose and treat drug-dependent adults with ADHD. One such study is presently conducted at the Clinic for Dependency Disorders in Linköping (Nyström et al., 2005). Until March 2009, 50 patients were included, of which 31 had amphetamine as their main drug of abuse (Tomas Trygg, personal communication, 2009). In most treated patients, slow-release methylphenidate (Concerta) was used. Abstinence from drug abuse during treatment was controlled by urine and hair analysis (Nyström et al., 2005). In a sense, one could view this treatment as a treatment of the drug dependency as well as of the ADHD, since the patients are usually very satisfied with the treatment and at the same time aware that treatment can only be carried on if they do not misuse drugs.

The following case history illustrates how ADHD treatment can work also as treatment for amphetamine dependency. Emil, like Helene, is very proud of his achievements and wants to be presented with his real name.

Emil, age 28

Emil grew up with his mother. His mother separated from his father when he was newborn. His father was an alcoholic with mental problems. Emil never got to know him and met him only five times before he died, when Emil was 18. He now wished he had known him better. He always missed having a father, and the men his mother chose to live with were no good in Emil's opinion. Most of them were alcoholics. When Emil was 18 his mother did meet a man, whom Emil could respect, but he died in an accident a few years later. Emil also liked his uncle, who was an amphetamine addict but still was good to Emil. His uncle committed suicide only 1 year after the death of his stepfather.

Emil was never very fond of his mother. He felt, and still feels, that she was unable to bring him up, particularly to set adequate limits for him. On the other hand, he was not an easy child. Already in nursery school he had to have his own assistant, mainly to protect other children, towards whom he could be very violent. He remembers always being more or less furious all through his childhood. He had no friends and the other children were not allowed by their parents to play with him. When he got angry, which was often, he could not control his impulses. He often hit other children, and as he grew older he often hit adults as well. He grew up to be a tall and strong boy, and consequently most people were afraid of him.

Emil was not successful in school. He had problems with concentration, so he missed out on a lot of subjects. Practical learning was easier, but he missed mathematics, English and subjects where you had to read texts almost completely.

He does not know any English, for example, which is very unusual, and a real handicap in Sweden.

Emil started to smoke cigarettes and inhale solvents about the age of 10. At 11, he tried alcohol, which he did not like. At 14, he tried cannabis, which he did not like very much either. At 15, he had his first encounter with amphetamine, at a private party. He took the drug orally, and this was a revolutionary experience in his life. Suddenly, his anger just fell off him, he could talk in a normal way to other people and he could control himself. He was happy. He was hooked immediately. To begin with he took amphetamine only on weekends and at parties but eventually he ended up taking it daily. He did not try injecting until he was 20, and he did not choose this mode of administration very often. He was too concerned about possible infections such as HIV and hepatitis and always made sure to have new injecting equipment.

Already at 16 Emil entered his first treatment, which was a small family-based unit with 5–6 boys with different and rather serious problems. He went to high school, with poor results in all theoretical subjects, and he took drugs, like most of the other boys, mainly amphetamine.

When Emil was 19 his mother took him on a boat cruise over the weekend. There he met a girl, Anne, who was to become his girlfriend for the next 8 years and the mother of his daughter.

Emil was admitted for military service and managed to serve 6 months until he was released due to drug abuse and assault of his girlfriend when he was on leave and high on drugs. Anne forgave him and he moved to the city where she lived and her mother, who tried to help Emil in various ways, helped him to find an apartment of his own, where he still lives. Anne never moved in with him. As a matter of fact, he has never let anybody into his apartment. He does not want anybody to see how he has arranged it. He feels he does not know how to decorate it properly.

Emil managed to get a manual job, and he was much appreciated there. He was basically never absent from work and he took amphetamine every day, in moderate doses such as 0.2–0.3 g/dose. He brought one or two doses with him to work. As he was not yet known by the police or criminal justice system, he was able to get a driver's licence and bought himself a car. He has always been meticulous about his personal affairs, keeping his apartment very clean and tidy, taking showers several times a day and keeping his finances in perfect order. During this period, he lived two parallel lives. With his wages, he paid his rent, his electricity, his petrol, his insurances and food. His amphetamine affairs were kept in a separate economy. He did not like to steal, so dealing drugs became his illegal occupation and he was disciplined and careful enough to get away with it. But in the end, he was not able to limit his drug taking in this manner and once he went binging on amphetamine for 2 weeks, with virtually no sleep. He did not go to work, and finally he was caught by the police after somebody reported him acting strangely at a petrol station. He was in a state of acute paranoid psychosis at the police station, but they released him after one night and he could go home and sleep. Because of this incident, he lost his driver's licence.

When this happened, Anne was pregnant with their daughter and she put an ultimatum to him. Either he would go into drug treatment or she would leave him. She had not been aware of the severity of his drug problem, and she felt he had been dishonest to her. So he went into treatment, for her sake. He entered a Minnesota treatment institution and stayed there for 8 months. After he had hit another client on an aggressive impulse, it was evident that he could not finish his treatment in this institution, so it was arranged with a small family institution, which worked for a few months.

By now Anne had finished their relationship. In fact, she did that a week after the baby was born. Emil had one week leave from the treatment institution in connection with the delivery, and he took amphetamine on the night before he was due back. That was the last straw for Anne. She could not trust Emil, and now with the baby she wanted nothing more to do with him. Emil was devastated about this, and in fact still is, but he decided that he would fight to get drug free to be able to at least have contact with his daughter.

By now Emil had learned about ADHD, and the more he heard the more he felt that this was his basic problem. He applied for an investigation and was put on waiting list. In the meantime, he once again entered Minnesota treatment and stayed there for almost a year. He had great difficulties with the programme due to his low ability to concentrate and to control his impulses. But now he had a goal. He knew he would not get the ADHD investigation unless he proved he could be drug free, and he was afraid what would happen the next time he relapsed. During his last relapse, he had taken heroin for the first time, and he had been really scared because he felt like he was going to die. He was also afraid that he would hurt somebody badly or even kill somebody because he often felt like that when he was binging on drugs.

Finally, he was investigated and started on medication. It took several months to try out the right dose for him. He now gets slow-release methylphenidate (Concerta) 144 mg in the morning and 72 mg at night, which is unusually high, but seems to be optimal for him. He can now control his aggressive impulses. He still gets angry, but he can step back and wait until the anger subsides. But life is still difficult for him. He now realises how much he has to catch up in order to live a normal life and to gain some confidence in himself. The investigation showed that he had an extremely low self-esteem. He is now enrolled in a job-training programme, and he has got his driver's licence back. He has started to read newspapers on the internet and follow the news on TV. He has very modest hopes for the future and takes one day at a time. He fights for his right to see his daughter. It is still difficult for Anne to trust him, although Emil has now been drug free for more than 2 years. He is very determined never to go back to drugs again. In his view, relapse is equal to death.

In Emil's case, the hope of investigation and treatment for ADHD no doubt was a strong motivational force to keep him in treatment and drug free. Now, on medication, he is able to 'think twice' before acting on impulses. This helps him to stay out of trouble and from relapsing in drugs when he gets frustrated.

Prospect for the future

In Sweden there is still political consensus on zero tolerance of drug misuse although suggestions to abandon the law on illegal drug consumption do arise. In EU, Sweden stands out as more restrictive on drugs than other countries, and there may be pressure to change this. On the regional level, there is always discussion about how much money to spend on prevention and treatment of drug misuse, and communes are sometimes tempted to save money on treatment of drug users, which is very expensive.

As for the pharmaceutical treatment of amphetamine we now have an anti-craving drug in naltrexone that still needs to be tried out in clinical practice. But since substance dependency is a chronic condition we will probably never be able to cure more than at best half of the heavy amphetamine users. Consequently, prevention will continue to be of utmost importance.

References

Bergsten, M. and Käll, K. (2007) Police interventions against illicit drug use among adolescents and young adults? A useful way of secondary prevention? Unpublished manuscript.

Ericsson, S., Widholm, L., Bränfeldt, L., Jönsson, E., Malmqvist, E. and Salamon Borg, M. (2001) Unga Män i Anstalt och Häkte. Kriminalvårdsstyrelsen.

Ersson, G. (2006) Missbruk och beroendetillstånd vid ADHD. Svensk Rehabilitering 3: 6–10.

Hibell, B., Guttormsson, U., Ahlström, S., Balakireva, O., Bjarnason, T., Kokkevi, A. and Kraus, L. (2009) The 2007 ESPAD Report: Substance Use Among Students in 35 Europen Countries. CAN, EMCDDA & Pompidou Group.

Jayaram-Lindström, N., Wennberg, P., Beck, O. and Franck, J. (2005) An open clinical trial of naltrexone for amphetamine dependence: compliance and tolerability. Nordic Journal of Psychiatry 59: 167–171.

Jayaram-Lindström, N., Hammarberg, A., Beck, O. and Franck, J. (2008) Naltrexone for the treatment of amphetamine dependence: a randomized, placebo-controllet trial. American Journal of Psychiatry 165(11): 1442–1448.

Jayaram-Lindström, N., Wennberg, P., Hurd, Y. L. and Franck, J. (2004) Effects of naltrexone on the subjective response to amphetamine in healthy volunteers. Journal of Clinical Psychopharmacology 24: 665–669.

Käll, K. (1997) Amphetamine abuse in Sweden. In: Klee, H. (ed.), Amphetamine Misuse: International Perspectives on Current Trends. Amsterdam: Harwood Academic Publishers, pp. 215–233.

Käll, K., Hermansson, U., Amundsen, E., Rönnbäck, K. and Rönnberg, S. (2007) The effectiveness of needle exchange programmes for HIV prevention – a critical review. The Journal of Global Drug Policy and Practice 1: 3.

Käll, K. I. and Olin, R. G. (1990) HIV status and changes in risk behaviour among intravenous drug users in Stockholm 1987–1988. AIDS 4: 153–157.

Socialstyrelsen (2007) Nationella riktlinjer för missbruks- och beroendevård.

Nutt, D. J., Fone, K., Asherson, P., Bramble, D., Hill, P., Matthews, K., Morris, K. A., Santosh, P., Sonuga-Barke, E., Taylor, E., Weiss, M. and Young, S. (2007) Evidence-based guidelines for management of attention-deficit/hyperactivity disorder in adolescents in transition to adult services and in adults: recommendations from the British Association for Psychopharmacology. *Journal of Psychophharmacology* 21: 10–41.

Nyström, I., Trygg, T., Woxler, P., Ahlner, J. and Kronstrand, R. (2005) Quantitation of R-(−)- and S-(+)-amphetamine in hair and blood by gas chromatography–mass spectrometry: an application to compliance monitoring in adult-attention deficit hyperactivity disorder treatment. *Journal of Analytical Toxicology* 29: 682–688.

Room, R., Palm, J., Romelsjö, A., Stenius, K. and Storbjörk, J. (2003) Kvinnor och män i svensk missbruksbehandling. Beskrivning av en studie i Stockholms län. *Nordisk alkohol- och narkotikatidskrift* 20: 91–100.

United Nations Office on Drugs and Crime. (2006) *Sweden's Successful Drug Policy: A Review of the Evidence*. Available at http://www.unodc.org/pdf/research/Swedish_drug_control.pdf.

Chapter 15

HARM REDUCTION AND AMPHETAMINES

Diane Riley

Introduction

This chapter looks at harm reduction strategies for amphetamine and other stimulant use and includes some international examples of good practice in programmes and policy. Any harm reduction strategy should be considered within the local social and cultural context in order for it to succeed.

Psychostimulant use in youth and adults can generally be categorised into five or six main patterns of use; these patterns may merge or change as circumstances or social networks do (Baker et al., 2004; Jenner and McKettin, 2004; NSW Health, 2005; Stubbs et al., 2004).

- *Experimental use*: part of normal youthful curiosity and risk-taking; most do not experience extensive problems or continue psychostimulant use.
- *Occupational use*: use is for the purposes of better/longer work performance such as that by truck drivers, students, restaurant staff and athletes.
- *Occasional use*: as exemplified by rave or club scene use; use is restricted to weekend or event-specific use (which may be infrequent or frequent).
- *Heavy, sessional use*: excessive or prolonged use over a short period of time, usually a couple of days.
- *Chronic use*: heavy and prolonged use.
- *Problematic use*: this is usually related to heavy, sessional use or to chronic use but may also occur with other patterns of use; it is often characterised by chaotic and compulsive (dependent) use, often associated with injecting drug use and sometimes with smoking of amphetamines (especially methamphetamine); such use results in psychological, social and often legal problems.

Patterns of amphetamine use and harm vary considerably in most countries in which use occurs and users come from all socio-economic groups, with a wide range of educational and cultural backgrounds (Baker et al., 2004; Darke et al., 2008; Jenner and McKettin, 2004; Stubbs et al., 2004; Weir, 2000). Because of these factors, there is a need for a wide variety of primary prevention and harm reduction strategies. Interventions need to be directed not only at drug user networks but also at recreational users who take do not see themselves as real 'drug users'. In addition, since many stimulant users are poly-drug users, multiple drug use and interactions (including with medications such as those for HIV) always needs to be considered as a possibility when designing harm reduction interventions.

Harm reduction education

Since so much psychostimulant use is experimental or social in nature, the emphasis of many interventions has been aimed at reducing the harm caused by this type of use (Darke et al., 2008; Stubbs et al., 2004; Weir, 2000). This has included provision of information on the effects and risks of taking psychostimulants (Baker et al., 2004). Harm reduction strategies include teaching early signs of problematic use, how to assist peers with problems and where help is available for individuals with problems (Dennis and Ballard, 2002). Many materials have been developed to give young people information on different stimulant drugs available, short-term and long-term effects, risks involved with use, suggestions about safer use and emergency procedures (see, e.g., www.hit.org.uk, www.dancesafe.org and www.ravesafe.org). The provision of sterile injection equipment is now also part of these harm reduction strategies in many countries. To reduce the risk of overdose, users are encouraged to not use alone and to call an ambulance as soon as unexpected and/or distressing symptoms occur.

In both primary prevention and harm reduction strategies, emphasis has been placed on information conveyed at schools, or raves and parties. To be really effective, harm reduction initiatives need to target more 'at-risk' groups such as street-involved youth. Stubbs and colleagues describe one attempt in Australia at targeting these areas involving the development of a psychostimulant-specific comic entitled 'On the Edge' since evaluation reports had consistently shown that comics are more successful than other print media in disseminating information to young people (Streetwize Communications, 2002; Stubbs et al., 2004). The development of this publication involved qualitative research with focus groups into the information needs of young psychostimulant users. The result was a language-appropriate comic addressing the issues of side effects (in particular drug induced psychosis), harm reduction techniques and treatment availability and accessibility which was distributed to gathering places such as youth centres and shelters.

In any primary or secondary prevention strategy, attention needs to be given to:

- providing accurate, unbiased information
- considering personal risk factors that may be associated with increased vulnerability
- teaching of coping and decision-making skills
- changing incorrect normative beliefs about the extent of use in a particular area or among a particular target population
- improving communication between young people and their parents, teachers and other adults

- providing regular updates so that information is accurate and recipients do not become too casual about real, current risks
- providing rewarding alternatives to substance use

Harm reduction interventions need to be tailored to the client's pattern of use and level of problematic behaviours. In general, those working with stimulant users recommend that all users be encouraged to practise safer sexual behaviours and use sterile equipment if injecting. They also recommend that all users be informed about the risk of neurotoxic effects and psychological and physiological effects of heavy use so that they can moderate or cease their use if problems are experienced (Baker et al., 2004; Darke et al., 2008). In order that they can stay informed or share information with stimulant using friends, users should be provided with a self-help guide that is relevant and accessible to them (see, e.g., materials by HIT and suggestions by Topp et al. (2002)).

In their review of psychosocial interventions with psychostimulants, Baker et al. (2004) noted that the recommendations regarding approaches to experimental psychostimulant users have primarily focused on reducing transition to injecting. Hall et al. (1993) recommended that for people at risk of experimenting with amphetamines, clinicians should discuss the hazards of injection, without exaggerating the risks of occasional low-dose oral use. For current users, advice to avoid injection and daily use is recommended. While there are no recommended safe limits for amphetamine use, Hall et al. (1993) have suggested that the risk of experiencing adverse effects of amphetamine use could be reduced by using it less than twice a week and using small amounts. Darke et al. (1994) have recommended that interventions to encourage safer use of amphetamines are needed to address misconceptions that injecting is more economical and healthy and to emphasise the vascular problems associated with injecting.

A number of suggestions for interventions with heavy users have been put forward, but these are based on general observation rather than on specific experimental studies (Baker et al., 2004). These include education about the purity of the drug, adverse consequences of heavy use, the need for moderation or cessation of use if adverse consequences are experienced, a false sense of psychomotor competence that may be produced when used in combination with alcohol, the need to avoid driving when using and the need to take precautions to reduce harmful side effects, such as obtaining the drug from reliable sources and using smaller amounts per occasion (see, e.g., Topp et al., 2002; Weir, 2000; and educational materials by organisations such as HIT).

Peer education

Peer education on psychostimulant use usually involves the use of peers who are credible, influential and have received training to help them to support and educate users to reduce the potential harms of stimulants use to themselves and others. There is limited information that specifically addresses the effectiveness of peer education in regard to stimulant use. Users who take psychostimulants at dance events are the target of organisations such as Dancesafe, which operates in Canada and the USA, and Ravesafe which operates in South Africa and several other countries. These are groups of volunteers that provide basic first aid, distribute information about street/dance drugs and safer raving and provide a place at parties where people can feel safe and secure, often referred to as a 'chill out' area. Another excellent example of harm reduction for young people (of all ages) is 'Venue Safety' from Australia, a harm minimisation strategy for raves and clubs which has been adopted by the rave community and municipal and public health authorities (www.venuesafe.com).

Because of the wide range of people using stimulants, a correspondingly wide range of harm reduction strategies is needed. Traditional peer networks are not enough; as noted above, approaches are needed which target people who do not consider themselves to be 'drug users' such as those who use drugs for occupational purposes or occasionally at recreational events.

Stimulant use during pregnancy and lactation

Not using drugs at all during pregnancy and while breastfeeding is preferable to use since these are times when both mother and child can be especially vulnerable to harm. Since women do use drugs at these times, they need to know about ways to reduce risks. In their review of stimulant use in pregnancy and lactation, Dean and McGuire (2004) suggest that following recommendations should be given:

- Even if a woman has used psychostimulants early in her pregnancy, there can still be benefits from stopping or cutting down later in the pregnancy, and women should be encouraged to do this.
- Pregnant psychostimulant users should be advised not to 'binge' during pregnancy.
- Pregnant psychostimulant users should be advised to reduce their use of other drugs, especially alcohol and nicotine
- If a woman is breastfeeding and using psychostimulants, then exposure of the child to the drug can be minimised by breastfeeding just before using, and not breastfeeding again for at least 2 or 3 hours

The guilt and shame experienced by many pregnant women who use drugs, combined with stigma, means that they tend to present later than other women for antenatal care and may try to hide their drug use. Both maternal and child health outcomes can be improved by early and non-judgmental antenatal care (Dean and McGuire, 2004).

Time of feeding in relation to maternal dose (Dean and McGuire, 2004)

If the drug is in an immediate release and not a sustained or controlled release dose form, the amount of drug transferred into the milk of a breastfeeding mother may be limited or reduced by the following strategies:

- If the drug is taken once daily, it should be taken around the time of the feed to allow the longest period of time to elapse until the next feed.
- It is not clear whether it is best to take a drug immediately before, during or immediately after the feed; whichever is most practical should be chosen.
- If the drug cannot be taken as a single daily dose, feeds and drug consumption need to be timed to allow the maximum possible time from administration to the next feed. This is usually best achieved if the mother takes the dose at the next feed. The mother should wait at least one half-life after the peak milk concentration is achieved before feeding again, as this will significantly decrease (by about 50%) the amount of drug excreted into the milk. Feeding away from the time of the peak milk concentration will minimise the infant's drug exposure.
- In practice, other factors such as chaotic lifestyle may influence a mother's ability to ensure breastfeeding occurs away from peak drug concentrations. Any clinical recommendations should take these factors into account.

Pill testing

Users of illicit psychostimulants need to be aware that the contents of the pills they are using are unknown. Strategies that can reduce possible harms of taking such include:

- not using alone, in case the pill has an adverse effect
- calling an ambulance as soon as unexpected and/or distressing symptoms occur
- not taking more than one pill at once

Testing of pills is questionable as a harm reduction strategy because it is unreliable and subjective (Baker et al., 2004; Winstock et al., 2001). Kits for testing pills cannot assess the purity of a pill or identify how much of an identified substance is in it and cannot distinguish between MDMA and similar but potentially more harmful substances (Winstock et al., 2001).

Substitution medications

Substitution therapies aim to replace harmful drug use with safer modes of drug use in terms of dose, route of administration and adverse effects. Effective substitutes may allow patients to stabilise on doses that prevent withdrawal and craving and to reduce the harms associated with illicit drug use. Lintzeris (2004) notes that attempts to replicate the model of opioid maintenance substitution treatment for stimulants date back to the 1960s, when dexamphetamine was prescribed in the UK as a substitution treatment for amphetamine-dependent patients. Advocates of this approach argue that such prescribing attracts and retains patients in treatment (thereby exposing them to counselling and harm-reduction interventions) and is effective in reducing their illicit stimulant use and injecting behaviours and enhancing psychosocial function. Critics have argued that any gains are outweighed by adverse events (e.g. psychosis, cardiotoxicity), persistent illicit drug use and widespread diversion.

Carnwath et al. (2002) reported that six out of eight patients with schizophrenia who had received prescribed dexamphetamine reduced amphetamine use and showed improved psychiatric health. There was no exacerbation of psychosis in any patient, while compliance with neuroleptics improved in most cases.

Mattick and Darke (1995) have suggested that amphetamine maintenance may be appropriate where amphetamine use is frequent (usually daily), attempts to achieve abstinence have been unsuccessful, dependence is evident, severe adverse complications have occurred and maintenance is likely to cause less harm than continued illicit use. Risks associated with maintenance include psychiatric and cardiovascular complications, particularly when additional illicit psychostimulants are consumed (see Chapter 6 of this book for full discussion of substitution treatment).

Some examples of good practice

HIT, Liverpool, UK

HIT has been in operation since the 1970s (when it was known as Mersey Drug Training and Information Centre). HIT conducts education and training about all psychoactive drugs but specialises in issues pertaining to dance and other youth culture. The organisation produces extremely high-level educational materials that are attractive as well as informative and which are designed around the interests of different genders and ages. The basic philosophy of the organisation is one of social marketing.

Crystal Clear, Vancouver, Canada

Crystal Clear is a participant-driven harm reduction project for street-involved youth who have experience with crystal methamphetamines and who are interested in improving their health and the health of their peers. The core activities of Crystal Clear include peer outreach, peer support, a peer harm reduction training and community involvement. In groups of two, Crystal Clear peers walk throughout the community and supply water, snacks, safer using information, service information and clean equipment (needles, filters, pipes, water). They also operate during hours when no other services are available to youth.

Home Nite Club, Sydney, Australia

Home Nite Club in Sydney established itself as a leader in club-based harm reduction, with the development of a comprehensive harm minimisation plan related to all aspects of its operation including security and health and safety initiatives. It implemented:

- the provision of chilled, filtered water free of charge
- custom-labelled water bottles with safety tips written by the National Drug and Alcohol Research Centre
- a purpose-built first aid treatment room including attendance of a qualified paramedic on club nights. The NSW Government has produced Guidelines for dance parties. This document provides organisers of dance events with comprehensive information and advice regarding all aspects of the responsible management of dance events. Included in these guidelines are responsibilities around security, harm minimisation, first aid and the safe disposal of needles and syringes

Good Practice in Psychostimulant Policy and Strategy, Australia

The Commonwealth of Australia has commissioned a number of projects under the National Drug Strategy aimed at addressing ATS use, including:

- an update of the National Drug Strategy Monograph Models of intervention and care for psychostimulant users
- the development of management guidelines for accident and emergency workers, ambulance officers and police officers on the management of acute ATS presentations
- a trial of cognitive behavioural therapy for ATS dependence following a pilot study that indicated this may be an effective intervention

Members of the Council recognised that a national approach to increased rates of supply and use of psychostimulant drugs was warranted and that projects were needed to advise frontline workers of the harms associated with psychostimulant use and manufacture and best practice responses (Ministerial Council on Drug Strategy, 2004).

Amphetamine, ecstasy and cocaine: a prevention and treatment plan 2005–2009 NSW Department of Health

The development of the NSW Health Amphetamine, Ecstasy and Cocaine Prevention and Treatment Plan is an acknowledgement that patterns of drug use are changing, requiring dynamic, evidence-based and innovative responses from the health sector in partnership with other agencies that are in a position to effect change. The Plan provides a framework to guide the health sector's response to the abuse of psychostimulants. The aim of the Plan is to reduce the harms associated with the misuse of psychostimulants. To accomplish this, six Key Activity Areas have been identified to guide action. These include:

- Information and Education
- Early Intervention
- Treatment Approaches
- Research, Monitoring and Evaluation
- Special Populations
- Partnerships.

References

Baker, A., Gowing, L., Lee, N. K. and Proudfoot, H. (2004) Psychosocial interventions for psychostimulant users. In: Baker, A., Lee, N. K. and Jenner, L. (eds), *Models of Intervention and Care for Psychostimulant Users*, 2nd edn. National Drug Strategy Monograph Series 51. Australia: Commonwealth of Australia, pp. 63–84.

Carnwath, T., Garvey, T. and Holland, M. (2002) The prescription of dexamphetamine to patients with schizophrenia and amphetamine dependence. *Journal of Psychopharmacology* 16(4): 373–377.

Darke, S., Cohen, J., Ross, J., Hando, J. and Hall, W. (1994) Transitions between routes of administration of regular amphetamine users. *Addiction* 89: 1077–1083.

Darke, S., Kaye, S., McKetin, R. and Duflou, J. (2008) Major physical and psychological harms of methamphetamine use. *Drug and Alcohol Review* 27(3): 253–262.

Dean, A. and McGuire, T. (2004) Psychostimulant use in pregnancy and lactation. In: Baker, A., Lee, N. and Jenner, L. (eds), *Models of Intervention and Care for Psychostimulant Users*, 2nd edn. Monograph Series No. 51. Australia: Commonwealth of Australia, pp. 35–50.

Dennis, D. and Ballard, M. (2002) Ecstasy: it's the rave. *The High School Journal* 85(4): 64–70.

Hall, W., Darke, S., Ross, M. and Wodak, A. (1993) Patterns of drug use and risk-taking among injecting amphetamine and opioid drug users in Sydney, Australia. *Addiction* 88(4): 509–516.

Jenner, L. and McKetin, R. (2004) Prevalence and patterns of psychostimulant use. In: Baker, A., Lee, N. and Jenner, L. (eds), *Models of Intervention and Care for Psychostimulant Users*, 2nd edn. Monograph Series No. 51. Australia: Commonwealth of Australia, pp. 13–34.

Lintzeris, N. (2004) *Pharmacotherapies for Illicit Drug Use*. London: The Medicine Publishing Company.

Mattick, R. P. and Darke, S. (1995) Drug replacement treatments: is amphetamine substitution a horse of a different colour? *Drug and Alcohol Review* 14: 389–394.

Ministerial Council on Drug Strategy (2004) *The National Drug Strategy 2004–2009*. Canberra: Commonwealth of Australia.

NSW Health (2005) *Amphetamine, Ecstasy and Cocaine: A Prevention and Treatment Plan 2005–2009*. Sydney: NSW Health.

Streetwize Communications (2002) *On the Edge.* Available at www.streetwize.com.au/publications. Accessed 15 July 2008.

Stubbs, M., Hides, L., Howard, J. and Acuri, A. (2004) Psychostimulants and young people. In: Baker, A., Lee, N. and Jenner, L. (eds), *Models of Intervention and Care for Psychostimulant Users*, 2nd edn. Monograph Series No. 51. Australia: Commonwealth of Australia, pp. 133–153.

Topp, L., Breen, C., Kaye, S. and Darke, S. (2002) NSW party drug trends 2001. *Findings of the Illicit Drug Reporting System (IDRS) Party Drugs Module.* NDARC Technical Report No. 136. Sydney: National Drug and Alcohol Research Centre.

Weir, E. (2000) Raves: a review of the culture, the drugs and the prevention of harms. *Canadian Medical Association Journal* 162(13): 1843–1848.

Winstock, A. R., Griffiths, P. and Stewart, D. (2001) Drugs and the dance music scene: a survey of current drug use patterns among a sample of dance music enthusiasts in the UK. *Drug and Alcohol Dependence* 64(1): 9–17.

Chapter 16

WHAT HAVE WE LEARNED: CONCLUSIONS ON TREATMENT

Diane Riley and Richard Pates

One of the purposes of this book was to examine the interventions for amphetamine-related problems that are available worldwide. Many practitioners are frustrated when working with amphetamine users because of the paucity of evidence of effective treatment. What is clear is that there are commonalities between countries on interventions but no universal agreement as to what the best treatments available are. This chapter reviews the other chapters and then summarises some management procedures selected from best treatment evidence in recent literature.

Evidence from the book

The chapters in this book have shown that there is a real rather than perceived problem worldwide with amphetamine. In most countries, the usual form of intervention is psychosocial in nature, such as cognitive behavioural therapy (CBT) or motivational interviewing (MI). In Canada, for example, Riley (Chapter 8) mentions a range of psychosocial interventions being used, namely:

- MI
- Behavioural therapy and CBT
- Contingency management
- Residential rehabilitation
- Therapeutic communities
- Self-help groups
- Family and multi-systemic interventions
- Residential treatment
- 12-step programmes

This is probably the full range of interventions (apart from substitute prescribing) currently available. But Riley concludes her chapter with, 'There is a pressing need to study and adopt new approaches to stimulants. As is the case with other chapters in this book, the interventions described here are far from uniform and no standard of treatment has yet been suggested to serve as "best" practice'.

In an extensive review of the countries of the former Eastern European bloc, Grund and colleagues (Chapter 13) write that despite and extensive problem, treatment *designed for* stimulant users is non-existent in this region, with the exception

of the Czech Republic, which might have the longest history of illicit methamphetamine use (some 35 years). The difficulty in finding workable, evidence-based
treatment for ATS dependence is not restricted to this region; little headway has
been made anywhere in developing effective treatment approaches. What is available for treatment in the Czech Republic is detoxification in conjunction with psychosocial interventions, with symptomatic relief provided by medication. Grund
and colleagues comment that few services provide after care and that many of the
services are based on abstinence treatment for alcohol problems and are largely
unsuccessful.

Käll (Chapter 14) comments that in Sweden most treatment of drug misuse
has been aimed at amphetamine misuse, since amphetamine has been the primary
drug for heavy users. She adds, however, that there is no specific evidence-based
treatment aimed at amphetamine misuse. The modern trend for treatment in Sweden
for heavy users is a 6-month inpatient programme with a 12-step emphasis followed
by several years of contact with Narcotics Anonymous (NA). For less dependent
users, CBT and MI on an outpatient basis are common.

In a discussion of the problems in Thailand, Cohen and McGregor (Chapter 12)
report that interventions have ranged from treatment in Buddhist monasteries
working with a combination of religious vows and meditation through use of
the Matrix Model, introduced in 1998 following a large upsurge in the use of
methamphetamine, to boot camps introduced as part of Thailand's infamous war
on drugs in 2002. These camps were mandatory treatment facilities run by the
military where life skills training and physical boot camp activities took place. The
programmes ran for 4–21 days and the number of people in treatment rose from
21 665 to 480 711 between 2002 and 2003, as a consequence of the mandatory nature of the programmes. Lack of follow-up meant that there was little information
about the efficacy of the programmes. The Matrix Model showed promising preliminary results with 80% of those remaining in treatment reported to be drug free
at follow-up. Comment was made about whether abstinence-based behavioural interventions, largely developed in the USA, translate well to an Asian culture: further
research is needed into this issue.

In another Asian country, which has had a long experience of amphetamine problems, Sato (Chapter 11) describes services available in Japan. The main provision is
through self-help facilities of DARC (Drug Addiction Rehabilitation Centre or 'da-
ru-ku' in Japanese) and NA; both work on a 12-step model of recovery. For patients
with psychiatric problems associated with their drug use, inpatient admission to
hospital is used with antipsychotic drugs prescribed and then, following discharge,
a return to NA. Sato comments that despite Japan's long history of problems with
amphetamine (over 60 years) no special treatments have been developed.

In a rich and thoughtful chapter on Australian responses to treatment (Chapter 9),
Shearer describes a range of interventions and settings. He notes that the main intervention is a CBT model of counselling as best practice from evidence-based
research. He also describes the need for differentiation between treatment for the
acute effects of methamphetamine intoxication and the chronic effects of methamphetamine misuse. Shearer also describes pharmacological interventions, Australia

being one of the only countries outside the UK to try substitute prescribing and the use of non-amphetamine-like drugs as substitutes. As Shearer comments, further research is needed into these methods, but it is clear that Australia is taking the treatment problem seriously and attempting to find best practice approaches.

In New Zealand, Wilkins and Sheridan (Chapter 10) note that unlike other countries injecting is not the most common form of use, with less than 15% of users injecting. Treatment is provided by Community Alcohol and Drug Services, where the most common form of treatment is psychosocial interventions with a small number of inpatient detoxification beds. Symptomatic medication is provided for problems such as insomnia.

The most comprehensive description of treatment in the book and the description of the most comprehensive treatment in use is that by Rawson. (Chapter 7) of the USA. The Matrix Model of outpatient treatment is a manual-driven treatment using a combination of well-researched and evidence-based interventions in combination. The interventions include individual counselling, skills building groups, relapse prevention and family education groups, 12-step meetings and social support meetings. This approach appears to be successful in the American context. Rawson and colleagues also discuss the use of contingency management, which they report is as effective as CBT in treating methamphetamine users.

Finally, the issue of substitute prescribing for amphetamine users is discussed by Pates (Chapter 6). The UK appears to be one of the only countries in the world where substitute prescribing of amphetamine takes place. The chapter describes a number of research projects around prescribing and the history of this type of intervention in Britain. It remains controversial but has been shown to reduce the use of street drugs and injecting, important indices of harm reduction. Australia is one of the few other countries where research is being carried out on substitute prescribing.

Psychosocial interventions remain the most common form of intervention ranging from counselling to the very structured matrix project. Many of the contributors discuss the need for further research into treatment for amphetamine problems and mention that most treatment services in their countries is aimed primarily at opiate users. Yet this disparity in treatment is clearly inappropriate when seen against the background of the problems that amphetamines cause both for individuals and for society. Much more work needs to be done to correct this imbalance.

The final part of this chapter is a summary of some management strategies for dealing with amphetamine and other psychostimulant problems as reviewed in recent literature.

Identifying and managing intoxication

Severe stimulant intoxication can cause aggressive, violent or difficult behaviour, as well as physical emergencies such as overheating. It can be very difficult to distinguish between psychosis induced by psychostimulants and a mental illness or a severe emotional disturbance. In their excellent review of stimulant intoxication,

Dean and Whyte (2004) recommend that the aims of the service provider should be to:

- provide a non-stimulating environment
- provide support and reassurance
- prevent users from harming themselves or others

This can involve:

- reducing environmental stimuli as much as possible, including removing the person to a quieter, cooler place and removing heavy or restrictive clothing
- avoiding confrontation or arguments while still allowing the person to talk
- approaching the person slowly and with confidence (showing that the situation is under control)
- providing reassurance that symptoms will pass with time
- encouraging supportive people to stay with them
- monitoring vital signs and mental state
- encouraging fluid intake

Management of acute psychostimulant toxicity

Dean and Whyte (2004) discuss the adverse effects of psychostimulants ranging from minor symptoms to life-threatening toxicity. They point out that although regular use or use of high doses increases risk of adverse events, many serious adverse events may occur even in the naive user. Early symptoms of psychostimulant toxicity include hyperactivity, restlessness, tremor, sweating, talkativeness, irritability, weakness, insomnia, headache and fever; vomiting, diarrhoea, cramps and anorexia occur in some cases. Agitation, hyperactive reflexes, confusion, aggression, delirium, paranoid hallucinations, panic states and loss of behavioural control may then ensue. Disorders of movements such as tics and tremors may also develop. In cases of sever intoxication, seizures, stroke and coma may occur. Severe hyperthermia can develop with risk of renal failure, multi-organ failure and death.

Dean and Whyte note that hypertension and tachycardia are common during stimulant intoxication and that more severe cardiovascular toxicity such as acute myocardial infarction can occur. They report that respiratory complications are common and liver injury is common if severe hyperthermia and/or vasospasm occurs; electrolyte disturbances and dehydration are common and metabolic acidosis occurs with severe poisoning.

Toxicity: assessment and management

Dean and Whyte suggest that clinical observation of potentially toxic signs and symptoms is more relevant than estimating the ingested dose of a drug. These include dilated pupils, often sluggishly reactive to light and flushed skin. They recommend that core temperature be monitored, as severe hyperthermia may develop, as well as serum electrolytes, renal and hepatic function and creatine phosphokinase; an electrocardiogram should be taken, with continuous cardiac monitoring in symptomatic patients.

Patients showing signs of stimulant intoxication-induced psychosis and aggression should be stabilised in a medically supervised setting for 2–3 days; antipsychotics and tranquillisers can be administered to reduce symptoms (Rawson et al., 2002). Dean and Whyte emphasise that treatment of psychostimulant toxicity requires prompt supportive care and careful use of medications. They also provide some suggestions for good management of psychostimulant toxicity as follows:

- Because the role of gastric decontamination after oral intake has not been established, ipecac-induced emesis is not recommended. Gastric lavage may be dangerous due to possible neurological and cardiovascular toxicity and activated charcoal is of doubtful benefit.
- Intoxication that is not complicated by other factors may need only observation and monitoring for several hours in a subdued environment, with supportive management, sedation and reduction of body temperature. Rapid cooling is needed if body temperature is above 41°C; this may be achieved through cooling shade, application of ice packs to neck, armpit and groin, dousing with water and fanning cold water immersion.
- If the person is extremely agitated or aggressive, drugs should be used to induce sedation. Sedation should be distinguished from rapid treatment of psychosis, which involves high loading doses of antipsychotics; the latter is not recommended in an emergency setting since high or frequently repeated doses of antipsychotics can cause side effects.
- Physical restraint alone is often not enough for users with acute behavioural disturbance and may cause harm if this disturbance increases; stimulant use may be a possible risk factor for sudden death of individuals being physically restrained. Sedation using sedative drugs provides a humane alternative and ensures safer, essentially physiological monitoring.

Behavioural problems

Violent behaviour is more common in chronic heavy users of stimulants than in occasional users, and risk of aggressive behaviour is increased by factors such as withdrawal from depressants. Dean and Whyte suggest urgent sedation may need to be used when there is a failure of other attempts to control the patient, when the patient is uncooperative, when the patient is at risk to themselves or others, and when there is a perceived need for medical intervention. They note that in some cases it may be difficult to differentiate between behavioural disturbance and potential drug-induced psychosis, but that the latter should not be considered a contraindication to urgent sedation.

Dean and Whyte point out that, in general, treatment of patients with psychostimulant-induced psychosis is similar to treatment of acute mania or schizophrenia and that the first thing needed is to create an environment that the patient perceives as safe. They note that acutely agitated or violent patients may need non-specific rapid sedation; the aim of such sedation is to control dangerous behaviour in order to allow better assessment and management (they caution that health care providers who provide sedation should have access to advanced airway assessment and management skills in case of adverse effects). The reviewers make the following comments about specific agents:

- *Benzodiazepines*: Research suggests that benzodiazepines should be the agent of choice when there is unlikely to be an ongoing need for antipsychotic medication after acute treatment; parenteral midazolam may be effective in controlling agitated or aggressive patients (Neave, 1994); there is little evidence for the superiority of lorazepam over other agents and it does not have a rapid onset of action.
- *Antipsychotics*: Haloperidol is frequently used for urgent sedation and causes less hypotension, fewer anticholinergic side effects and less decrease in seizure threshold than do other neuroleptics, but it is not the most sedative of these. There is however much disquiet about the use of haloperidol in this context among treatment professionals. Droperidol is a fast-acting antipsychotic, rapidly eliminated from the body, but the Cochrane Review of droperidol for acute psychosis concluded that this area is under-researched and well-conducted clinical trials are needed (Dean and Whyte, 2004).
- *Combination regimens*: Studies support the use of benzodiazepines and antipsychotics in combination as safe and effective options and seem to indicate that combination therapies are superior to single-agent regimes, though this may be because patients in the combination group receive a greater total dose of drug than those in a single-agent group.

Serotonin toxicity

Serotonin toxicity is caused by an increase in the activity of the neurotransmitter serotonin (5-hydroxytryptamine, 5-HT). Serotonin toxicity can be the result of a combination of antidepressant medications, atypical antipsychotics or psychostimulants, particularly MDMA (Vuori et al., 2003). According to Dean and Whyte, serotonin toxicity is a triad of clinical features: (1) autonomic signs, (2) neuromuscular changes and (3) altered mental status; the combination of certain well-defined clinical features (clonus, agitation, diaphoresis, tremor, hyperreflexia, hypertonia and high temperature) is sensitive and specific (Dean and Whyte, 2004). The clinical course of serotonin toxicity ranges from mild to potentially fatal, with serious cases showing muscle rigidity, coma, hypertension or hypotension. They recommend the following:

- Treatment should involve prompt supportive care and judicious use of specific agents, with general supportive measures for severe forms including IV fluids/volume resuscitation, antipyretics, external cooling, muscular paralysis with neuromuscular blocking agents, mechanical ventilation and sedation with intraveneous benzodiazepines.

- Standard measures should be used for secondary cardiac arrhythmias or seizures.
- In cases of serious serotonin toxicity, serum electrolytes, glucose, renal function, creatine kinase levels and electrocardiogram should be monitored.
- In more severe cases, hepatic function and arterial blood gases should also be monitored.
- Muscle rigidity should be controlled.
- For patients who develop such conditions as coma or cardiac arrhythmia, more specific measures are needed (Dean and Whyte, 2004).

Psychostimulant withdrawal and detoxification

A withdrawal syndrome is a cluster of symptoms, lasting for a meaningful period of time, which impairs functioning to a clinically significant degree. Although it is now generally accepted that there is a psychostimulant withdrawal syndrome, the literature on psychostimulant withdrawal is inconsistent and of variable quality. In their comprehensive review, Jenner and Saunders (2004) found no studies that describe the natural history of amphetamine withdrawal among dependent individuals and that the process is still poorly understood. There is some agreement, however, that the psychostimulant withdrawal syndrome is unlike the withdrawal syndromes associated with depressants, in which effects are the opposite to those of the acute pharmacological effects of the drugs. A number of symptoms of the psychostimulant withdrawal syndrome appear to be the same as those of the acute intoxication effects such as agitation and hyper-arousal.

Many users of psychostimulants experience a 'crash' or brief period of recovery that can last for a few days following binge use. Jenner and Saunders point out that this recovery period does not in itself constitute a clinically significant withdrawal syndrome, but is a process of recovery from a period of CNS over-stimulation and is usually characterised by excessive sleeping and eating and irritability of mood. They suggest that such a recovery period may be compared to the experience of a 'hangover' from alcohol, which is recognised as time-limited and not a withdrawal syndrome in itself. The incidence, severity, course and subjective experience of the withdrawal syndrome depend on the following:

- the severity of dependence
- duration of use
- frequency of psychostimulant use
- potency of psychostimulant used
- duration of action of psychostimulant
- the presence of other physical or psychiatric disorders
- psychosocial factors

According to Jenner and Saunders, psychostimulant withdrawal is characterised by signs of CNS hypoactivity such as lethargy, slowed movements and poor concentration that are interspersed with agitation and insomnia, the result of depletion of monoamine neurotransmitter stores and alteration in brain structure (Cho and Melega, 2002; Jenner and Saunders, 2004). Clinical studies of amphetamine withdrawal are far few, following cessation of daily use of amphetamine, users report fatigue, inertia, an initial period of hypersomnia followed by protracted insomnia and an onset of agitation, usually within 36 hours of cessation, that lasts for between 3 and 5 days, with mood disturbance ranging from dysphoria to severe clinical depression (Jenner and Saunders, 2004)

Jenner and Saunders recommend that the person should be monitored throughout the course of the withdrawal using observation charts such as the Amphetamine Withdrawal Questionnaire, a 10-item self-report instrument designed to detect severity of withdrawal symptoms (Jenner and Saunders, 2004). Ratings of the subjective experience of withdrawal symptoms, particularly agitation, sleep disturbance, depression and symptoms of psychosis, are used to determine need for medications. The reviewers, however, point out that pharmacotherapy for psychostimulant withdrawal is of limited value and that there is no evidence that tapered withdrawal from psychostimulants is preferable to abrupt cessation. They also caution that while psychostimulant withdrawal is rarely life-threatening, users with serious depression may become suicidal. Psychotic symptoms seen in the acute intoxication/toxicity phase may worsen during the early stages of withdrawal: an SSRI or tricyclic antidepressant may be prescribed if necessary, with careful monitoring. Jenner and Saunders note that since relapse to psychostimulant use is common, care should be taken when prescribing SSRIs due to the as toxicity associated with increased serotonin levels. Antipsychotic medication such as phenothiazine may be prescribed in the short term (1 to 2 weeks), but if psychosis is severe or persistent, psychiatric assessment is needed along with general psychosis management and treatment.

References

Cho, A. K. and Melega, W. P. (2002) Patterns of methamphetamine abuse and their consequences. *Journal of Addictive Diseases* 21(1): 21–34.

Dean, A. and Whyte, I. (2004) In: Baker, A., Lee, N. and Jenner, L. (eds), *Management of Acute Psychostimulant Toxicity in Models of Intervention and Care for Psychostimulant Users*, 2nd edn. Monograph Series No. 51. Australia: Commonwealth of Australia, pp. 35–50.

Jenner, L. and Saunders J. (2004) In: Baker, A., Lee, N. and Jenner, L. (eds), *Psychostimulant Withdrawal and Detoxification in Models of Intervention and Care for Psychostimulant Users*, 2nd edn. Monograph Series No. 51. Australia: Commonwealth of Australia, pp. 35–50.

Neave, G. (1994) Midazolam for acute agitation in the psychiatric patient. *Australian Journal of Hospital Pharmacy* 24: 356.

Rawson, R., Gonzales, R. and Brethen, P. (2002) Treatment of methamphetamine use disorders: an update. *Journal of Substance Abuse Treatment* 23: 145–150.

Vuori, E., Henry, J. A., Ojanpera, I., Nieminen, R., Savolainen, T., Wahlsten, P. and Jantti, M. (2003) Death following ingestion of MDMA (ecstasy) and moclobemide. *Addiction* 98(3): 365–368.

INDEX